ENEMIES WITHIN

ENEMIES within

The Cold War and the AIDS Crisis in Literature, Film, and Culture

JACQUELINE FOERTSCH

UNIVERSITY OF ILLINOIS PRESS
URBANA AND CHICAGO

Manufactured in the United States of America
c 5 4 3 2 1

∞ This book is printed on acid-free paper.

Library of Congress Cataloging-in-Publication Data
Foertsch, Jacqueline, 1964–
Enemies within : the Cold War and the AIDS crisis in literature, film, and culture / Jacqueline Foertsch.
p. cm.
Includes bibliographical references and index.
ISBN 0-252-02637-3 (alk. paper)
1. American literature—20th century—History and criticism.
2. Cold War in literature.
3. Cold War—Social aspects—United States.
4. Postmodernism (Literature)—United States.
5. AIDS (Disease)—United States—History.
6. AIDS (Disease) in motion pictures.
7. Postmodernism—United States.
8. AIDS (Disease) in literature.
9. Cold War in motion pictures.
I. Title.
PS228.C58F64 2001
810.9'358—dc21 00-011199

Contents

Acknowledgments vii

INTRODUCTION: *Five* Minutes to Midnight—What Is a Postmodern Plague? 1

1. COUNTING DOWN—TO CATASTROPHE OR CURE? 9
   Bomb Scares: Two Epidemic Eras
   History Repeats Itself: The Cold War as Mirror to the AIDS Crisis
   History Reproduces Itself: The Cold War as Blueprint for the AIDS Crisis
   Talking Cures: Metaphor, Metonymy, and the Location of Illness in Language
   Exploding Cures: The Irradiated Metaphoric

2. *FOUR* CORNERS OF A CRISIS: GENRES OF PLAGUE TEXTS 36
   Before, Beyond, and Within: Where We Are in Our Plague Texts
   Forward, Backward, and Over Again: Two Views of the Primal Scene
   Boxed In by Our Fears: Four Plague Genres
      Backward Glances: The Pre-epidemic
         Inward Glances: The Pre-AIDS Autobiography
      Steps Sideways: The Alterapocalyptic
      Two Small, Deserted Islands: The Preapocalyptic and Extraepidemic
      Deathbed Dictations: The Intraepidemic
      Forward Lunges: The Postapocalyptic

3. *THREE* POINTS OF SIGHT: GENDER IN PLAGUE TEXTS 94
   Danger Zones and Other Postmodern Myths
   Plague Texts and the Feminine
      Presence and Absence in Nuclear Literature
      Positivity and Negativity in AIDS Literature
   Textual Triangles

Bombshells and Basket Cases: Gendered Bomb/Gendered Illness in Nuclear Texts
Tantrums and Time Bombs: Gendered Illness/Gendered Bomb in AIDS Texts

4. *TWO* TAKES ON A SCARE: CINEMATIC PLAGUE TEXTS AND THEIR REMAKES 162
The Return as the Repressed: Plague Film Remakes
Incredible Shrinkage: Having the Phallus/Be(com)ing a Penis
Parasites with Submarines: Some Small, Sick, Scientific Spies
Panic in the Streets of San Francisco: Cross-Metaphoric Treatments of Plague Themes
Kids These Days: The Oedipal and Extra-Oedipal in Remake Relations
Not *The Blobs* but the Blobs

CONCLUSION: *One* Fine Day—Toward a Realization of the "Eutemporal" 189

Notes 193
Works Cited 219
Index 235

Acknowledgments

This book came into being with the critical support of the multiple anonymous readers serving the editorial boards of journals that have accepted (and rejected) parts of this work and, of course, the experts in my field consulted as commentators on this manuscript by the University of Illinois Press. Although I cannot refer to them by name, they were the primary critical audience for the later forms of this project and have shaped it importantly and effectively. At Illinois, Richard Martin, Theresa L. Sears, and August Gering have provided wonderful editorial assistance and support. My thanks to all of them.

I owe an even greater debt to this project's earliest readers, who added nurturing encouragement and invaluable friendship to their incisive critical responses: Annette Trefzer read early drafts of this book in its dissertation form and encouraged its continued development; Frank Edington Durham's training in physics and interest in literature-science interdisciplinarity enabled his valuable perspective; Molly Anne Rothenberg's pointed and detailed response provided indispensable guidance; and Geoffrey Galt Harpham has shepherded this project from its earliest paragraphs and responded helpfully and willingly to ideas and drafts at every stage of its development. His analyses, especially of the grotesque in literature, and analytic methods played an essential role in the formation of this work and model the rigorous inquiry it has sought to emulate. I am grateful to all four of these teacher-philosophers for their careful, constructive interactions with this work and for their examples of scholarship and brilliance, which continue to inspire me.

Assistance of a more amorphous but still priceless quality has come from the communities of scholars, activists, and friends with whom I have been privileged to associate in the several years of this project's development. At Tulane University, Sandy Haro and Jan Mulvilhill provided clerical and technical support for it in dissertation and early manuscript stages. Jill Buchanan, Kristina Busse, John Dudley, Dietmar Felber, Julia Hodges, Bess MacInness, Jennifer Maier, Lee Miller, and Molly Abel Travis are Tulane friends and colleagues who created a stimulating environment while I was among them and provide wonderful memories now. Laszlo Fulop, David Larivierre, Darla Rushing, Claire Ryan, Roxanne Smith, and Mike Stasio are New Orleans friends who also made my life there so very enjoyable. Hallie Stein Gorup, Leslie Richardson, and Kathryn Duncan will, I know, always be "there" (in New Orleans and beyond) for me.

At Auburn University, Paula R. Backscheider and Miriam Marty Clark have given valuable advice to assist me in the final publication stages; Marc Silverstein has read and responded helpfully to a portion of this project. A large group of friends have formed a receptive space for the production of my work and delightful diversion when a break from work is required: Philip Acree-Cavalier, Dan Albergotti, Jon Bolton, Diane Boyd, Chris Campagna, Marian Carcache, Alicia Carroll, Lou Caton, Tim Dykstal, Delia Fisher, Patsy Fowler, Bonnie Gerard, Marie Gibson, James Goldstein, Eric Hayot, Margaret Hundleby, Christian Gregory, Colleen Hamilton, Chris Kiersted, Marta Kvande Kiersted, James C. McKelly, Keith Perry, David Peterson, Constance Relihan, Gary MacDonald, Ann Marie Mann Simpkins, Margaret Smith, Susanne Thomas, James Truman, Joseph Walker, Frank Walters, Jodi Wyett, Hilary Wyss, and Jake York. To them, their spouses, and families go my gratitude and love. Most of all I thank my family, especially my beloved aunt, Sr. Jordan Dahm, OSF, a scholar, community leader, and joyful servant, for all she has taught and given me, and my "nuclear" grouping—Richard, Philomena, Christine, and Michael—whose interest, encouragement, and love comfort and sustain me always.

Finally, some words of gratitude and admiration for the courageous clerical and medical staffs of the Infectious Disease Inpatient Unit and HIV Outpatient Program at New Orleans's Charity Hospital, and especially for the heroic men and women served by these facilities. The pizzazz and grace with which they face their daily battles with terrifying illness and death will always amaze and inspire me. This book is dedicated to them and to the memory of the many angels I encountered there, now sorrowfully lost to HIV/AIDS.

• • •

Earlier versions of portions of this book appeared as "The Bomb Next Door: Four Postwar Alterapocalyptics," *Genre: Forms of Discourse and Culture* 30.4 (Winter 1997): 333–58; "Not Bombshells but Basketcases: Gendered Illness in Nuclear Texts," *Studies in the Novel* 31.4 (Winter 1999): 471–88; and "Angels in an Epidemic: Women as 'Negatives' in Recent AIDS Fiction," *South Central Review* 16.1 (Spring 1999): 57–72.

INTRODUCTION

Five Minutes to Midnight—What Is a Postmodern Plague?

> Illness has changed in the last fifty years, during the transition from modern to postmodern times. We fall sick from unheard-of ailments, we pass through undreamed-of treatments, we die in unsettling new ways and places.
>
> —David B. Morris, *Illness and Culture in the Postmodern Age*

In January 1980, on the eve of the Reagan-Bush decade of societal dismantling and abandonment, the "Atomic Scientists" who have published their world-watching *Bulletin* since the dawn of the nuclear age nudged their doomsday clock from 9 minutes to midnight, where it had been set since 1974, to the 7-minute position. The "clock," actually only an upper-left quadrant whose menacing features dominated the cover of the *Bulletin* from 1947 until the mid-1960s, has been reduced in size and moved to the inside pages, yet it remains a widely consulted barometer of the stability or chaos of the global nuclear situation. In 1980 this chronometric surge was an indictment not of Reagan, whose "evil empire" was as yet more rhetoric than realization, but of the Carter administration—its deadlocked arms discussion with the Soviets and both superpower leaders' persistence in acting like "nucleoholics." The clock's minute hand began a forward drift in the mid-1970s, following the "détente decade" (1960–72)—during which it had hovered at a relatively free-breathing 10 or 12 minutes to midnight—and after the Strategic Arms Limitations Talks (SALT) broke down at a Moscow summit.

Yet the clock's move forward at the dawn of the "me decade" was an equally telling prediction of things to come, as the nuclear stockpiling that propelled Reagan's economy and politics during his first term encouraged a similar buildup by the Soviets and resulted in heavy deployment of missiles throughout Europe by both sides. Margot A. Henriksen points to a wealth of responses to the threat of the bomb in the early 1980s, after several decades of seeming acceptance or indifference to atomic power;[1] and perhaps in conjunction with this increased awareness, the clock moved from 7 minutes in 1980 to 4 minutes a year later and then to 3 minutes—where it had been in 1953 after both the United States and the U.S.S.R. successfully detonated their first hydrogen bombs—in 1984.[2] The new cause for alarm was the rapid escalation of the Reagan-Gorbachev showdown, a near-termination of arms negotiations. The clock remained at 3 minutes to midnight for the duration of Reagan's second term and, as if loosened by a global sigh of relief, fell back to 6 minutes in January 1988, on the eve of his ultimately less powerful successor's presidency.

By the time the Berlin Wall was felled by the youth and otherwise outraged citizens of East Germany in fall 1989, the *Bulletin*'s clock, still at 6 minutes, was poised to reflect a new era of détente. Hailing not only this momentous upset but concurrent (however embryonic) victories for democracy in South Africa and Tiananmen Square, the clock setters reversed the minute hand to the 10-til position, then to the unprecedented 17-til outpost a year later, with the signing of the U.S.-Soviet Strategic Arms Reduction Talks (START) treaty. A modified clock design accompanied the minute hand's retreat from the zone of the fourth quadrant; instead of a magnified view of "the last" 15 minutes, an entire clock face was visible, although the clock's designers, wary of too much optimism, continued to depict five-minute markers for the 9 through 12 positions only.

• • •

As stated above, the clock registers, in part in spite of itself, not only the endless oscillations between nuclear buildup and disarmament by the reigning superpowers but also the greater social tides—Reagan's powerful presidency, revolution in China, apartheid in South Africa—that oversee our chances of survival. In its pages, the *Bulletin* has addressed other, related issues of environmental health and the poverty of third-world nations, the ways in which all of these seemingly separate fields interrelate and affect our ability to avert global disaster. Although the issues of AIDS and HIV have never been a focus of the *Bulletin* (or a factor in the movement of the doomsday clock), we must note the remarkably accurate reading of this newer but concurrent crisis as is provided in charting the clock's progress as well: a leap toward midnight in 1980, when the virus was first discovered and hit the national consciousness in tidal waves; another surge forward in 1981, when the disease gained greater recognition but also drew more homophobic hysteria; the precarious 3-minute setting that shadowed the late 1980s and marked the zenith of government indifference and underfunding of AIDS treatment and research, the spread of misinformation in the media, and skyrocketing infection rates in affected populations worldwide. The discovery and distribution of AZT in the late 1980s, the subsequent passage and funded support of the Ryan White Act, and the current administration's positive stance on the rapid development and Food and Drug Administration (FDA) approval of cutting-edge medical treatment coincide with the doomsday clock's recent easing back from the brink of destruction in the specifically nuclear register. Indeed, the development and markedly successful testing of the promising protease-inhibitor drug class may prove to be the worldwide HIV community's own fallen Berlin Wall: in the coming months and years, we will learn of the longer-term success rates of these drugs; in the present moment, we can only hope that these recent discoveries are indeed as revolutionary as they seem.

Yet while the clock has remained at the 17-minute mark through much recent global upheaval—ethnic conflicts in the dissolving Yugoslavia, resurgent communist voices in Russia and its breakaway republics, threats from the biological warfare machinery of Iraq—this reprieve has been only temporary. In June 1998, the nuclear arms testing that resulted in a showdown between India and Pakistan goaded the *Bulletin*'s editors into advancing the minute hand once more, to the 9-minutes-to-midnight mark, the biggest jump in thirty years. Likewise, HIV continues to threaten its original and now newly affected populations. African-American men, women of all races, teenagers, and even young gay men who, we might think, should know better than any of us, face rising infection rates; budget shortfalls in the United States and the general inability to meet this disease's worldwide funding needs threaten to cancel any recent gains in medical technology. In addition, these new treatments, even if they continue to show promising results, are so prohibitively expensive that only the minuscule few who can afford the cost of obtaining them may ultimately benefit.

Thus our doomsday clock, inching once more onto a forward course that may mark the beginning of another nuclear buildup, chronicles in indirect fashion the equally concerning, lingering threat of AIDS. That these crises may be much closer to midnight than any clock has begun to show—indeed, that they are composed of the volatile matter that could send their respective hands spinning toward 5 minutes, 3 minutes, even midnight itself in less than a moment's notice—define these crises as postmodern nightmares, as the "epidemics" of fear, hostility, hysteria, and global threat that plague our postmodern times. In the shadow of this clock, life in the postbomb era itself is an endless counting down, an awareness of time and the momentousness of its movement toward midnight that bothers our dreams, diminishes our ability to care and love, and exacerbates our fears in the face of biological and environmental crises into hysterical searches for scapegoats and enemies within.

• • •

This study will consider the cultural conditions that have formed in these waning moments before midnight and, specifically, the status of these remaining drops of grace as they are horded, squandered, and increased through the literary and cinematic offerings of this era. The cold war, with its legacy of nuclear conflict, disarmament, and energy-related environmental hazard, and the more recent AIDS crisis will form the poles of this inquiry into late twentieth-century existence, our perception of these five minutes we inhabit as it drives us toward paranoia and hostility but also in search of cures and peace.

Throughout, I will make frequent use of two terms that are indispensable to this study: "postmodern," which, as a theoretical and cultural concept, fundamentally shapes our understanding of life (and time) itself ever since the bomb itself; and "plague," a decidedly premodern concept that conjures up images of old (ineffective) science and medicine, old styles of public policy, and old-time religion. Modern rejuvenations of this latter term may seem equally incongruous with the slant and purpose of this study, as the term has been deployed as a weapon by some religious fundamentalists who have read AIDS itself as a "plague upon" multiple populations deemed deserving of such punishment. Yet "plague" is as necessary and appropriate to this study as "postmodern"; in fact, despite its medieval history and flavorings, the term "plague" is a consummately postmodern one. Notwithstanding the efforts of science or city managers in medieval times or religious conservatives today to use the term and the occasion it represents to castigate, divide, and banish, the profound *infectiousness* of "plague" has always rendered such efforts largely futile, instead forging among members of seemingly opposed groups an identification and a relationship that is life-threatening or life-sustaining.

While we might find the term "plague" naturally gestating in our more recent AIDS era, recall that "contamination" represented an equally palpable fear during the atomic/cold war period and is still an issue of significant importance with respect to nuclear hazards of all kinds. Despite multiple medical and social advancements throughout the twentieth century, fears of plague have not been eradicated by science, politics, or religious fervor but have instead spawned a *plague of fears* that worsens the crises attending any period of true biological threat and fuels the fires of mistrust and misinformation in contexts where this threat is nonexistent. It is the postmodern that allows (or forces) all of us to recognize the ways we are affected *and infected* by every episode of epidemic suffering in the postbomb era and, perhaps more importantly, the ways in which the fears of the survivors (healthy, so far) among us are more infectious and destructive than any actual environmental disaster or virus ever could be.

In chapter 1 I establish in detail the parameters of these postmodern plagues and make the case for the strong resemblance and profound interrelation between them. While bound to consider these plagues to some degree as political, historical, and medical phenomena, as a practitioner of literature and language studies I focus primarily on the language surrounding and arising from these periods, specifically literary and cinematic texts, through which we, as users of language, "contract" but also exacerbate or alleviate the continuing effects of these plagues. To that end, chapter 1 concludes with an in-depth consideration of basic linguistic structures, metonymy and metaphor and the supplemental dynamic between them, as they describe and complicate our more complex conceptions of illness and explosion—and our hopes for surviving these. This chapter is helpfully influenced by Susan Sontag's comparative analyses of tuberculosis, cancer, and AIDS in language and history, and her work is extensively considered at this point as well.

In chapter 2 I enlarge upon this concept of the "postmodern" by considering a central theme in postmodern theory that is also vital to a genre-based reading of plague themes—the spatiotemporal. I begin with a thematic analysis of four plague genres controlled by spatial and temporal markers: postapocalyptic and alterapocalyptic nuclear texts, pre-epidemic and intraepidemic AIDS texts. I then investigate several significant examples from these genres—novels, plays, and auto/biographical accounts—as they are defined and clarified by my spatiotemporal generic distinctions. In the course of these delineations, I pause to examine and finally reject two problematic subgenres within plague texts—the preapocalyptic and the postepidemic—for their oversimplified treatments of war and illnesses, their reliance on an impermeable boundary separating healthy from ill that is only a dangerous delusion.

I name this impulse to purge and homogenize the "utopic" based on the problematic ways this trope has been employed in literature since Sir Thomas More's *Utopia* and in conservative political ideologies for even longer. Certainly, utopia as a literary genre suffers from a preachy, pedantic quality that is likely to put off and bore a readership unable to maintain interest in the story of a world completely devoid of conflict or complication. Often the positive message utopia would send is lost on readers who, literally, cannot see the problem with the society set up as an instructional model. And for all of its potentially progressive, inclusive ways, utopia is an engineered, perfected space that demands of the imperfect humans occupying it conformity to the strictest standards, with failure to adhere to these eliciting a sentence of expulsion.[3] While moral standards of generosity, fairness, nonviolence, and love should be goals for every society, we know that "morality" is defined quite differently by many in the mainstream of developed nations and that the wall of the utopia island resembles in recent times the demarcated map of the United States espoused by the likes of David Duke, with racial, ethnic, sexual, and political minorities securely partitioned off from the "white nation" that is Duke's—and many others'—dream.

Likewise, the *physical* ("aryan") perfection that is often part of the utopic agenda cannot be enjoyed by everyone equally, especially with the sick redefined as moral "failures" and expelled in similar fashion. Certainly the *dream* (the utopic fantasy or "no-place") of a world without the sick or the threat of contamination is much easier to construct out of lies to a trusting public or divisive legislation than to transform into a lived *reality.* Pundits from the far right who advocate, for instance, the marking and seclusion of homosexuals or HIV-positive individuals promote their dangerous dreams of "a world without AIDS," a utopic space that is, in reality, a nightmare. As David B. Morris has incisively observed: "One measure of change in the postmodern era is the degree to which utopian thought—in emphasizing the solitary, secular, individual body—has expanded the role of health from by-product [of progressive social practices] or metaphor to highest social good. Health no longer refers . . . to the ideal social state that generates it but instead signifies the perfection of a single private self" (139).

In chapter 3 my emphasis on "plague" is found in my concentration on the biological as opposed to the theoretical, the affected and afflicted bodies that inhabit significant literary texts and the text-producing bodies (i.e., authors and readers) inhabiting cold war and AIDS-era contexts. Introducing the concept of triangularity, which I find essential to consideration of gender in plague texts, I analyze the originary feminine-masculine oppositions found in these to be shortly, inevitably disrupted by a triangulating third term. I proceed to examine the various triangles, romantic and otherwise, evident in these texts and compare triadic configurations as offered by early and late postmodern authors. In the remainder of this chapter I consider the densely interrelated imagery of these plague themes, the ways in which nuclear literature and AIDS literature *each* form powerful alliances with *both* image repositories under discussion here—gendered images of illness and of the bomb. As I move thematically instead of text by text in chapters 2 and 3, novels and plays with multiple meanings for this project will be found "exploded" over the course of several discussions from one chapter to the next and sometimes within the same chapter. In this manner I am only enacting the reading of exciting literature that rewards multiple returns to it with new understanding each time. I hope also with this method to strengthen my attempt to knit the relationship not only between these plague periods but between the significant thematic concerns defining them.

In chapter 4 I turn to cinematic examples from these two eras, considering cold war and AIDS-era cultural artifacts at their most interrelated: through the phenomenon of the cold war original and the AIDS-era remake. The remake relationship allows for an especially close comparison of discourse and influence from one era to the next, and the pattern created by the repetition of one film by another creates an illuminating picture, one that is potentially capable of alleviating plague's negative effects. Here I examine a range of plague-film styles and remake relationships, relying on psychoanalytic, feminist, and semiotic film theories to illuminate the important generational ties between these films and the eras into which they were born.

My conclusion will return briefly to the "enemy" as I have described it all along—the utopic impulse that promises safety and survival for the healthy few and encourages the abandonment of the ill and disempowered through the offer of these false promises. The (e)utopic as beautiful *space* must be substituted, I argue, with the concept of a *(e)utemporal:* not a "no time" but a "better time" that includes not only everyone now existing in our space but the space (our struggling planet) itself. As time is fluid, uncontrollable, and universally shared, it is a contagion that is simultaneously a cure—forcing an awareness of the limits of our "five minutes" on earth that in turn elicits thoughtful and healing efforts to ensure and improve the five minutes of those who will come after.

1

Counting Down—To Catastrophe or Cure?

BOMB SCARES: TWO EPIDEMIC ERAS

In describing two postmodern events—the cold war at its hottest from 1945 to 1962 and our own current era of devastation by AIDS—as *plagues,* I may have "sickened" both a good deal more than is correctly the case. I could have chosen a less dramatic term, such as "epidemics" or "outbreaks," and perhaps excluded the earlier event from the discussion altogether, since the cold war never actually made anyone sick (aside from a relative few above-ground testing victims in the American West, the South Pacific, and perhaps the outlands of the former U.S.S.R.). Also, I may have overestimated the significance of the sickness caused by AIDS, as the syndrome gets disproportionate attention from the news media, while the less-trumpeted cancer and heart disease always were and always will be much more widespread killers. In response I must defend my use of this term, as it contains all the political and discursive depth necessary to describe not the biopolitical phenomena themselves but our *collective affliction by and response to* them—literarily, cinematically, culturally—in their respective periods. Thus the cold war spawned a plague, not of communism or of bomb-related illness, but of paranoia, xenophobia, and red-baiting that took on witch-hunt proportions. Likewise, the AIDS era will be remembered not for its *epidemic* of HIV but for its *plagues* of homophobia, germophobia, racism, and classism.[1]

Indeed, these debilitated states of fear, hostility, and ignorance have arisen in response to a demonstrably devastating, notoriously indiscriminate physical threat. In the earlier era we faced the possibility of a nuclear-induced "epidemic" of cancer and radiation-related injuries—widespread contamination that would wipe out whole sections of geographically proximal populations as if it were a contagious disease. Politicians up through the Reagan and Bush administrations have spoken of "winning" a limited nuclear attack, the likes of which would cause millions of fatalities from radiation sickness and unprecedented cancer death rates; in the immediate postwar period this situation seemed even more imminent, and society geared itself up to survive such an event in a fit of hysteria that obscured the futility of its efforts. Even now, in days of relative peace, the threat of nuclear meltdown from mismanaged, ill-maintained reactor sites threatens the populations and environments of hundreds of thousands in developed countries; in the United States this threat is almost always directed toward poor and powerless communities whose dependence on nuclear-industry-based livelihoods or the resulting devaluation of property keeps them tied to a place that may be deadly to themselves or their children. In the AIDS era the frightening and disfiguring conditions caused by the virus and the high mortality rates that characterized the disease in the 1980s, as well as our growing awareness of the virulence and resilience of countless "emerging" viruses in the 1990s, have been a cause of deep concern. Since the 1970s, increased media coverage of medical scares like toxic shock syndrome, Legionnaires' disease, Lyme disease, "mad cow" disease, and especially AIDS has led us to regard the world as invisibly but fatally toxic and to regard our own bodies as permanently besieged yet hopelessly underprepared for defense.

Yet in the immediate postwar period fears of unknowable enemies, and equally unrealistic dreams of destroying them, caused an anti-"red" craze that did more damage than communism in the West ever did, while virulent homophobia, virophobia, and classism infect the seronegative among us today. In both periods an exaggerated fear of succumbing has forced us into paranoid isolation and finally powerlessness against the biological danger at the root of each crisis. Jonathan Schell concludes that the nuclear threat (afflicting us yet) has caused our capacity for love to diminish as our capacity for destruction expands: "it has tended to withdraw to a mental plane peculiarly its own, where it has become an even more solitary affair: impersonal, detached, pornographic" (*Fate of the Earth* 158).[2] As the love Schell describes is Freud's Eros in particular, the archetypal foe of the death drive, his diagnosis applies equally to the AIDS crisis: put off in many respects by the sexual nature of the disease, we have forsaken all physical contact, withdrawing our hand from those who need it most.

In both cases, then, I am describing as plague not the actual illnesses around which each period developed but the web of political, social, and discursive reactions to both that have been so widespread, so psychologically and societally debilitating, that no term can overdramatize the problem. In one respect our fears have been in response to a nonexistent threat, revealing them as that much more deforming: neither communism nor nuclear attack during the cold war were at our back door in the manner it was commonly believed; and neither AIDS nor homosexuality can be "caught" by shaking hands or sharing a classroom with HIV-positive or gay individuals.[3] Having said this, I do not wish to imply that in all other respects the threats of nuclear destruction and AIDS are not imminent and globally significant, to be fought against with every effort; nor will I suggest that these plague-like societal reactions could have formed or can be fully understood outside of their relationships to the illnesses themselves.[4] The illnesses have spawned the plagues, which in turn only worsen the effects of the illnesses, binding both ever more tightly in the same fatal knot.

• • •

In describing these two world-threatening events as *postmodern,* I may be attempting to "linguify" both in a way that might jettison the material reality of their damaging effects, as well as the body itself, into the realm of inconsequence. Perhaps I am being trendy and theoretical about two issues that defy all efforts to theorize, that stop us silent—if not dead—in our tracks due to the magnitude of the destruction that attends both. Doing so, I run the risk of conflating the related but not identical issues of theory and practice, suggesting that ideas, couched sensitively enough, have a life of their own outside activism. In response to this even more valid critique, I would point out the illuminating potential of defining these biological threats as decidedly postmodern conditions: not only do significant similarities that may help us contextualize and thus better understand both appear; examining the linguistic components of each will demonstrate indisputably our fundamental relationship, as language users, to these entirely "communicable" diseases, preventing us from closeting them into a seemingly contained, removable realm and forgetting our urgent responsibility to erase them from our experience.

In the appendix to *The Archeology of Knowledge,* Michel Foucault determines that the "ponderous, awesome materiality" of language manifests itself in our inclination to be "enveloped in words, borne way beyond all possible meanings by it," to feel "there would have been no beginnings: instead speech would proceed from me, while I stood in its path—a slender gap—the point of its possible disappearance" (215). Here language is likened to its presumed opposite—the material conditions of history itself—and the properties that each borrows from the other redefine both in specifically postmodern terms: seen as language, history manifests a fluidity and timelessness (ahistoricity); seen as history, language reveals itself as an influence on world events as decisive as captured territory or the assassination of a king. Emphasizing just this dissolution of categories in our first postwar conflict, cold war journalist John Sharnik writes that the "cold war is an anomaly with no precise starting date" and no initiating "incendiary event," the likes of which have characterized every other major conflict (5). And while politicians may insist that the cold war is over, new threats of a nuclear dimension present themselves every day, as nuclear technology circulates the globe, questioning, if not dissolving, any notion of a conclusion. Thus the cold war is an example of one of Foucault's language "envelopes," surrounding those who are living through it as if it consisted of tangible events while, like all other envelopes, containing in fact only the letters, written documents, and communiqués that are its events instead.

In *Libra,* Don DeLillo's novel of the Kennedy assassination, a CIA operative plots an attempt on the president's life that will look like the work of Castro loyalists: "We do the whole thing with paper. Passports, drivers' licenses, address books. Our team of shooters disappears but the police find a trail. . . . We script a person or persons out of ordinary pocket litter" (28). Later in the novel the character of Oswald (coming across as a crackpot to even his own communist compatriots) is discouraged by the Fair Play for Cuba Committee from opening a "branch office" in New Orleans, although "they were nice and polite and made spelling mistakes and anyway the important thing was the correspondence itself. He would keep everything. These were his papers. . . . Besides he didn't need New York's backing to open an office. He had his rubber stamping kit. All he had to do was stamp the committee's initials on a handbill or piece of literature. Stamp some numbers and letters. This makes it true" (313). Displaying these scraps of his record as a loyal communist to officials at the Soviet embassy in Mexico, Oswald is confounded by their refusal to permit him to travel to the Soviet Union. He insists that "documents are supposed to provide substance for a claim or a wish. A man with papers is substantial" (357). Of course, we are to read Oswald's inner monologue ironically in one respect and, in another, to disdain the false pretenses of this paper hero, a nobody desperate to break into history. Meanwhile, it is Oswald's own papers and the papers of political theorists (he is an avid reader of the communist classics and U.S. military handbooks) that send him around the world in search of a utopic society and then home to Dallas among the reams of the Texas Schoolbook Depository where his own paper trail will align itself perfectly with the one being created by the CIA. Thus Oswald, in all the ways he is historically significant, is made of paper—his own, the CIA's, the pages of DeLillo's novel—yet out of these papers flies the bullet that "broke the back of the American century" (181).

Likewise, the AIDS crisis began from no locatable incendiary event, as its origin is thus far indeterminable and may have begun its course of destruction in the thick of our response to another worldwide epidemic: the perfection of a polio vaccine.[5] However, even this "origin" refers only to its introduction to human history; its life as an organism unto itself may well be as old as the planet. Also, an absolute end to AIDS is highly unlikely, even if a vaccine is discovered, as viruses and bacteria are uncannily postmodern in their ability to mutate into resistant strains and then, after years or decades of dormancy, return at an opportune moment. We see that the tuberculosis bacterium affecting so many AIDS patients with near-deadly effect is an especially relevant example.

In "The Plague of Discourse: Politics, Literary Theory, and AIDS," his inquiry into the relationship between language and history (figurality and literality) in AIDS discourse, Lee Edelman points out that even gay- and HIV-affirmative groups like ACT UP try to borrow scientific certainty in their "mathematical" equation "Silence = Death." This authoritative claim to the literal, however, is hopelessly undercut by the equal sign's deep attachment to the figural, specifically the metaphoric: "Though Silence = Death is cast in the rhetorical form of geometric equation . . . , the fact remains that the equation takes shape as a figure, that it enacts a metaphorical redefinition of 'silence' and death" (311–12). Edelman concludes that "the truth of such equations can only pass for truth so long as we ignore that the literal must itself be produced by a figural sleight of hand" (312). Similarly, S. C. McCombie has pointed out the resemblance between an "AIDS" designation and the classically postmodern instability of the sign: "To have 'AIDS' one must have some other disease, such as *Pneumocystis carinii* pneumonia or Kaposi's sarcoma. . . . But a person with HIV infection who becomes ill and dies does not have 'AIDS' unless evidence for one of these or number of other conditions is found. *Thus, 'AIDS' is defined in relationship to other known diseases*" (13; emphasis added).

The ways in which this AIDS designation slides along the surface of one diagnostic signifier to the next bears a marked resemblance to the extreme *superficiality* of the infectious process itself: viral particles are attracted to *the surface* of CD4 cells and dock with appropriately "dressed" host cells in a complicated surface-point interlocking process. Furthering the seeming two-dimensionality of HIV (in fact the virus particles are spherical) is our understanding that they are *not* alive, do not "reproduce" but "replicate," like a wall full of Warhol Marilyns; an oft-used analogy for an infected cell is that of an HIV "copy machine." Discursive terms like "messenger RNA," "transcription," and "translation" define the virus's most insidious skills—its ability to invade, transform, and co-opt functions in the healthy cell. Deftly manipulating cellular surfaces, HIV cells are masters of disguise, inserting themselves into healthy host cells and masquerading as bodily allies that the immune system misrecognizes and allows to proliferate. At other points in the infectious process, HIV particles latch onto the surfaces of healthy cells, reconstituting their surfaces so that the cells appear to be bodily enemies, soon destroyed by this same confused immune system. The linguistic elements in these postmodern events—their insubstantiality, figurality, continuity, immeasurability, and superficiality—bring out their likeness to language itself, infecting us through our very positions, universally held, as users of language.[6]

As materiality, the linguistic components of the cold war and AIDS have caused, even created, historical events with all the force and effect of more traditional incendiary events. Communications theorists Lynn Boyd Hinds and Theodore Otto Windt Jr. argue that not only was the cold war *fought* with language but for the most part it was *created out of* the inflammatory political speeches, news reports, and telegrams that preceded the military and economic maneuverings that are historically associated with the cold war. Hinds and Windt, as well as Sharnik, allude to the decidedly performative nature of Winston Churchill's "Iron Curtain" speech delivered at a Fulton College commencement after he had been voted out of office. Harry S. Truman was in attendance that day, and the otherwise obscure moment turned out to be "history-making" in the most radical sense. Sharnik notes that the speech that described an iron curtain[7] as having descended "from Stettin in the Baltic to Trieste in the Adriatic" was heard in the British Foreign Office as "disastrous" and "warmongering," while Stalin himself called it an "invitation to war" (26). Specifically, the address effectively divided into two entrenched and opposing camps a postwar world that most had seen as shifting, multilateral in objectives, and at least generally reflecting the World War II groupings of Axis and Allied powers. Instead, "now there were but two sides. . . . In this ideological dichotomy there was no middle ground. The sharp division was a paradigm in which European nations were already either on one side of an iron curtain or another, and the other nations of the world had become the battleground to determine on which side they would eventually fall" (Hinds and Windt 93). While Churchill may have only been describing what he observed (or, more precisely, what his fears had caused him to imagine), it was the verbalization of these fears in such a politically charged context that transformed his remarks from benign description to menacing prescription.

Likewise, the role of language in worsening and in some cases creating the ill effects of the AIDS crisis has been documented by multiple AIDS cultural theorists. Simon Watney argues that people with AIDS (PWAs) have suffered almost as much from media mistreatment of AIDS as they have from the disease complex itself. Citing numerous instances of outright homophobic journalism in British magazines, newspapers, and television shows, Watney finds AIDS, as a hot story, is "'good' news" for journalists and newscasters whose work, as always subject to consumer interest, "is thus inexorably caught up in the larger discourse of retribution against gay men" (82). Cindy Patton has also worked extensively to debunk media-created myths about AIDS, such as "AIDS madness," an alleged cognitive deterioration that "provide[s] the popular imagination with a pseudoscientific basis for the longstanding fears of the psychologically impaired homosexual or the crazed junky" (*Inventing AIDS* 28). For both Watney and Patton, the media's economically motivated construction of "victims" out of patients, "tragedy" out of heroism, and "innocence" solely out of the profiles of middle-class, married, and drug-free PWAs creates false realities for gullible, frightened readers.

In addition, the red tape of public- and private-funding bureaucracies—Medicaid, Disability, Aid to Families with Dependent Children (AFDC), life or health insurance companies, and viatical settlement organizations—is, of course, a language-made obstacle directly threatening the survival of PWAs. The disease process being what it is, many HIV-positive individuals fail to qualify for medical disability because their symptoms are not visible enough; others with limited education have trouble filling out public aid forms, maintaining personal records, and even understanding dosage instructions printed on their prescriptions. Meanwhile, language—education and outreach—is also one of the most effective treatments we can offer those at risk or already infected: a clever advertisement or provocative poster can do almost as much to save lives as can current drug regimens; a generous funding policy, even a kind word, can mean the difference between suffering and survival.

Thus it is these postwar crises' consummate relationship to and definition by the *postmodern*—language-created and language-controlled—that have caused their simultaneous transformation into historical, political, and cultural *plagues.* The discursive hype attached to communist ideology, the nuclear threat, homosexuality, and HIV/AIDS takes on its own life as soon as it ignites, obscuring a core biological threat that is either something completely different or, for many of us in so many respects, entirely nonexistent. Alarmingly, the more fanciful and ephemeral (exaggerated, hysterical, incorrect) the language surrounding and constituting these biological phenomena becomes, the more powerfully negative the real-world effects they produce. Thus does language circle back to do the work done by weapons-based and germ warfare in earlier periods: it creates hostility, misunderstanding, even suffering and death, directing its destructive valences toward the receivers of words and policy and back against language makers and language users themselves.

HISTORY REPEATS ITSELF: THE COLD WAR AS MIRROR TO THE AIDS CRISIS

Remarkably, featured players in both these postmodern crises share similar profiles—as victim, carrier, invisible enemy—in plague discourse, causing us to consider even further the nature of the relationship between them. Chris Glaser observed several years ago a correlation between the fear of suspect symptoms, anxiety, mistrust, and survivor guilt felt by persons with HIV and these same emotions as experienced by Japanese *hibakusha* (nuclear bomb survivors), as evidenced by Robert Jay Lifton's research. On the other, more ubiquitous side of the coin, McCarthyites during the cold war, according to Cindy Patton, were able to link the perceived threats of communists and homosexuals through "us[ing] medical and military imagery interchangeably: reds and queers were alternately diseases and invasions. . . . Although homosexuality was less overtly discussed (though much alluded to), communism and faggotry were well established as threats to U.S. security" (*Sex and Germs* 88).[8] In *Libra* (an AIDS-era comment on the cold war), the World War II fighter pilot David Ferrie is an interesting variation on Patton's theme—heroic and patriotic (yet a co-conspirator to treason), openly homosexual, and a real "sicko" in every respect. Ferrie (could history have named names more serendipitously?) suffers from alopecia universalis, a total lack of body hair, and resembles unfortunately "something pulled from the earth, a tuberous stem or fungus esteemed by gourmets" (29), while his efforts to disguise the condition are only more disconcerting: "He winced all the time in front of the mirror as he pasted on his homemade eyebrows and mohair toupee" (29). His physical appearance is comical and unkempt, his apartment filthy and dark—an emblem of the disordered "crimes against nature" he perpetrates there against young, resisting men (Oswald included). Significantly, he is obsessed with cancer and the search for a cure, his bookshelves sagging with the weight of medical textbooks and autopsy reports, his conversation laced with the terminology and graveyard humor of a complete oncophobe. He tells his secretary, "I'm a walking sandwich board for cancer" (67) and claims that "once you set out consciously to cure the disease . . . you run the risk of catching it" (46). He refers snidely to "Comrade Cancer," shading medical and political hysterias into each other, and blasts the FBI for its intrusive ways: "They're on you like the plague. Once you're in their files, they never leave you alone. They stick to you like cancer" (45). Although the reader senses that Ferrie is finally just another member of the ensemble of freaks and outsiders populating this historical drama, his obsession with grave illness, his own physical peculiarities, and his frequently unrequited homosexual advances *mark* him as a special case—a creep even within a company of creeps and in multiple respects the villain of the piece.

Indeed, these two groups—reds in the earlier period and gays then and now—have been marked and mistreated in similar ways. Both communists and gay men (even most of those who are HIV-positive) move relatively inscrutably through the "general population."[9] The ultra-right's greatest fear of both these groups was/is their near-invisibility, the impossibility of spotting them at a distance and taking cover or taking revenge. Acceptance of Joseph McCarthy's otherwise ludicrous red-baiting and the protracted and wide-ranging intrusion into various Americans' private lives by the House Un-American Activities Committee (HUAC)—but also the flourishing of covert operations by both the CIA and FBI during this period—stemmed from the public's inability to tell a red from a patriot and take comfort in these stable categories. Pat Buchanan's call in 1983 to quarantine those infected with HIV, William F. Buckley's insistence that HIV-positives be marked with tattoos, and recent efforts in Congress to remove HIV-infected servicepeople from their posts *before* they have shown the first signs of illness have created an "insidious" invisibility for HIV infection in its early stages, suggesting that this illness, stealth bomber that it is, is a potential weapon that must be guarded against with a preemptive first strike. These views represent a modern-day McCarthyism, suspecting subversives in the least likely places, stirring up frenzy over a nonexistent threat.

Reds and gays have long been considered infectious in that communists were thought to be recruiting members among the idealistic and dissatisfied in this society, some of whom lived in your own backyard, and homosexuality (let alone AIDS), considered to be catching, is, according to Eve Kosofsky Sedgwick, the root of straight men's "homosexual panic"—a common and astoundingly effective legal defense of unprovoked verbal and physical gay bashing (*Epistemology* 19–20). Likewise, Lee Edelman argues that early nineteenth-century hate crimes against homosexual men were deemed by those who witnessed them inevitable and even proper due to "the brutalizing effect on the populace of any public discourse on sexual relations between men" ("Seeing Things" 93). What both theorists describe then is a perceived "infection" of the observer with gay sexuality *through observation alone* that allows these bystanders to turn violently—and legally—against their victims.

It is significant that, inside the head of his character Jack Ruby (who is constantly asking the strippers who work for him, "do I look like I'm queer to you?" [*Libra* 250]), DeLillo uses sexually suggestive language to describe Oswald's "contamination" of Ruby in the aftermath of Oswald's murder: Ruby "is miscast, or cast as someone else, as Oswald. They are part of the same crime now. They are in it together and forever and together. . . . He begins to merge with Oswald. He can't tell the difference between them. . . . Oswald is inside him now. How can he fight the knowledge of what he is?" (444–45). Interestingly, it is impossible to assign with certainty an identity to either "he" in this passage's final question, enmeshing Oswald and Ruby even more inextricably within each other's histories as well as within classically homophobic ruminations on "the knowledge of what he is." The homophobia is only worsened by the figuration of the man inside another man as an infection or cancerous growth whose violent eradication (Ruby's murder of Oswald; straights' crimes against gays) is therefore justified.

This decidedly postmodern fear of the infectious enemy—an enemy so close yet so unrecognizable that he may not only be on my home turf but may even be myself—defines the peculiar shape of the postmodern scare: no longer identifiable by racial or ethnic markings, this new "enemy within" has been since the cold war and continues to be the subject of intense investigation by medical and political "experts." Policymakers feeling threatened by these invisible enemies have redefined subjectivity itself by expanding their definition of the subversive to its widest, safest margins, reclassifying those they suspected not according to the relatively visible, definable lines of what they *did* but to amorphous, indefensible suggestions of who they *were.*

In the first volume of *The History of Sexuality,* Foucault describes the enormous change that occurred in our understanding of genders and sexualities when, late in the nineteenth century, the "homosexual became a personage, a past, a case history, and a childhood, in addition to being a type of life, a life form" (43). Earlier identified by the performance of individual *acts,* most of which had nothing to do with the taking of one's own sex as object choice, the class of the invert was expanded yet solidified in one move: now this population was, because much less definable, potentially much larger; yet this did not prevent the proliferation of discourse from physicians, psychologists, and legislators that had the effect of situating and containing this new type by the very power of discourse itself. David Halperin argues that the invention of the term "homosexuality" a little over a century ago—which allowed science and society to identify and taxonomize that which it defined and marked—was the "*appropriation* of the [gay] human body and of its erogenous zones by an ideological discourse" (25).

Likewise, a clause included in Truman's "Loyalty Program," an instrument for policing communist activity at home during the 1950s, enabled similar containment through expansion—an expanded definition of "red"—when it defined disloyalty not only as subversive *activities* but as having suspect *associations* as well. Hinds and Windt note that "such loose language opened the proverbial Pandora's box for investigation. [It] lifted people out of time, out of history" (168). The executive order that included this reclassification effectively dissolved the relatively stable category of subversive acts. One no longer had to do something to be investigated by HUAC; one could be guilty *by association.* This introduced the idea that one could be and not be a communist at the same time, that one could "contract" the ideology without even knowing it, while sitting around the dinner table with friends. The difficulty in identifying actual disloyalists and keeping accurate records of their activities incited fears of widespread "contamination," a red "plague" to match the horrors of its biological predecessors throughout the centuries—if not in terms of human casualties, at least in terms of its presumed debilitation of society.[10]

Fredric Jameson's theory of the populist tendency in postmodernism reveals some characteristics shared, if not by communists and gays themselves, then by their corresponding contexts, the nuclear and AIDS crises. He opposes the distinctly welcoming impulse in postmodern art to high modern architecture, which imposed an elitist aesthetic on the humbler buildings around it, slumming them in comparison. We find an epidemiological analog to modernism in the gentrifying tuberculosis strain that, says Susan Sontag, imposed a sensitivity and refinement on whomever it visited (35). In marked contrast, exposure to neither radioactive material nor HIV is understood to improve one's social status in this respect. It is the lower classes who would be affected first in the event of a meltdown in impoverished rural areas and those trapped in burned-out inner cities who would be threatened most in a nuclear attack; likewise, AIDS downclasses even the formerly middle class and well-to-do, as PWAs who used to hold good jobs with excellent benefits lose these and multiple other social privileges and suddenly find themselves waiting in lines and suffering the indignities associated with state-sponsored social and medical assistance. Their economically less fortunate counterparts, who are used to bearing these and related trials, suffer an even further downgrading, having now to accept "sick" and "contagious" in addition to the other burdensome labels (such as "homeless" or "addict") attached to them by the system that has been set in place to help them. Thus, while Jameson applauds the postmodern aesthetic for embracing the "common man," the thoroughly undesirable biopolitical realities of the postmodern, in their equally strong grasp of those least able to fend them off, must be lamented instead of lauded.

Additionally, we may observe the analogous *relationship between* each pair of terms under consideration here: as the nuclear is to cancer, so AIDS is to HIV. In each pairing there is a discursive and a biological component—a large, language-made cloud of an "issue" subjected to much theorizing by the press and professionals among the preapocalyptic and/or the uninfected, covering over the root of the discussion, the illness that is confined to the region of the unsayable. Even though Jacques Derrida, writing for a special "Nuclear Criticism" issue of *Diacritics,* determined that the nuclear is "the name of nothing . . . the pure name, the 'naked name'" ("No Apocalypse" 31), there is hardly a dearth of discursive material, even in his own essay, attempting to get some sort of fix on the nature of the nuclear. It is an eminently theorizable—or, as Derrida says, "fabulously textual"—subject, as theories are, with a handful of notable exceptions, our only way of understanding nuclear catastrophe thus far. Nuclear theorists William Chaloupka and Peter Schwenger are, in separate works, influenced by Derrida's mandate that peace-loving liberal arts practitioners intervene in this crisis that, far from being outside their fields, belongs more to them as textual interpreters of that which can be only text or else the end of textuality, than to any others: "nuclearism is no longer the interpretive province solely of realpolitik" but must be undertaken by nuclear critics who "expose nuclearism's presumptions . . . in an unprecedented way" (Chaloupka xiv). Yet this fascinating issue, so clarified by theory, so dependent on theory for many forms of its existence, tends to obscure its reason for being—fears of cancer and a "cancer" of fear, both of which continue to plague us even though the cold war is "over."

Sontag has found that cancer's "shameful" geography—its propensity to attack the breast, the colon, the prostate, and so on—prevents us from treating (in both senses of that term) the illness with plain language. "Any disease that is treated as a mystery and acutely enough feared will be felt to be morally, if not literally, contagious. Thus, a surprisingly large number of people with cancer find themselves being shunned by relatives and friends and are the object of practices of decontamination" (6). Likewise, the news and entertainment media tend to speak of this issue only when it wears a happy face: that of the survivor; the "fighter" (even when the battle is all but lost); the plucky, baseball-capped ten-year-old on his way to Disneyland; the scientist speaking cautiously but reverently of wonder drugs bringing lab rats back from near-death. Especially when newscasters and journalists take up the subject of the nuclear threat, it is always in terms of a *political* crisis originating between nations or factions, as the *biological* crisis that is the nuclear's immediate and inevitable aftermath is simply too much for words.

Although at first AIDS and HIV seem to describe the same phenomenon, to be much closer in meaning than a pair like the nuclear and cancer, "AIDS" moves further from the actuality of HIV with each new discovery about the virus.[11] I disagree with Sontag's assertion that the equally horrific geography (and biography) of AIDS has condemned it to the shunning and avoidance cancer receives (103–4); in fact AIDS has continued to affect mainly marginalized populations in U.S. society, enabling the news and tabloid media to speak freely and frequently on this subject, to "investigate" the crisis as noisily and intrusively as their readerships demand. Press coverage about AIDS, so much of it exaggerated fearmongering, is part of what Paula Treichler has defined in "AIDS, Homophobia, and Biomedical Discourse" as an "epidemic of signification"; it has only worsened the already-negative image of gay men, intravenous drug users, poor minority women, and the racial "others" populating Asia and Africa in "mainstream" America's imagination.

Meanwhile, in the medical and patient communities most affected, the term AIDS becomes more and more archaic, as the "syndrome"—the unexplainable mystery—that originally defined this disease complex begins to break down and dissolve. Healthcare providers speak of "HIV patients," or even just "positive patients"; and shortly thereafter it is the various specific conditions—Kaposi's sarcoma (KS) or *Pneumocystis carinii* pneumonia (PCP), cytomegalovirus (CMV) retinopathy or cryptosporidiosis—that form the basis for dialogue among doctors, among the HIV-positive themselves, and between members of both groups.[12] While "AIDS" is easier to remember, quicker to pronounce, already associated with all the attention-getting, perhaps lifesaving stories of the past fifteen years (Rock Hudson, Ryan White, Magic Johnson), we should be working to convert to the new language that new knowledge has created for us, since the discrepancy between the two terms is in fact endangering lives: in a state of denial and relative sound health, HIV-infected individuals have in some cases determined that they are "only" HIV-positive, do not actually have AIDS, and continue to engage in unsafe sexual practices that may threaten others and hasten the progression of their illness; unaware of the many differences between a diagnosis of "AIDS" and "HIV" uninformed patients may entertain and even act on suicidal thoughts or refuse the medical and lifestyle regimens that can indeed prolong their lives.

Associated with the failures of medical science and social support structures throughout the 1980s, "AIDS" is indeed a death sentence we have hopefully begun to move beyond. At this point the term remains meaningful only in the context of state-sponsored aid, which is allowed to individuals who meet the criteria for "full-blown AIDS" and denied to those in a rather arbitrarily circumscribed "pre-AIDS" situation. HIV-positivity, in marked contrast, is a way of life, a diagnosis that enables health maintenance and increased knowledge for patients and their care providers and may one day be treatable as a chronic but survivable illness that never reaches an AIDS-like final stage. Surely, the proliferation of overexcited discourse surrounding both cancer and HIV does not lessen the persisting "unsayability" of either but only drowns out the silence of fear and suffering that are their roots.

HISTORY REPRODUCES ITSELF: THE COLD WAR AS BLUEPRINT FOR THE AIDS CRISIS

Our current situation—that is, our shared experience of and response to AIDS—not only resembles significantly but also *emerged directly from* its midcentury predecessor in several ways. First, the cold war period has been defined by Peter Radetsky as a "golden age of virology,"[13] ushered in by John Enders's 1949 success with growing viruses in living tissue cultures—an event essential to Jonas Salk's discovery of an injectable polio vaccine in 1955.[14] Despite the success of this earlier effort against a deadly virus, evidence has surfaced linking the move of HIV from simian to human populations to this very vaccine development process. Jeremiah Creedon argues in the *Utne Reader* that it was the gestating of the oral forms of the polio vaccine in HIV-infected monkey kidneys that may have been the origin of AIDS's contact with humans, after these contaminated vaccines were ingested by children. He theorizes that the story has been disavowed or ignored thus far because the medical establishment will not admit the possibility of its playing a role, however unintentional, in releasing the virus into the human population. One even more controversial theory, from Mirko D. Grmek, posits that HIV emerged "from a mutation stimulated by—the experimental atomic explosions" (qtd. in Kruger 209). Grmek describes this theory as farfetched but seductive, playing on deep-seated fears "by coupling disasters symbolizing today's twin peaks of horror" (209).

Cindy Patton points out that the study of immunology flourished in the early 1960s, providing a holistic version of health with the appropriate westernized trappings of science, which "nicely mirrored the growing perception of the human being as being precariously perched in a world ecology" (*Inventing AIDS* 59). Patton notes that whereas virology focuses on and discovers the problem in the invading microorganism, immunology looks, in a way that resembles "Cold War paranoia," toward the body for the cause and cure:

"Immunology provided the grammar for shifting dominant metaphors of disease from offense to civil defense. Increasing concern with domestic unrest . . . demanded that our immune systems should conform to a policing and confessional ideology" (60).[15] I will be arguing throughout this study that the conditions prevailing during the cold war have come to characterize the AIDS era as well, so that the body remains precariously placed and as susceptible as ever to immunology's depiction of it as on the defensive, yet badly defended.

Within the cold war period are also the origins of a "golden age of homophobia" that reaches yet into our current period and has only barely begun to show signs of abating. Patton notes that "during World War II . . . countless lesbians and gay men relocated to urban industrial centers to be inducted into military service or work in military related fields" (*Sex and Germs* 124) when the desperate need for manpower forced the army to accept soldiers of any orientation. The end of the war and the alleviation of the personnel shortage allowed the military to return to its criminalizing, pathologizing stance toward homosexuality. In 1949 the newly created Department of Defense issued a strong policy against homosexuality; and in 1951 the Uniform Code of Military Justice included a specific ban on sodomy. Alan Bérubé has pointed out that while technically subject to an antisodomy rule included in the Articles of War of 1916, gay soldiers were allowed to remain in the armed forces during the war and excelled in not only stereotypical duties such as clerks, court stenographers, and chaplain's assistants but also in traditional masculine positions such as tank drivers, pilots, and cannoneers (57–58). We may infer that it was in part the fear of communism itself that exacerbated fears of *any* invasive outsider and led to the stiffening of antigay military policy that remains in effect to this day.

Beyond these several generational ties, the cold war has imposed itself on the collective consciousness and defined to a significant degree our experience of all succeeding postmodern plague periods,[16] the AIDS crisis included. Derrick De Kerckhove posits that "because of the bomb we are all experiencing the psychological conditions of wartime permanently" (78), and Jonathan Schell describes our increasing apathy toward survival, finally manifested as zombie-like indifference to all social problems, as "a second death." Sontag describes AIDS as the latest casualty of the cold war, finding our ultimate indifference to endless threats and weapons proliferation to have desensitized us to the plight of AIDS patients and all segments of humanity with special needs: "Apocalypse is now a long-running serial: not 'Apocalypse Now' but 'Apocalypse from Now On'" (*"Illness as Metaphor"* 176).

Again, the work of Don DeLillo provides relevant and provocative illustration. Several of his characters are fascinated by, yet disturbingly inured to, scenes of catastrophic destruction as found in alarmist, isolationist literature or among the sensationalist offerings of lowbrow television programming—due no doubt to the horror and fearsomeness of "reality" itself in the post-bomb age. In his early novel *End Zone,* Gary Harkness is a gifted but directionless defensive lineman recruited to a desolate college campus in north Texas whose other major source of identity and pride is its Reserve Officers' Training Corps (ROTC) program. Gary audits ROTC classes but performs in them better than the enrolled students due to his morbid fascination with postnuclear narrative in its goriest detail. When he is encouraged by Major Staley to join "the wing" and consider a military career, Gary protests that he is only "interested in certain areas of this thing in a purely outside interest kind of way. Extracurricular. I don't want to drop H-bombs on the Eskimos or somebody. But I'm not necessarily averse to the purely speculative features of the thing" (157).

This desire—not for a role in the realization or aversion of Armageddon but instead for an anonymous and unobstructed ringside seat—is arguably more perverse than that of the war-charged patriot but one that DeLillo's characters occupy in rapt submission. In *White Noise,* Jack Gladney's entire family succumbs to what Eugene Goodheart (borrowing from Saul Friedländer) calls the "kitsch of death": "DeLillo's characters (like us) comfortably watch 'floods and mud slides, emptying volcanoes,' while eating 'take out Chinese'" (124). Says DeLillo, "Every disaster made us wish for something bigger, grander, more sweeping" (69). Daniel Aaron has pointed out that "the creepy David Ferrie [of *Libra*] finds thoughts of bombs heart-lifting (as do, to their dismay, Gary Harkness and Jack Gladney)" (79). More recently, in *Mao II,* Karen is a former disciple of the Reverend Sun Myung Moon, engaged in the effort to deprogram herself, yet transfixed by televised scenes of mass-fanaticism and self-destruction. Quickly these narrative moments of Karen watching shift to an intense and detailed examination of the scenes themselves—a crush of wild fans at a soccer tournament, chaos around the coffin of the Ayatollah Khomeini—so that readers are forced into the position of horrified yet fascinated voyeurs, a position most of us no doubt readily accept. To complete the effect, DeLillo intersperses full-page but grainy reproductions of these various scenes of disaster (including the mass-wedding of thousands of "Moonies" at Yankee Stadium, in which Karen is depicted as having taken part) among his chapters so that the reader can/must "watch a little television" between the narrative episodes yet must intently scrutinize the pictures to make sense of them, becoming as engrossed and distracted as the zombified Karen. In an interview with Anthony DeCurtis, DeLillo acknowledged in his work "an apocalyptic feel" and an "intimation that our world is moving toward greater randomness and dissolution, maybe even cataclysm," asserting that "this reality has become part of all our lives over the past twenty-five years" (66). While DeLillo dates the start of this slide from the Kennedy assassination, his incisive and disturbing vision stretches back easily to include the cold war from its very inception.

• • •

This reality reflected so luridly on television sets throughout DeLillo's universe is indeed both outrageous atrocity and thoroughly ingrained matter of course. Multiple "bad habits" settled into—and originally justified in the name of democracy—during the cold war have grown and worsened in succeeding decades, causing and exacerbating our most current plague period of AIDS. For example, cancers and viruses have both emerged to some degree as late capitalist side effects: environmental disasters introduced to nonimmune populations in the process of military-industrial exploitation of the planet. While they are no less physical—that is, harmful—in nature, they are by no means "naturally occurring," as each new disruption of an ecosystem inevitably releases destructive organisms into atmospheres unequipped to fend them off. Sixty to 90 percent of carcinogens come from exposure to unkind material in our environment, many of these related to energy sources such as electricity and nuclear power. Jonathan Schell notes that due to aboveground nuclear testing in the 1950s and 1960s, the per capita dose of radiation is 4.5 percent above the natural background level for the United States (*Fate of the Earth* 12) and that traces of the radioactive isotope strontium-90 are detectable in the bone tissue of every person alive (62), a phenomenon likewise due to atmospheric testing. More recently, the ever-expanding hole in our atmosphere's ozone layer, due in large part to the pollution from auto emissions and big industry, increases daily our exposure to carcinogenic ultraviolet rays.

Similarly, viruses (especially many previously unheard-of and deadly strains) are theorized as being traceable to the manipulation of rain forests and other tropical regions where they were formerly maintained in an undisturbed, dormant state. Writing in the *New Yorker,* Richard Preston calls AIDS "the revenge of the rain forest. [It] is arguably the worst environmental disaster of the twentieth century, so far" (62). He goes on to explain that the development and exploitation of delicate South American and African ecosystems have shaken loose and sent traveling a multitude of organisms that the human population has no immunity against. In addition to industrially produced carcinogens, another cause of cancers is now understood to be viruses themselves—viral oncogenes—circulating in the environment or as part of a cell's inherited predisposition. Thus this viral assault on the general population by big business and the military may lead to a proliferation of both cancers and viruses, even recreating the possibility of a contagious "cancer epidemic" similar to the widespread carcinogenesis that would result from any level of nuclear attack.

Not only have diseases themselves been engineered inadvertently (or not) since the industrial boom of the cold war, but those who will be stricken and those who will survive may also be part of a larger plan. Sontag has observed that the "white flight" phenomenon from cities to suburbs in the immediate postwar period may have been due to middle-class fears of contagion in close quarters in big cities, leaving the inner-city poor to their own resources (74). Expanding this reading even more interestingly, Dean MacCannell attributes the same phenomenon to an unofficial but widely held understanding that a nation could be impervious to nuclear attack if it could render its cities (the main target of bombs) "expendable" by abandoning them to the "undesirable" element.[17] MacCannell cites James Bryant Conant, a presidential adviser and president of Harvard in the 1940s and 1950s, as the mastermind behind this demographic shift, which he and others in power sold to the American public as the rediscovery of rural roots that had been lost. Also, recent cultural critics have described the waning interest in AIDS treatment and prevention as racial minorities and intravenous drug users become the primary infection populations in the United States. Thus not only the illnesses but their recipients, the sick themselves, are in a certain respect cultural constructs, numbering among the multiple deleterious "byproducts" of global expansion for which big industry and Big-Brotherism are yet to claim responsibility.

You will note that I have just referred to a sick person, a patient with AIDS or environmentally induced cancer, as a "cultural construct" and "byproduct." I use these terms with terrific misgivings, as I fear this kind of linguistic situating may lend itself to the undercutting of actual patient experiences in unforgivable ways. I have always felt that there is a certain point, past sweeping demographics and the minutiae of cell biology, at which the phenomena we are grappling with escapes the barrage of theorization that reds and gays, the nuclear and AIDS, cancers and viruses cannot. This threshold marks the place of that which will not generalize itself to any theorizable degree, will not fit itself out for neat debate or resolution, and exists no doubt in sharp proximity to bodies themselves. While we can theorize "the body" until the cows come home, actual bodies, especially sick bodies or bodies in pain, may respond to no discursive gesture beyond the silence of sympathy.[18] As the poet Carolyn Forché has stated in a nuclear context, "there is no metaphor for the end of the world and it is horrible to search for one" (qtd. in Stone 68); and Sontag is disturbed by our inability to talk plainly about illness, denouncing all metaphoric manipulations of actual cases and reading any silence surrounding these as unwarranted shame. In her view this linguistic sidestepping is an illness itself, a sign of our dis-ease with what we at this point cannot—but must—learn to deal with honestly.

Yet I argue that the untheorizability of that most physical component of sickness or pain makes our silence at the final stage inevitable, incontrovertible evidence of, as performance theorist Jeanie Kay Forte argues, "the limits of theory . . . which [are also] . . . the limits of language" (439). Elaine Scarry's helpful formulation conceptualizes the problem: pain is "that which cannot be denied and that which cannot be confirmed" (9), and Forte adds that pain resists, and thus destroys, language by "reduc[ing] its subject to a state anterior to language. . . . It resists language because it has no object, no referential content" (440). While the diseases that I am here associating with postmodern plagues are in certain forms highly *communicable,* there is an absolute limit to our ability to *communicate* with the pain and discomfort that attends their physical manifestations.

By contrast, we must recognize that communication at some level is essential to all healing or preventative processes, and we must examine just those modes of "linguistic sidestepping" that Sontag denounces but that may not only be our lesser evil but our best hope. As Mary Ann Caws asks, considering a response to the nuclear crisis (and certainly countering Forché), "How to deal, in words, with what is most serious, except with metaphors?" (60). Turning now to an in-depth examination of language at its own limit, I would like to explore the viability of metaphor, or the literary in general, as a cure for the illnesses confronting us. As it may well be the last point of contact between two ultimately separate spheres, metaphor in its profound communicability is a source of unity and strength, a contagion that is in fact a cure.

TALKING CURES: METAPHOR, METONYMY, AND THE LOCATION OF ILLNESS IN LANGUAGE

The depth of the hysteria generating postmodern plague is determined by the condition of the *barrier* perceived to separate healthy from contagious, patriot from traitor, straight from queer: the more difficult we feel this barrier is to locate, erect, or maintain, the more virulent the reaction against those suspected of belonging on the other side. Perhaps it is conceived of as a straight line dividing health from sickness or safety from threat; perhaps it is an encircled or otherwise solidified *zone* within which the healthy remain, safe but restricted, or the sick are deposited in ever-growing numbers, as the effort to decontaminate the outer world can never stop. It is significant that Sir Thomas More's Utopia is an *island* before it is anything else, its difficult-to-access boundaries essential to its development and preservation of untainted, perfected society. The utopic desire for boundaries that hold ignites the rhetoric of the reactionary right throughout the cold war and AIDS eras, with destruction of these seen as equivalent to apocalypse. Significantly, the countertradition of dystopia (about which much more will be said later) rejects the dream of the island and the sustainability of the barrier, which more often than not is a prison wall. These are fantasies perpetuating a false reality that, seen beyond, will dissolve, enabling a fairer outcome for all concerned.

This barrier separating "me" from "not me," and especially from the chaos threatened by the removal of this barrier, is considered in some theories of illness and language through the discussion of *metaphor* and its various linguistic counterparts—the literal, realism, or metonymy. In a worthy effort to free patients (with cancer, AIDS, or tuberculosis) from the cordon sanitaire enforced by hysterical segments of society, Sontag, for instance, views metaphor *as* this dividing line, a distancing mechanism that allows those who employ it to shun, neglect, and objectify those forced onto the other side. Sontag denounces the conglomeration of metaphors surrounding tuberculosis, cancer, and AIDS, singling out for special critique "military" metaphors like "a war on AIDS" or "wiping out cancer in our lifetime." Like other recent critics,[19] Sontag is disturbed by the proliferation of terms that relegate these illnesses to the status of other, foreign intruder, enemy. She points out correctly that this divisiveness conflates the patient with her illness and solidifies the opposition as an ever-diminishing group of "us"—untainted and intact, at least as of our last checkup. Language (or, more specifically, the speaker of language) is incapable of isolating the ailment from the ailing and must therefore work to ban illness-as-metaphor from circulation entirely. Sontag, then, speaks not only of illness as metaphor but of *metaphor as illness*—a defect of every user of language, augmenting the misery and sometimes hastening the demise of those truly afflicted, that we must work together to purge ourselves of and recover from collectively.

Geoffrey Galt Harpham's investigation of illness ("the grotesque") as represented throughout the modern period in part concurs with Sontag's argument that metaphor marks the presence of illness in language. Harpham describes metaphor as a disseminator of the grotesque in language, as a principle of corruption and dissolution that is evident in the "grotesque crushing together" of elements perceived as insoluble in their literal ("pre"-

metaphoric) state. Harpham's examples are the grotesque sensations produced by momentarily literal readings of the metaphoric statements "Hector is a lion" and, even more bizarrely, "you are a typewriter." The metonymic, a casual, associative relationship between entities that allows the boundaries of each to remain intact, is closely related to the literal in this schema and is—in classic supplemental fashion—both opposite to and essentially included within the metaphoric function. In a nonrealist text like Thomas Mann's *Death in Venice,* says Harpham, Aschenbach's entire world becomes contaminated by metaphor, a bleeding of inner into outer worlds (and vice versa), represented finally in Aschenbach's own corpse dissolved into the death state.

Thus, while for Sontag metaphor constitutes the dividing line between healthy and ill, for Harpham metonymy (or realism) fills this role, enabling the *break* that opposes the impure and chaotic *blend* controlling metaphor.[20] Also in opposition to Sontag, who implies that it is possible to remove metaphor from language, Harpham sees in its degenerative activity an "extraordinary sense of 'inevitability'" (132). He is helped to this understanding by his reading of Derrida, who argues that "language is originally metaphorical" (*Grammatology* 271) and, as origin, *is* "nature," the natural state from which language arises and toward which it tends, however impure, tainted, or ruined this origin may be. Interestingly, whether metaphor is seen as the enforcer of health (but linguistically dispensable) or the mark of illness (but linguistically inevitable), both Sontag's and Harpham's arguments offer effective tools for the dismantling of the barriers separating "us" and "them."

To the degree that information is vital to survival in these toxic times, metaphor continues in deconstructive fashion as the mark of illness that in fact enables this survival. In the course of my own thinking about AIDS and the nuclear, of my investigation into the discourse surrounding them, I have seen the ways in which vivid metaphors—those of "street talk" as opposed to "straight talk," to loosely borrow Samuel Delaney's formulation—can make plain the complicated scientific processes—How does a nuclear reactor work? How does a virus take hold in a cell?—that a relative nonexpert like myself would find difficult to envision otherwise. When a recent writer on the history of viruses, admittedly producing for popular consumption, describes a virus's "invasion" of a cell as "commandeer[ing] and recast[ing] the now doomed cell to make replicas of its own form" (Radetsky 7), he is clarifying a complicated process involving RNA, DNA, ribosomes, and cellular activity that is difficult to comprehend and nearly impossible to retain without these "visual" aids. Metaphoric clarification like this informs instead of confuses a lay reader, allowing understanding of basic cell-biological functions, processes of infection, methods of transmission—whatever information she may be in search of. These metaphors are not exaggerations of the event, as healthy cells are indeed surrounded and taken over by tumor or viral cells in an infectious process. In even more popular media, headlines featuring a confrontational metaphor enlist the emotional, sometimes even the financial or legislative, support of a flag-waving, victory-loving society like our own, which thrives on its role as the "good guy" in the war against anything we would call subversive. Metaphor's ability to colorize and narrativize can be said to "fictionalize" an account of an illness in a way that brings it home more realistically than ever.[21] Involvement like this personalizes the crisis for individuals who had heretofore considered themselves outside of it, leading them to take precautions against the illness themselves and generate a sympathetic attitude toward those already affected.

• • •

Interestingly, Derrida, who above emphasizes the metaphoric, blended, "impure" quality of all language, insists elsewhere on a "break" in language, a separation from "the origin" that he characterizes questionably as "the violence" of the letter.[22] But the differences between "illness" and "violence" (the blend and the break) are many and vital; and here Sontag, especially in her distaste for the military metaphor, must be reconsidered and redeemed. For violence insists on the sort of false binary that Derrida rejects throughout his work—that between "me" and "not me"—due to the outward thrust implicit in the term itself. Violence is done *by* one *to* another, directed "over there" like an artillery shell or grenade. Yet as these older forms of weaponry become all but extinct in the postmodern age, so the concept of violence that configured them belongs as well to bygone days: warfare throughout the modern period left the effects of violence behind it—broken glass, dead bodies, blood and gore. In marked contrast, the bombings of Hiroshima and Nagasaki, while beginning in violence (the blast itself), "ended" (continue still) in illness, spreading radiation sickness and elevated cancer rates over large and unpredictable distances, inflicting emotional and psychological devastation on a national scale over the course of generations, and fueling a worldwide, cold war paranoia that produced the bitter fruits of Stalinism and McCarthyism and forced a nuclear stockpiling and breakdown in international relations that we may never move completely beyond.

Where violence is divisive and destructive, illness is democratizing and transformative. In its indiscriminatory victimization illness negates categories of villain and hero and renders efforts to isolate the sick from the healthy morally suspect and inevitably worthless; in its essential infectiousness it travels not unilaterally or bilaterally but multilaterally and with stealth. Only its devastating symptom complex, its unerasable trace, is visible after its visitation is complete. In its boundary-dissolving capacity to blend sick cells with healthy ones, to mirror life and death processes so well that they are indistinguishable, to reduce (once-healthy) "me" to the status of (now-ailing) "not me"—illness is the condition of the metaphoric; and metaphor is, to our detriment (and, finally, to our benefit), the condition of postmodern illness.

EXPLODING CURES: THE IRRADIATED METAPHORIC

As theorists in the above discussion debated whether metaphor functioned as a falsely constructed dividing line or as a principle of dissolution and corruption (that line itself divided and destroyed), so nuclear theorists have sought answers to similar questions in recent debates. If the "break" of metonymy in the above discussion separated (again, falsely) realms of health and illness, here it may promise a difference between "clean" and contaminated zones of life but may also describe a policy of nuclear "containment" that, however difficult to enforce, is essential to planetary survival. Here the "blend" recognizes the impossibility of securing safe zones in the wake of nuclear detonation and recognizes the densely imbricated relationship between bombers and those being bombed. Conversely, it may describe a principle of "expansion" and Westernization that should be resisted by both the "Westernized" and the Westernizers themselves. As I trace the multiple connections between the nuclear and metaphoric activity in language, I will ask questions similar to those above: Under which conditions is the metaphoric defined as "health," a sane nuclear policy and a proper respect for people and planet? Under which conditions is it defined as "illness," our least favorable position with respect to global survival? When is it a sign of hope, and when must it be read as the end of all signs, of language's (civilization's) ability to recoup and go on?

Mary Ann Caws begins a discussion of the literary and the nuclear by stating that our relationship to "what is most serious" is metaphoric; yet her literary model is not centrally metaphor but the surreal. Nevertheless, it is the metaphoric quality of the surreal that she finds most encouraging, even though she does not name it as such. She determines that "the metaphors and images of surrealism at its best are oxymoronic combinations of clashing elements from different realms in view of a violent and revolutionary separation" (62), when in fact the notion of a "surrealistic metaphor" is entirely redundant: this surrealism, very close to Harpham's grotesque, is a supplemental relation between seeming opposites, emphasizing the boundary destroyed. In the parlance of the nuclear, says Caws, the surreal is "where fission meets and is met by fusion, . . . [where] by violent separation and reshuffling mental and material, new substances are created as old elements split apart and join differently, about a new and nuclear center" (64).

While Caws reads the surreal (and hence metaphor) as the solution to the bomb, Derrick De Kerckhove discovers the metaphoric in the bomb itself. "The only possible value of the nuclear armament is metaphorical, not actual," he argues, pointing out that beyond deterrence, the bomb in its inception was already "such a prodigious aggression on our biocultural responses" that we must understand ourselves not to have averted it but to have lived through it (75). Having recognized that "the bomb is, technically speaking, completely redundant" (75) and learned the lesson of the damage caused by such aggression—De Kerckhove uses the word "education" often—we may proceed alongside the bomb yet at the same time beyond it in a damaged but strengthened state. Finally, the opposition between Caws's more traditional reading (the bomb as illness) and De Kerckhove's more radical one (the bomb as cure) resolves itself on one level as complete agreement, in that both look for a solution, a source of healing, in the metaphoric.

If De Kerckhove's surprising delineation of the bomb not only as a cure but as an "educator" and something of a planetary savior seems not only radical but implausible, perhaps that is due to his inattention to the full nature of metaphor, its inclusion of the literal ("the grotesque crushing together") as a permanent precursor to the figural reading(s) that emerge. With the "metaphor" of the bomb, we must consider the actuality of occurrence *as well as* the specter of such, while De Kerckhove recognizes only the benefits of the latter: "the nuclear bomb has become, quite unexpectedly, the greatest communication medium mankind has ever invented, not for information but for transformation . . . not the destroyer . . . but the transformer" (72).[23] It is as if its moment of actualization, that which closed off the modern era and opened up the postmodern one, also changed the function of the bomb itself from modern destroyer to postmodern "great communicator." In its eternally suspended state, its language is no longer violence but language itself, and it is this state of threat, this metaphoric condition of not being and having already been that will, according to De Kerckhove, save the planet.

De Kerckhove asserts that the bomb as metaphor in fact creates a metonymic relationship, erects a barrier, between the West and the rest of the world, specifically stating that it has effectively contained Western expansionism. Yet this idea is implicitly reversed throughout his subsequent argument, as De Kerckhove touts "the westernization of the planet" and "networking" (wiring the world from Western power sources), as accompanying benefits of "nuclear communication." Thus we are to accept and even embrace the collectivizing effects of the bomb, including the extremely problematic notion of the Westernization of the planet. Not only is this a most bizarre depiction of a better world, but in relationship to my immediate argument we see that this binary opposition between containment and explosion collapses in De Kerckhove's own drawing of the situation. Only by ignoring the fullness of the structure of metaphor, present inadvertently everywhere in his essay, can De Kerckhove maintain the categories of theory and actuality, transformation and destruction, education and annihilation as discrete. When fully recognized, however, metaphor replicates the fission/fusion properties of the nuclear in the break/blend of its own structure, subjecting all reified categories to rapid dissolution and including its opposites in a way that dissolves the category of "categories" itself.

Derrida, whose ideas are once again relevant here, defines metaphor as it informs the nuclear as uncontrolled *repetition,* a dangerous "allegoriz[ing]" or "domesticat[ion of] terror" ("No Apocalypse" 21) that will lead to catastrophe. Our habit of discerning patterns in history, of deriving lessons out of the past, says Derrida, is an efficient means toward progress but is just as often a misrecognition of a genuine break with whatever we have known before. If, then, as Ronald Reagan tried to do, we introduce the principle of "prevailing" in a nuclear conflict, we will have blended an aging, vestigial aspect of warmaking, in which winning was a feasible goal, into an absolutely new version of war; in short, we would be acting historically when what we were potentially dealing with was the end of history. Here, then, Derrida equates metaphor with a misrecognition of the magnitude of destruction that the nuclear stands for; as was often the case in *Of Grammatology,* particularly in his denunciation of metaphor's ability to "simulate immediacy," Derrida finds the metaphoric controlled by the blend to be a condition of illness—not of the body but of society poised on the brink of annihilation.

Yet the blend-as-break (not simply repetition, but the blurring of one historical period with another) that more accurately characterizes the metaphoric is figured several times throughout Derrida's "No Apocalypse, Not Now,"[24] most significantly in his definition of "textuality," of literature itself, which is fundamentally defined by this double move: a "form of archivizing" and a "form of law" (26); that is, textuality is an accumulation of texts that dissolves distinctions (the blend) and a form of distinguishing or separation that permits comprehension (the break). Late in the essay Derrida defines literature as "not . . . possible without (1) a project of stockpiling, of building up an objective archive over and above any traditional oral base; (2) . . . the development of a positive law implying authors' rights, the identification of the signatory . . . , the distinction between the original and the copy" (26). It is this double condition, resembling so closely the double movement of the metaphoric that for Derrida describes literature itself, that informs its textuality and marks it (no matter what its century) as "belong[ing] to the nuclear epoch, that of the crisis and of nuclear criticism" (27).

Thus it is Derrida's definition of literature itself, and not his version of "metaphor," that partakes most fully of the metaphoric principle and, while identified as belonging to the nuclear age, works endlessly, inevitably against the nuclear threat, the end of textuality that is also the end of life on earth. Metaphor is more rightly, then, not the illness but the cure, the antidote to total destruction that links it in significant ways with Caws's surreal and, elsewhere, Frances Ferguson's nuclear "sublime."[25] All of these literary devices are employed to do battle against the threat of annihilation at some level, yet only those are fully armed that are entirely coincident with this double action of metaphor that controls and empowers them.

• • •

As with the presence of illness in language, we see that the thematic of the nuclear in texts is the subject of spirited, sometimes dissonant debate yet is consistently illuminated by an understanding of the mechanism of the metaphoric. As some theorists read metaphor as cure or illness in language, so others determine whether its presence is a sign of, a method for, deterrence or apocalypse. I contend that these several debates are resolved in a proper understanding of the doubling, deconstructing movement of "the metaphoric," its ingestion and reconfiguration of the break and the blend that only seem to be separate and opposite. Of course, I have been arguing throughout this chapter that in important and illuminating ways the cold war and the AIDS crisis are not only linguistic constructs, as is metaphor itself, but also both metonymically related to (i.e., generationally descended from) each other and vital and provocative metaphors for each other. In classic supplemental configuration, these plague periods' multiple differences not only suggest and enable their shared features but generate and richly reward our simultaneous study of both. While it is vital to plot the metonymic or "generational" relationship between these two eras, this mapping[26] along a horizontal plane must be understood as only the first step: folding the map in half upon itself reveals the even more telling patterns repeating in both eras, the metaphoric ("blueprint") relationship between them, which fosters greater understanding of both periods and perhaps one day will provide the ability to minimize or prevent future plague crises. Throughout the remainder of this study I will examine both the principles of metaphor (which includes metonymy) and the problematic, largely mythical movement of metonymy (the boundary that holds) as a solitary principle, where these are posited in multiple roles—as violence, illness, deterrence, and cure—and throughout various literary and cinematic examples from the last five decades of the twentieth century. Again, it is the emphasis on these fundamental linguistic structures that I hope will show the many ways all of us, dependent on these for our very speech, thought, and subjectivity, are equally dependent on the successful containment and cure of the postmodern plagues surrounding us.

2

Four Corners of a Crisis: Genres of Plague Texts

BEFORE, BEYOND, AND WITHIN: WHERE WE ARE IN OUR PLAGUE TEXTS

On the back cover of the 1988 Vintage International edition of Alan Hollinghurst's *Swimming-Pool Library*, the editor's synopsis/plug describes the book as "a darkly erotic novel of homosexuality before the scourge of AIDS," assuming it into a subgenre of AIDS literature known as the "pre-AIDS" novel. Produced during a peak period of gay-related diagnoses and deaths from this disease, the novel nevertheless manages, according to its publicist, to recreate the lavishness and unfettered sexuality of a time before HIV and its effects had ever been heard of. In addition to Hollinghurst's novel, Peter Cameron's collection *One Way or Another* and his novel *Leap Year* and George Whitmore's *Nebraska* may be said to belong to this growing body of texts. To describe these texts, as they have all been, as "pre-AIDS" and not simply "para-AIDS"—coinciding but not conversing with the epidemic—is to acknowledge the extreme infectiousness of HIV, not only biologically but psychologically and discursively as well: how to form a narrative that takes place during these years, describes centrally the triumphs and tragedies of urban gay men, yet travels its path *alongside* the AIDS crisis, remaining immune to it throughout? The answer—that it is impossible to do so—is embodied in the terminology of "before the scourge" or "pre-AIDS," which admits finally that the only place from which to talk about gay life without including the effects of AIDS *is* before, in the prehistory of this disease's own life span.

We should not, therefore, designate as "pre-AIDS" gay-authored works actually written before the virus manifested itself in the early 1980s, since this term infects and designates all texts we name with it as "positive" anyway: to include the word "AIDS" in the generic marker is to acknowledge the menacing cloud these novels are all written in the shadow of, all in helpful ways respond to, all to some degree defend against.[1] In other words, they are AIDS novels (and at the same time anti-AIDS novels) that attack "from the rear," from before or behind the advent of AIDS, and obliquely, speaking all the while they describe something else about the crisis itself in significant, though perhaps unwitting, ways. In an important respect, then, these gilded, sometimes golden recreations like Hollinghurst's, of days of unlimited sexual freedom and cultural consumption, are strikes against the devastations of AIDS, an important and vital source of "treatment" for an audience whose medical alternatives often fail.[2]

How then to refer to other AIDS texts such as Paul Monette's novel *Afterlife,* Larry Kramer's drama *The Normal Heart* and short story collections such as Edmund White and Adam Mars-Jones's *Darker Proof* and Mars-Jones's *Monopolies of Loss,* which plainly acknowledge their "positive" status, completely structuring their narratives around the drama that already is diagnosis of, survival with, and succumbing to the ravages of AIDS? In what ways do the characteristics and strategies of the "intraepidemic" differ from those of the "pre-epidemic," and what does it mean when we change our plane of relationship to these texts from the temporal (the "pre") to the spatial (the "within")? Before answering these questions, we should observe the several ways in which the cold war and nuclear literature that I will examine here may be read according to quite similar spatiotemporal designations.

Specifically, the "postapocalyptic" refers to a genre of novel (and in many cases a genre of film) depicting a world that has sustained, perhaps immediately prior or centuries earlier, worldwide nuclear conflagration. These narratives may be characterized by the presence of an arid and ruined landscape, few and radically altered survivors, and an atavistic, kill-or-be-killed code among the survivors that structures and directs the plot. In popular fictions (e.g., the *Mad Max* trilogy starring Mel Gibson) they are overlain with the trappings and hardware of science fiction, yet there are more complex examples that rely less on space-age toys and weaponry and more on examining the internal and interpersonal experiences of these postapocalyptic survivors as well—Russell Hoban's *Riddley Walker*[3] and Raymond Briggs's *When the Wind Blows* being among those I will discuss in detail.

Like the pre-epidemic text, the postapocalyptic seeks release from its present age, yet this time its attachment to (or infection by) the disaster of its origin is intentional and is integral to its effect: whereas pre-AIDS narratives offer curative escapism in their return to better times,[4] the postapocalyptic offers aggressive aversion therapy, through head-on collision with and a sprawling land on the other side of what, thanks to works like these, will hopefully never happen—global holocaust. By depicting postnuclear worlds so horrific and unrecognizable as to give the most hawkish among us nightmares, these texts attempt to head off the disaster they depict through the very telling of their stories. Thus, although temporally manipulative like the pre-AIDS text, the postapocalyptic shares even more features with the intraepidemic, braving (and forcing us to brave) events of devastation and working through these graphic narratives to create awareness and tolerance for the survivors of AIDS and nuclear technology as well as intolerance for the ever-worsening conditions that perpetuate both of these postmodern crises as issues of societal concern.

Meanwhile, postapocalyptic's less easily recognizable corollary, the *alterapocalyptic,* works in many of the same ways as does the pre-AIDS text and includes, I would argue, a variety of well-known early postmodern novels that deal, however indirectly, with the devastation of nuclear war and the potential for worldwide political oppression and dictatorship that was often regarded as its alternative. Works such as George Orwell's *1984,* Ray Bradbury's *Fahrenheit 451,* and, more recently, Margaret Atwood's *Handmaid's Tale* and Paul Auster's *In the Country of Last Things* all describe worlds that have averted universal catastrophe but at great price. Human life has been spared, but the threat that this situation could be reversed at any time haunts a society controlled by oppressive dictatorships, curtailing freedom and opportunity for those beneath them. The controlling state apparati are largely ideological instead of repressive; nuclear violence and traditional warfare are curtained offstage, paraded only occasionally in demonstrations against an unknowable enemy, while the social avenues of control such as work, family, home life, and personal relationships are policed to the nanometer. As far as this threat is understood, then, as a specifically nuclear one, these novels, like the pre-AIDS texts, speak effectively, however indirectly, against the larger, unspoken threat as well.

Note that between these two subgenres of the apocalyptic we feel that same spatiotemporal slide—from the temporal (the "post") to the spatial (the "alter"). Neither of these pairings can be understood as opposites or halves of one whole due to the diagonal movement we are forced to make from one category to another. Finally, the spatiotemporality connecting these subgenres defines my interface with the texts themselves and the contexts surrounding them and has produced the range of positions I may occupy as reader and respondent. For I, too, as artifact of the postmodern period, attach to the themes of these stories primarily on a horizontal (spatial) plane, temporal conditions being largely out of my control: I am fixed, therefore, in a post–cold war, intraepidemic, preapocalyptic moment, yet the array of subject positions that constitute my present moment—HIV-positive and HIV-negative, gay and straight, victimized through race or class by the hazards of nuclear waste and reactor sites—exist within highly permeable boundaries that may allow me in or pull me in (depending on how one looks at it) under any number of circumstances.

Note, however, that once again the metonymic (my present spectrum of available identities) is as easily and necessarily understood as the metaphoric (the realm of permeable boundaries) and that the nature of my shared ground with each of these subject positions is best highlighted in terms of a temporal situating: I am not HIV-negative but much more accurately only *pre*-positive,[5] perhaps not so much straight as *pre*–lesbian consciousness, certainly not so much uncontaminated by the water and land around me as *pre*-habituated to this danger zone, as the zone moves closer to my present *space* all the *time*. Thus my own position as commentator on and participant in these postmodern texts/events is consummately mediated by the spatiotemporal; it is a definitive aspect of postmodern plague narrative as well as a chief conceptualizer of my relationship to it.

FORWARD, BACKWARD, AND OVER AGAIN: TWO VIEWS OF THE PRIMAL SCENE

In his essay "No Apocalypse, Not Now," Jacques Derrida seeks to restore the temporal to an age that has allowed the progress of history to accelerate to such a degree that it is almost entirely "out of time." In an effort to equalize the relationship between (i.e., rediscover the interrelationship that has in fact always constituted) the spatial and the temporal,[6] Derrida emphasizes the importance of time and timing, of turning back the clock to relive a particular moment a little more slowly and much more sensibly. The argument resonates not only with his no doubt deeply felt interest in planetary preservation but also with a theoretical concept that has always interested Derrida, that of repetition itself. The pleasure of repetition as it is discovered and elaborated on by Freud is the subject of intense focus throughout the latter portion of Derrida's *Post Card* and has influenced other critics of Derrida and of the nuclear, most interestingly Peter Schwenger in *Letter Bomb.*

Yet both Derrida and Schwenger-reading-Derrida come to conflate this temporal concept of repetition with what is in fact its opposite, the spatial movement entailed in "the return,"[7] and in the same move elide this latter term's more radical and "dangerous" associations. Both align repetition with pleasure, specifically with "mastery" of a sexual, masculine nature, and with the repetitive "game" of narrative itself—fort:da!—that constitutes the psychic makeup and, by their extended arguments, encourages the continuation of global existence. Yet narrative's forward movement from "fort" to "da" cannot be experienced more than once (i.e., as *repetition*) without there being an intervening and enabling *return* or reassembling of the initial game dynamic, from "da" back to "fort." Denoted here, then, is the originary, even "primal" positioning of the return—not the repetition that aligns itself with masculine prowess in bed but that to which it is implicitly opposed throughout these theorists' arguments,[8] the passivity of "turning over" and being mastered that characterizes queer male sexuality.

In "Seeing Things," Lee Edelman has argued incisively for just this primacy of the turning back and the "turning of backs"—for Freud, for Derrida, and for all subsequent understanding of the mechanisms of sexuality and meaning. He points out that for all the emphasis on repetition as definitive of Freud's terminal sexuality or state of sexual "health," the return itself is fundamental to an understanding of the movement of the unconscious. Edelman writes that in this way Freud's theories "define a psychic experience in which the most crucial and constitutive dramas of human life are those that can never be viewed head on, those that can never be taken in frontally, but only, as it were, approached from behind" (95). Not only is the mirror stage itself controlled by this "behindsight," but Freud's case of the Wolf Man, Edelman reminds us, although depicting a child's witnessing of sex between man and woman, is a scene envisioned as coitus a tergo; and this viewing leads not only to the Wolf Man's later anal-erotic fixation but to the recognition that in Freudian terms, "the primal scene is always perceived as sodomitical . . . [which] designates male heterosexuality, by contrast, as a later narcissistic compromise that only painfully and with difficulty represses its identification with the so-called 'passive' position" (101).

Late in the essay Edelman reads Derrida's own witnessing of the "primal scene of philosophy," depicted on a postcard in the Bodleian Library gift shop that shows Plato standing behind, and thus seeming to dictate to, Socrates. This scene plays out, says Edelman, "a vertiginous reversibility of positions" (110) of the kind that fascinated and haunted Freud. Edelman is quick to point out the overtly sodomitical content both of the postcard itself and Derrida's reading of it: "'I see *Plato* getting an erection in *Socrates*' back' [Derrida] writes, 'and see the insane hubris of his prick, an interminable, disproportionate erection . . . slowly sliding, still warm, under *Socrates*' right leg'" (110). Edelman notes that this "vertiginous reversibility" is profoundly disturbing to Western philosophers who encounter it, as it upsets the "spatio-temporal positions on which Western philosophy rests" (110).

Edelman's effort to define sodomitical sex not as deviant from but constitutive of "normal" sexual development and the rules of social discourse that follow from it is evidenced as necessary in light of Schwenger's own reading of this same postcard. Interestingly, Schwenger too understands that what we know we know only in hindsight, that all writing is "written on the back" in distinctly postcard-like fashion. Yet his emphasis on language and purely linguistic forms of knowledge jettisons the homoerotics from this moment in *The Post Card,* forcing a reading that reveals their Derridean primacy as well as the Freudian fears of castration and loss they elicit. Schwenger notes that "the ambiguous image on the Bodleian postcard gives rise to some playful speculation on Derrida's part: Plato is shoving through the back of the chair a massive phallus, which emerges under Socrates' right leg; he is taking Socrates out for an excursion in a wheelchair; he is pushing off on a skateboard.... All this play contributes to a serious argument about deconstructive play, ... the multiple interpretations ... [that] call into question expectations of understanding and mastery" (140). Schwenger's citation is decidedly different than Edelman's. Whereas Edelman lingered over and enjoyed Derrida's homoerotic "emissions," Schwenger drains them of their charge by rushing through the moment, then heaping on the decidedly desexualized images that follow—the afternoon meanderings of old men and the innocence of children's games. Finally, his association of this sort of "play" with a loss of "understanding and mastery" effectively severs the masculine heterosexual powers of repetition developed earlier in his study from what is an inevitable but by no means enviable position of unknowing, engaging in child's play, the so-called stunted development and inherent passivity also associated with gay sexuality.

Thus while both are indebted to and accepting of Derrida's Freud-influenced theories, Schwenger and Edelman position themselves in otherwise opposite ways. For Schwenger, the mastery of repetition, the constant movement that s(t)imulates (straight) male sexual activity, is both a metaphor of (nuclear) explosion and its opposite—the motion that leads to planetary preservation. On the other hand, for Edelman, it is the turning back and the decidedly queer sexuality resembling this move that represents the explosion of sexuality as well. But for Edelman this explosion—the queer sex act and the recognition of our primal queerness that is to burst into and thus terminate the psychoanalytic scene—is already the cure as well, the moment of social healing and psychic peace that is forever held in abeyance by the heterosexist biases that have structured life.

John M. Clum has argued that "in a gay culture now rightfully obsessed with a killer plague, remembering becomes a central act" and that "memory and desire are poignantly intertwined" (649).[9] While Edelman has theorized elsewhere specifically about AIDS, we may understand that the return as he describes it here is not only fundamental to a theory of queer sexuality but one of reading AIDS-related texts as well: for while nuclear apocalypse is still in our future, that is, it allows for steps that may still be taken *forward*, the AIDS crisis is radically, devastatingly upon us; that there is no more forward movement that may be taken before it; and that at present the chief restorative direction is *backward*—through recollection of our own primal queerness, which will enable a more sympathetic, effective treatment of gay sufferers of this disease, and through a return to earlier decades and centuries that recall exuberantly the limitless past of gay history that in important ways ensures its own limitless future.

BOXED IN BY OUR FEARS: FOUR PLAGUE GENRES

Backward Glances: The Pre-epidemic

Hollinghurst's *Swimming-Pool Library* begins and ends without a single reference to AIDS or HIV yet is useful as a response to the crisis by being its own backward glance, an artifact of the "present" (the AIDS era), which casts its glance steadily and unapologetically toward two vital and inspiring pasts—one immediate and the other ancient. The title makes a connection most relevant to a study such as this, between bodies and texts, coming together productively in the concept of "the type": a swimming-pool library redefines the swimmers therein as various, but always readable books. While at one point in the narrative Lord Nantwich is embarrassed by a seller of gay pornographic postcards and acknowledges regretfully, "he had read me like a book" (214), the swimming pool "reading matter" referred to in Hollinghurst's title is of a "type" that is successfully secretive and thus vibrant and subversive, whose codings form a language that excludes and thus defends against unsympathetic outsiders while expanding and enriching the bonds within the community that speaks the language. On a more literal level, the title refers to the conflict confronting the central character: as "prefect" or librarian of the swimming facilities at his boys' school years earlier, Will Beckwith recognizes yet attempts to resist the role he is inexorably destined for—that of curator and chronicler of "the swimming-pool"—the setting and facilitator of gay life. Content at first to merely swim with the flow—of the sex and leisure his wealth affords him—Will finally learns that the reading of texts is the key to the full freeing of his sexual identity yet also to the truth about his own ancestry of homophobia and persecution.

In the story, Will and his friends recognize the connection between ancient gay cultures and their own postmodern one, enjoying the luxurious swim-and-gym life at the thoroughly upscale and straight-seeming Corinthian Club and delighting in the authentic Roman bath that undergirds (but also undermines) the powerful position (literally, the mansion) of Lord Charles Nantwich, Will's aging suitor. As was likely the case within enclaves of scholar/lovers in ancient times, few women are present in Hollinghurst's world, while Will and his young friends enjoy the attention of the group of old men that Charles brings into their lives, even if ultimately eluding their advances. The wizened looks of many of these aging characters and their chronic, alarming symptom complexes[10] recall vividly the wasting and illness that afflicts end-stage AIDS patients and highlight, in contrast, Will's unstoppable youth and energy. Meanwhile, Will eventually must depend on Charles to provide the link to Will's own past and an important third era of "ancient history" that brutally interrupts the "gay affirmativity" of ancient and modern times: the sexually repressed, racially oppressive reign of Victoria at home and in the colonies.[11]

Will at first resists but finally acquiesces to the scholarly project Charles foists on him, reading and transcribing Charles's diaries, written during his years of service in the British Empire's army. Ironically, Charles describes his career of colonial exploitation as a more innocent time: "Oh there will never again be a time of such freedom. It was the epitome of pleasure. When I sink back into the mood of those days, & then think of what happened afterwards I am amazed" (131). It is impossible for us (if not for Will) to ignore the dual valence of this nostalgic regret. Finally, Will's very act of reading (and our reading of *his* story) forces him and us into the position of having to recognize a lost and innocent past and, perforce, a comparatively bleak and tragic—epidemic—present age.

As Will immerses himself in Charles's biography, he comes to understand the importance of the backward glance, of historical awareness and his own implication by historical circumstance. The diary recreates a friendship between the young Charles and a black servant named Taha that eventually turns erotic and disruptive, mirroring the relationship decades later between Will and the chef at Wick's (who turns out to be Taha's son) and between Will and Arthur, a dark-skinned lover whom Will fetishizes for his skin color much the way Charles and other colonizers did their own black conquests. Thus Will is likened to his oppressor-forebears in this respect, due no doubt to his failure to understand his own history and catch himself in the act of repeating its mistakes.

In addition to the racial bigotry suggested here, violent suppression of homosexuality is documented in Charles's account and, during the climax of the novel, is revealed to have emanated from the policies of Will's own grandfather, a virulent homophobe with much power to wield during Victoria's reign. Will's discovery that homosexual oppression is part of his own blood line, that is, his ancestral heritage, constitutes what I believe to be a remarkably fertile analog to AIDS as a shaping force of history in this text: while Will believes for most of the novel that homophobia is a "violence" done to gays "out there"—removed from his past and present experience—his final understanding of this injury as within—not only inflicted directly, insidiously *on* him but as emanating directly *from* him—redefines it irrevocably as blood-borne "illness" instead, a condition of contagion and the dissolved boundaries between "me" and "not me" that is principally definitive of the viral event and the epidemic that follows from it.[12]

A final historical document, a decades-old home movie featuring one of the men from Charles's own past—near the end of his life then but still campy and demonstrative before the camera—and viewed with surprise and admiration by a group of young and old men at novel's end, is a final display of the powers emanating from bodies as text (here, film instead of "type") that performs a service to a threatened gay culture: it is the recomposition (and self-composition) of an "old" man as vibrant, young, and sexual again, a "dead" generation at once rejuvenated and eternally youthful, promising an "immortality" not only to those in the film but to those watching it who themselves may never reach the end of long, natural lives.

Like Hollinghurst, George Whitmore in his novel *Nebraska* makes interesting, AIDS-suggestive use of the concept of illness shared by blood (in families), of illness as a condition that remains a secret for years, even to the one who has it. Both tell triumphant stories of gay men triumphing *through* stories—the finding, accepting, and telling of them in these young men's own voices. However, the protagonist of Whitmore's novel has little in common with the British upper-class twentysomething featured in Hollinghurst's work, as fourteen-year-old Craig is embedded, even trapped, within an impoverished extended family in 1950s rural Nebraska and faces, to use the social worker's expression, an entirely different set of issues. While we might read even gay protagonists of a privileged class such as Will's as suffering injustice and misunderstanding at the hands of family and society, the case Whitmore offers in *Nebraska* is so severe that the sexual inner conflict experienced by the narrator, central to the stories of many other gay authors, is often the least of this boy's worries.

At the beginning of the novel twelve-year-old Craig suffers a violent blow from a speeding pick-up truck, breaking his arm, requiring stitches and much superficial healing, and, worst of all, losing a leg. His selfish mother and sisters confine the boy to his bed for months, palliating him with painkillers and afraid (but also unwilling to bear the cost) of allowing him to embark on the physical therapy program he desperately needs. At one point, a young, well-schooled "County" visits the family and insists they dispose of the pain pills and begin the physical therapy. Aunt Eileen, however, who "used to be a practical nurse" and thus feels free to overrule this advice, "saw the doctor to the door then when she came back she fetched that little bottle out of the wastebasket and saw to it I took my noon dose with orange juice" (26). The physical rehabilitation is postponed for months, and when Craig finally begins, he has "muscles like Jell-O from being in that bed too long and sores up and down my backside" (52). Much of the narrative emanates from the feverish and frustrated vantage point of Craig's ill-suited sickbed and later, even more horrifyingly, from the confines of his estranged, kidnapping father's demented care. At these and many such junctures in the novel we cannot help but let more vital—indeed, more urgently biological—concerns than those of his sexual coming-of-age define him and our response to him.

In fact our understanding of Craig as sexual (as having the "leisure" to be sexual) comes a good bit *after* our understanding of him as physically compromised, emotionally bereft, and denied the essentials that boys his age enjoy, including commerce with friends and an education. At one point his mother finds a handkerchief smeared with semen and commands Craig to never produce such a laundry item again, yet even at this point the heterosexualized (even if not heterosexual) reader might make the incorrect assumption that Craig is jerking off to female fantasies (i.e., he is straight until proven "guilty"). In fact Craig mentions "dates" as an adolescent and "having a girl" as a young man and even loses his virginity to a female prostitute, although the session does not go well. Thus Craig's homosexuality, the identity we feel he eventually finds himself through, is not *born* with our earliest understanding of him but comes to us (and perhaps to him) later in the story and therefore may seem less than absolutely "natural"—when in fact this is the very thesis Whitmore ostensibly tries to make.

Even more problematically, this sexuality is pathologized in a way anathema to the typical gay-affirmative text, as it is suggested to be either a product of the overbearing, largely female, dysfunctional family life Craig seeks to extricate himself from or of the "tainting" influence of a charismatic uncle who indeed loves Craig but whose suggestive touching of him is the first *observed* instance of homosexual desire in the boy. Thus gay desire seems derived from, instead of being born into or even grown into, seeming to confirm the worst suspicions of those advocating the total separation of gays and children. In this unfortunate, and likely inadvertent way, Craig's homosexuality makes of itself a metaphor for the contagion of HIV as has been forced innumerable times in the mainstream, homophobic media.

Later in the novel this uncle is punished for his "crime," (trumped-up charges that Craig unwittingly reinforces in court testimony) by surgical neutering that leaves him asexual but boyishly content. The neutering seems to have included some lobotomizing as well, since Uncle Wayne without his testicles is not more outrageously feminine but seemingly moderately retarded. This utterly unjust mutilation, largely unexplained by the novel (as are many of the other injustices suffered here), seems a product of mid-1950s rural-doctored Nebraska, forcing the socioeconomic circumstances of these characters once more to the fore. In a relatively enlightened California setting, Craig still struggles with his emerging gay identity, and only in the novel's final pages does he begin to fear and then accept that he actually "is one." This less-than-exhilarated embrace of his sexual self is coupled with his somewhat curious sexual object choice—sleeping, disabled, blood-related Uncle Wayne instead of the alert, available, obviously caring Vernon, who was Wayne's former lover and now sole caretaker.

It is in this pathologizing of gay sex and the overarching socioeconomic deprivation that postpones and almost prevents Craig's sexual awakening that we find our most vivid concessions to the AIDS crisis in Whitmore's text. HIV has indeed had both these negative effects on gay men's lives—forcing them to fend off once more the ugly notion that homosexuality is unnatural and contagious and depriving them of the quality of health care necessary to live longer, healthier (more sexual) lives due to the high cost of its treatment. Despite the many ways in which this novel is indeed a triumphant narrative of sexual awakening, beginning and ending long before AIDS can ever touch these characters, the crisis that plagues living in and writing from this present age infects the text nevertheless.

For entirely different reasons[13] Joseph Dewey describes this novel as "the most significant journal of our plague years" (33), and I would certainly agree that *Nebraska* is central to the challenge to this crisis that is waged at the literary level. Craig struggles to overcome obstacles that are, as I argue, representative of the very injustices AIDS causes contemporary gay men to suffer, and he ultimately succeeds. He is freed of his oppressive family, secure in an environment of men who love or will no doubt come to love him, and well on his way to accepting and enjoying his identity as a gay man at the very threshold of an era of sexual exploration and liberation. Even before this last scene, however, Whitmore's text is redemptive at every moment, as it is Craig's narrative voice—engaging, insightful if limited, riveting in its no-frills, native strength—that is allowed to tell the story, make every mistake and discovery throughout, and shape our entire perception of his world. That Craig keeps *talking* and talking wonderfully, despite the multiple setbacks and sometimes life-threatening trials he endures, leads us to understand that he will not only endure but flourish.[14] His continual and ever-strengthening talk about himself must be understood as one more version of this backward glance that preserves an unapologetic gay identity in the midst of a devastating crisis.

Despite the escapist-sounding title of Bo Houston's *Dream Life,* this novel technically belongs to a more overtly AIDS-related genre, since several of its characters mention AIDS, ailing friends, and the trials of safer sex. The book achieves a complex aura of a dreamed past, however, in frequent, extended flashbacks of "more innocent" times, and AIDS belongs only to the future for well over three-fourths of the story. As in Whitmore's novel, youth is a protagonist here, as the past narrative depicts the childhoods of both young Jed and middle-aged Hollis (Holly) Flood. Even more pointedly than in Whitmore's novel, deprivation and a miasma of pathology prevail thematically; even though Holly seems financially cared for as a child and Jed's family has much wealth, both "boys" suffer from tremendous lack—of father figures, of motherly love and attention, of friends who understand them, and, as Holly says at one point, even "of myself" (115). As in situations of actual poverty, this emotional impoverishment leaves both susceptible to multiple ills: Holly walks with a cane, wheezes and coughs constantly, and is addicted to his painkillers (so that even medicine is an illness here), leading the reader to believe that he is much older than he actually is. Holly's mother is grotesquely mentally ill, his associate Julius talks constantly about sick and dying friends, and on a plane trip Holly and Jed notice a long visit to the restroom by a young woman and theorize that she has gone in there to deliver a baby and then flush it down the toilet: "she finally came out. . . . She was holding her arms around her stomach. Her face was red and sweaty and the ends of her hair were stringy and damp" (78).

Jed is loved by Holly for his embodiment of youth and vitality, yet even he in the course of their travels suffers an intense and disorienting bout with fever that, Jed feels, causes Holly's devotion to diminish somewhat—as it might have, had the diagnosis been sexually transmissible. Likewise, the episode delays their next move, exposing them to capture by authorities (as their trip is impromptu, Jed is a minor, and the charge against Holly of kidnapping is not entirely false). Even once he has recovered, the specter of illness threatens their relationship, as Jed at one point questions Holly's unsafe sexual practices. As the two have become lovers by now, Holly problematically dismisses Jed's concerns, arguing "God wouldn't be so cruel as to give me AIDS. Not after everything else he's given me" (142). Yet unlike the blasé attitude characterizing HIV transmission in some extraepidemic novels (which I criticize later in this chapter), Holly's unwillingness to practice safer sex has genuine repercussions here: after this confrontation, Jed leaves the house and soon thereafter makes a new circle of friends. Jed begins to feel "disgust" for Holly and to resent his selling of Jed's sexual services to various tricks around town—not so much for financial gain as for Holly's own sexual gratification. In the novel's "present" narrative, Holly speaks elegiacally about his "lost" boy, and we realize that, while Jed has simply grown tired of the older man and run off to San Francisco, Holly has in part "lost" Jed to AIDS as well—to the unrealistic attitudes that advanced the demise of their relationship.

We should note a pattern in these texts produced by gay men that explore the importance of history and a shared cultural past, positioning themselves as "pre-AIDS" yet profoundly AIDS-literate as well, a pattern that further defines the effects they produce: Hollinghurst's, Whitmore's, and Houston's "fictions" all function interestingly as *autobiography* as well, that is, as a construction of a gay life before or apart from theirs that in multiple significant ways represents their own, or their own community's, experience. Hollinghurst creates a "clone" protagonist who reflects the look and lifestyle of countless gay men in Western postmodern cultures (including his own), while Whitmore and Houston speak for "deprived" classes of gay Americans who face especially difficult barriers to the development of a sexual identity. The distinction between "me" and "not me" (here autobiography and fiction) that I have been challenging throughout is dissolved again in these pre-epidemic texts, speaking powerfully for one but as well for all—again drawing strength from recourse and reference to the resilient, inexhaustible "type."

To what end this narcissism, this love affair with the (text as) mirror that seems a baseline condition, a chronic yet life-sustaining "symptom" of gay lives? In *Homographesis,* Edelman warns against separating this narcissistic or passive tendency from and opposing it to "activism" as "anti-sex" advocates such as Paul Monette and Larry Kramer have at times called for. This nondifferentiation between the self and mirror *as* definitive of gay subjectivity, Edelman argues, is just as effective a form of AIDS activism as is picketing a Food and Drug Administration (FDA) office or staging a march on Washington. This "narcissism," which is "the very non-differentiation from which the active [heterosexual], masculine subject, in what [Edelman] would call his narci-schism, differentiates himself" (108), must be reclaimed as an activist pose by the gay community. The gay activist must challenge by refusing to replicate the dominant subject position that equates the active mode (desire for and pursuit of the Object) with the "good fight" and passivity (surrendering oneself to *be* the Object) with a lost or abandoned cause.

Thus, to imbue a text about "something else" with all the properties of the mirror as well constitutes, through indulging in or succumbing to the malady of narcissism, a vital form of activism that is all the more effective for belonging so specifically to an identifiably gay culture. To write a "gay story" that in no uncertain terms professes also to be one's own story is a textualized version of coming out that unites these writers and their subjects in a community that is as politically powerful as the Stonewall rioters'. I would point out that the autobiography or textual mirror is, like many other central terms to emerge here, controlled by the metaphoric, a metonym for gay culture that is simultaneously a metaphor for the gay subject himself, a breakdown of the boundary between the subject and his image that resembles so strongly, says Edelman, the nondifferentiation that precedes the psychoanalytic mirror stage.

Inward Glances: The Pre-AIDS Autobiography As far as this mirroring in/of texts is a potent form of activism, even AIDS activism, "pre-AIDS" texts that are explicitly autobiographical may be read as even more vivid pronouncements against the crisis. Paul Monette's autobiography of his early life, *Becoming a Man,* and Edmund White's autobiographical novel *The Beautiful Room Is Empty* portray the lives of young men stumbling through the early stages of sexual identity formation, succeeding thoroughly in artistic and intellectual pursuits but only in sharp contrast to the confusion and loneliness their queerness within homophobic society produces. Both tell stories of stifling if privileged youth, solitude and repression during years in the Ivy League, and eventual triumph in coming out to selves and early lovers. White even offers an oblique but heady recreation of the Stonewall revolt that gave birth to an entire culture.

Within Monette's and White's texts is not a single mention of AIDS or HIV, as this term is anachronistic (and thus powerless) among the recreated narratives of beat culture and the vituperations, now only echoes, of J. Edgar Hoover (of all people) and Cardinal Spellman. That these stories stick close to events and details of these earlier decades allows their authors and readers to begin and complete a gay story, to end a "life" without its "dying" of AIDS-related causes. Their culminations are not in death but coming out, in the actual triumph of gay culture as a whole in the late 1960s and early 1970s and of countless gay men and women since then. Their unassailable vitality constitutes these texts' highly effective challenge to (at the same time it is an acknowledgment of) the devastation of AIDS.

In the enlightening and entertaining *Who Was That Man? A Present for Mr. Oscar Wilde,* Neil Bartlett constructs a pre-epidemic text that is autobiography, historical biography, and the most productive exploration of the body-text metaphor of all those examined here. Also, as with all the other pre-epidemic texts being discussed, Bartlett casts a backward glance not only to the era immediately preceding the advent of AIDS but also (as with Hollinghurst) Victorian England as it celebrated and then destroyed the great Oscar Wilde. Early in his work Bartlett specifically equates his historical research with writing and thinking on his own life: "Biographies are best written when their subject is dead. Are you dead, that is, has your life stopped changing? Are we dead, that is, have we arrived in a city whose gay culture we now have only to buy and enjoy? Is your favourite hero 'dead,' that is, has his role as a source of information, inspiration, and wardrobe suggestions been exhausted yet?" (25). That "you" (the reader), "we" (gay culture), and "your favourite hero" (the eternal Wilde) are not only not dead but, thanks to the work of texts like Bartlett's, literally (at least literarily) incapable of dying suggests, then, that "biography" shall not (perforce cannot) be written and that this story of "us" will be about the ostensible subject Oscar Wilde but inevitably also about Bartlett himself—and, by extension/infection, not only his entire gay readership but also straight readers who are brought through their very action of reading into the history this "story" is all about.

Through cataloging and analysis of a rich closetful of nineteenth-century "types"—"Flowers," "Faces," "Possessions," "Pretexts"—Bartlett's chief aim is to define Wilde himself (and all other gay men) *as* "type"—in all senses of that word. As slavish imitators of each other's styles, gay men have produced through history recognizable codes of dress and manner that allow them to communicate secretly and effectively in the midst of a homophobic society. The codes alleviate the "symptom"—the psychological burden and sometimes resultant physical maladies plaguing gay men that a heterosexist science has declared manifestations of their "aberrant" sexuality.[15] In fact, Bartlett argues, any symptoms actually suffered by nineteenth-century homosexual men much more likely resulted from the enormous secret they labored all their lives to contain: "All of [Wilde's] characters are in terror of being discovered. Their elegance of diction is only a front; anything rather than speak the truth. They sweat, they talk with revealing hysteria about the *secret of life*" (93). Thus this typecasting of themselves along such strictly identifiable lines is read here as the cure to life itself—the existence that is not able to be lived—an early form of coming out that did not find more effective corollaries until late in this century.

Another way to define "type" here—as the letter of a text itself—provides not the means by which to cure "living" but those to treat illness and death, that is, HIV and AIDS, in the best way we so far know how. In an inspired moment Bartlett reminds us that the word "camp" comes from the French *se campre,* which means to pose or compose oneself as for a picture. This thoroughly refined ability of gay men to compose their own lives and identities out of the "details"—the possessions, luxuries, and stories of their contemporaries and gay men before them—allows them a position that is as blatant a "forgery" as the green carnation Wilde sported in his own day but that they nevertheless themselves "forge" and therefore control. Derrida's assertion that "there is nothing outside the text" (*Grammatology* 158) may remind us of the tenuousness of our own subjectivities, while this tenuousness is for Bartlett and Wilde a chief strength, the textuality that, because it is without beginning (is unoriginal) is also without end.

When Bartlett writes, "They found their peers not in other men but in other texts" (199), he means that in Wilde's time and now the safest, most accessible form of gay identity consists of reading about the lives of other gay men, the dynamics and devices of gay sexuality. In this sense the border that separates text from body remains intact, an effect of societal persecution and now epidemiologic necessity that prevents gay bodies from freely mingling without repercussion. Yet also we note that body and text are inextricably bound, that the eroticism of texts emerges from their roles as substitutes for bodies while the neverendingness of the body stems from its ability to be recreated and read as text. It is our ability to read "type" as body and text that constitutes Bartlett's fullest response to the crises of gay history.

But what about the crises of the future? What specifically is Bartlett saying about AIDS in the midst of his discourse on nineteenth-century British history? Interestingly, his own move toward naming and dealing with the current crisis is as careful and tenuous as were Wilde's toward his own, and the text pushes gently but firmly out of the pre-AIDS genre and into the current moment in its final pages. The first oblique reference we find is an ironic reference to "Safe Sex" (170); thirty pages later the metaphor of "infectious prose" (208) continues this train of thought. Then the oblique but somber references begin to snowball: "These are certainly dark times" (218); "a fatal, sexually transmissible disease" (219); "our crisis" (220). Finally the term AIDS is named (221) and is followed immediately by Bartlett's apt summation: "We are born late. Much of my life didn't start until I was nineteen. . . . For many of us 'born' late, the lack of a past, of history is not felt as a lack. Too eager for the future to look back. I used to think I had no need of history, no need to look to Wilde's London for information" (221). This, of course, is exactly the position of Hollinghurst's Will Beckwith, and Monette mirrors Bartlett's subject position when the author/protagonist of *Becoming a Man* admits to having had "no past," only realizing the importance of claiming one much later. Monette, already writing "later"—that is, with an eye toward the approaching end of his own life—begins with an understanding of this lost past as a source of deep regret. It is "the childhood" without which one is bereft of the early vital experiences of innocence, simple pleasure, impervious security, without which one, as child, has no existence. Of course Bartlett's text is in homage not only to Wilde but to the very reversal of this assumption that history is unnecessary. Thus we may read the backward glance as not only curative of the ailments of a closeted existence but as our most successful treatment to date for a future that rests in mortal danger: "born late," gay men must retrieve their past to "complete" their lives—that is, *conclude* them, if necessary, however unwillingly or prematurely, in a manner that is entirely their own.

Steps Sideways: The Alterapocalyptic

We can observe the many empowering effects attributable to the pre-AIDS text in the course of the previous discussion: text as body, which is at the same time reproducible, indistinguishable, indestructible; text as treatment, which eases personal and societal suffering from AIDS by connecting readers to narratives, characters, and other readers; text as mirror, which allows for activism but on one's own, culture-specific terms. The pre-AIDS text is sexualized and sexually charged, as is so much to come from the culture that produced it, and is therefore attached to what is most vital and regenerative in the body, its sex drive. This vitalizing deployment of the pre-epidemic text is in marked contrast, however, to the fragility Derrida attributes to the text when threatened with nuclear apocalypse;[16] and Peter Schwenger, in his study of nuclear literature, notes that postmodern words explode "in spite of themselves"—in imitation/anticipation of the bomb (xvi).

Nearly all of the cold war and nuclear texts I examine in this chapter will demonstrate that tendency toward paralysis and collapse as is described by Derrida and other nuclear theorists. While the language of the *post*apocalyptic indeed exhibits the fragility described by Derrida, that of the *alter*apocalyptic will suffer the opposite condition—being heaped up and overburdened with so much multiple meaning that it quickly becomes paralyzed and impotent. Language in this genre suffers a bloating and an inertia, a hypermetaphoricity that, like cancerous cells out of control, quickly chokes off the original organism. Thus a "yes" or "no" or a surreptitious glance bears so many vectors of implication that it is impossible to interpret. We have moved momentarily, therefore, from a Derridean lexicon to one developed by another French postmodernist, Jean Baudrillard, who describes more than once the condition of postmodernity in markedly similar terms: "Tentacular, protuberant, excrescent, hypertelic: this is the fate of inertia in a saturated world. To deny its own end through hyperfinality—is this not also the process of cancer?" (*Fatal Strategies* 13). In the alterapocalyptic universe, illness has not been averted merely because nuclear catastrophe has, as the strain of living in its never-waning shadow only sends its symptoms "underground"—resurfacing seemingly without cause in the tic, the outbreak, the paranoia and madness. In the ailing social states of these texts, the protagonists struggle to break through to meaning but remain for the most part trapped in language.[17]

Indeed the characters of these novels are trapped in many respects. We saw that pre-epidemic texts are powerful, gay-affirming "backward glances," that is, histories and memoirs of earlier times that nevertheless face the present-day situation with implicit, sometimes subversive strength and effect. The alterapocalyptic text, in contrast, cannot "go home again": as Baudrillard himself has asked, "By what miracle could we go back in time to head off [history's] disappearance?" (*Fatal Strategies* 15).[18] And Jonathan Schell has pointed out in *The Fate of the Earth* that to return to the prenuclear state would entail no less than a rewriting of history, a disarming of matter itself and our nondisposable understanding of its properties. Likewise the alterapocalyptic cannot—indeed, dare not—go too far into the future, lest it encounter nuclear catastrophe and transform itself into the postapocalyptic, a genre constituted by entirely different methods and purposes. Also, the alterapocalyptic hangs back from a far-in-the-future designation so as to maintain its relevance to modern readers. Patrick D. Murphy has pointed out that "hugging close to the shore of present time" enables dystopian authors to "enforce a cognitive function and didactic purpose" in their fiction (27), and several readers[19] of the novels under consideration here have pointed to these narratives' positioning in the near future or even in the "exaggerated" present as a source of their power and meaning.

Finally, spatial configurations define these texts more significantly than do temporal manipulations: in addition to their being alternatives to our world, they contain within them alternative worlds of their own—mysterious and alluring offstages that act as both unspeakable menace and avenue of escape. While these novels, then, do not look *backward* or *forward*, their characters can crane their necks to the *right* and *left*—sensing themselves in hostile territory and always on the lookout for an escape, perceiving the world (as they have indeed been forced to perceive it) as controlled by strict oppositions of right and left, repressive and progressive political convictions that tear their worlds apart.

I said above that the "offstage" in these texts is both a threat to what security their characters possess and a tantalizing avenue of escape. In the offstage the repressive forces maintain the thinly veiled bomb, often referred to as "war" or "the enemy" but visible behind these puppet terms as the only form of destruction yet unleashed on a global scale—nuclear destruction.[20] As was the case during the actual cold war, this frightening outer territory is often exaggerated, if not imagined entirely, in an effort to keep citizens trapped in a prevailing ideology instead of discovering this other world to be remarkably similar to their own (if not a much-improved version of it). Thus these terrifying outer worlds, when finally penetrated, are often discovered to be liberating, revolutionary spaces where bands of insurrectionists are already gathering force. Even when the outer worlds are relatively bleak and disorganized, the very occupation of them is an act of resistance to the repressive forces that would posit a singular world—not a duality or, more likely, an aggregate of varying positions but a single-minded, all-encompassing monolith—opposition to which equals extinction.

To the degree that the forces in these novels are capable of closing off competing versions of their worlds, successfully depicting the bomb as the only alternative out there, they are equally able to manipulate and encumber language in a way that traps and discourages their inhabitants even more thoroughly. In four novels that significantly represent the alterapocalyptic,[21] I will examine the role of this offstage as it houses and showcases the nuclear threat as well as reveals an avenue of escape that will mean either liberation or undoing for these novels' inhabitants and the ever-weakening language that sustains them. I move here not in chronological order of publication but from the most open and hopeful among these texts to the darkest, most despairing, dystopic and "tongue-tied"; the farther along this scale a text finds itself, the more effective is its depiction of the nightmare that is complete totalitarianism and the more memorable and arresting the offstage to the alterapocalyptic space—as both astonishing horror and ungraspable dream.

• • •

Paul Auster's *In the Country of Last Things* is the least despairing of the alterapocalyptics in these several respects: the outside world is theoretically accessible and only recently departed from,[22] the language of a less repressive time has been at least partially preserved, and the disorder defining the characters' lives, desperate and dangerous as these may be, is largely unmonitored, resembling the circumstances of Orwell's unencumbered "proles."[23] Indeed, both escape and meaning can be had in this country—for a price. Here money (or whatever bizarre commodity does its work on a given day) is retained from a stabler time, and the fact that it still has value not only within its nation of origin but in other, less fearsome places—that is, is still in communication with the outside world—indicates that the boundaries of this "country of last things" are penetrable and thus dissolvable. Indeed, the very title of the novel reminds us that this place, hellish as it may be, is still only a "country," not an entire "world."

Anna Blume has recently arrived here in search of her brother, a reporter on assignment who disappeared over a year ago. She carries with her this brother's picture, and the fact that she is able to retain such hard evidence, such an incontestable correlation between a signifier and a signified, signals again that this world has not (yet) severed itself completely from the world of meaning. However, Anna says in the letter to her brother's editor, which constitutes the entire narrative, that this place has a fearful tendency to suck you in, that the mounds of garbage and debris she walks over daily offer numerous possibilities to trip, disable, and trap her there permanently.[24] The landscape writhes with such ambushes, as there is nothing left but garbage—all valuable possessions such as decent shelter and nutritious food having disappeared long ago—and the gangs of thugs who struggle for control over this or that rubbish mound. Finally Anna realizes that it is not only things that are in desperate need of retrieval but the meanings that were once attached to them as well: "How can you talk to someone about airplanes, for example, if that person doesn't know what an airplane is? It is a slow but ineluctable process of erasure. . . . Entire categories of objects disappear—flowerpots for example, or cigarette filters, or rubber bands—and for a time you will be able to recognize those words, even if you cannot recall what they mean. But then, little by little, the words become only sounds, a random collection of glottals and fricatives, a storm of whirling phonemes, and finally the whole thing just collapses into gibberish. The word 'flowerpot' will make no more sense to you than the word 'splandigo'" (89). As these words disappear, those remaining become overburdened and sluggish, tumorous with extra meanings they cannot support, and soon fail. Anna cannot communicate to anyone her ideas for escape, and she ultimately has "to give up the idea of going home" (89). The gaps these disappeared words create cut off communication and leave "each person . . . speaking his own private language" (89)—a condition of total separation and irrelevance to each other as is created by the purely metonymic, here a condition of illness and death for a society.

Interestingly, the monetary unit for which this various junk is sold is the "glot," reinforcing the notion of a unit of currency that is also a unit of speech or meaning. It is in fact meaning that these denizens hoard and trade and hope will last them through the winter or, in Anna's case, until she reaches the border of another land. Thus, while the reference to a "country" in the novel's title offers the comfort of an identifiable (thus ultimately traversable) boundary, it is countered a good bit by this notion of "last things," of a place that sucks up matter as does a black hole, infinitely increasing the scope of its space and density until no escape is possible. Indeed, Anna's brother, lost somewhere in this very same country, with his clever sister armed with photos and information about him in pursuit, may as well have wandered into the wilds of another planet for all the good a search after him will accomplish.

As her ties to that original, outer world grow more and more tenuous, Anna stumbles on two other "withouts" in the course of the novel that lead her into significant and healing love relationships. Both of these are actually "withins," secret and somehow protected enclaves of people like herself that foster acts of resistance, however minimal, and support and sustain those who find their way there. The first is a library of Jewish scholars, miraculously untouched by repressive governmental policy; the second is a hospice for the injured and starving who make their way to its doors. Not surprisingly, both of these offer Anna only temporary refuge, as she is at one point kidnapped from the library and eventually the hospice collapses at the hands of looters and suspicious authorities. At novel's end, a party of escapees makes its way to the border on the authority of some falsely obtained traveling papers. Anna prays that they will still be worth something when they arrive at the crossing, yet we can hope that, so long as there is still such a thing *as* value in this country, something will be able to be traded for their freedom.

Interestingly, the territory they have lit out for bears a striking resemblance to the very "labor camps" that are used as threats by the authorities—"a place west of the city" where life may be "better than it is in the city" (32). All we know of these camps is that hard work is involved—but no doubt there is hard work in store for the escapees in whatever land they happen into. Yet as open as the future may be to them, there is at this point no going back. Anna never meets up with her brother, and no mention is made by novel's end of returning to "you," the brother's editor to whom the entire letter/novel is addressed and who remains in Anna's country of origin.[25]

The "outside" of Ray Bradbury's *Fahrenheit 451* is also "within"—within language itself and the books that are sought out and torched to ashes by the "firemen" of the censoring and repressive government, books that are destroyed because they provide dangerous avenues of escape. While the chaos of Auster's novel afforded its characters a measure of freedom that enables their ultimate release, Bradbury's world is overordered and deadly silent. There is no conversation or expression of emotion, only the mindless babble of prefabricated entertainment to fill in the devastatingly quiet background. Late in the novel the protagonist, Montag, tells the old scientist Faber,

"I could feel [a revolutionary urge] for a long time, I was saving it up, I went around doing one thing and feeling another. It was all there. It's a wonder it didn't show on me, like fat" (116). At this moment Montag realizes that the double life one must assume in order to survive under this book-burning regime results in a doubling of all meaning, a "fattiness" or tumorous overgrowth of experience itself that is actually visible on the body.[26] While Montag feels himself weighed down by the simultaneous urge and inability to revolt, his society deems words themselves as overburdensome and steadily removes them from circulation. While Montag feels sickened by the weight he carries, the ruling order perceives him as sick—deranged and disruptive, punishable by death—when he begins to shrug off this weight.

In an effort to maintain social health as it is now defined, the residents of this society keep quiet. They stay at home or in small, benign, blithering groups, policing each others' speech through eavesdropping and more sophisticated surveillance methods afforded by new technology. Montag's wife, Mildred, is the chief representative of this silenced population,[27] opening her mouth only to regurgitate the tritest clichés—that is, to say nothing at all. She describes a new interactive television script she is about to read, as a daytime drama plays out on three walls of their living room:

> "Here for instance, the man says, 'What do you think of this whole idea, Helen?' And he looks at me sitting center stage, see? And I say, I say—" She paused and ran her finger under a line on the script. "'I think that's fine!' And then they go on with the play until he says, 'Do you agree to that, Helen?' and I say, 'I sure do!' Isn't that fun, Guy?"
>
> [Montag] stood in the hall looking at her.
>
> "It's sure fun," she said. (18)

Mildred's words, while giddy and effusive, are meaningless—exactly as the regime that controls her leisure time (and in fact she has no other kind) would have it. In contrast, Montag's words are few but pregnant with the meaning they seek to hide but eventually cannot. Even his silences, the look he gives his wife in the above scene, for example, are so swelled with suppressed meaning they eventually explode, revealing his disloyalty to the book-burners who control him and marking him for demolition by these forces.

I would add that the offstage in this novel works in ways remarkably similar to those I have outlined above. From a radio that "hums somewhere," the threat of a "war" that "'may be declared any hour'" (30) keeps the population distracted from making war on its own repressive government. Near the end of the novel Faber describes "walking camps" down by the railroad tracks where scholars and thinkers meet, but Montag only catches up with them after the pseudonuclear conflagration at novel's end. They relieve the words they store within their minds of their pent-up, piling-up significance by sharing them with each other. The knowledge contained by these men flows out, easing the embolic state that threatened each of them, and the words they memorize and store in their brains are thus restored to their true weight, their true significance, stabilizing the pressure that nonexistence was forcing on them.

Once again, as with Auster's novel, the "without" (or offstage) not only exists but is eventually reached, ensuring a relatively upbeat outcome for the novelistic characters who reach this place. In Margaret Atwood's *Handmaid's Tale,* the offstage is both maddeningly present and ultimately unreachable. It initially threatens the omnipotence of Offred's suffocating universe but ultimately offers her no refuge. Early in the novel a group of Japanese tourists penetrates (quite easily, we must assume) this repressive, strictly stratified Republic of Gilead, which has entrapped Offred and women like her—who have retained their fertility in the wake of "ecological devastation"[28]—in its menacing clutches. The pernicious den mother Aunt Lydia warns that "the Republic of Gilead . . . knows no bounds. It is within you" (31). Yet these "Westernized" strangers in short skirts, open-toed shoes, and pink toenail polish parade themselves before the starved handmaids, causing, one might think, intense frustration, envy, and murmurings of mutiny among the women who glimpse the conditions of the outside world.[29]

The society Atwood depicts is nevertheless so confining that Offred and her companion Ofglen cannot even admit to having seen these sensational things on penalty of severe punishment. The uniform they wear includes a large white headdress that makes looking up burdensome and acts as a blinder for all peripheral views, ensuring that the handmaid's vision is limited and directed downward. Likewise, they cannot admit to wanting to be seen, as one of the tourists asks to take their picture, and the interpreter accompanying them, widely understood to be a government spy, asks if they would mind this too much. Like the loaded words that clog the arteries of Bradbury's universe, this simple question is really a trap. Offred knows that proper handmaids cannot stand to be looked at, that the official doctrine equates being looked at with unsanctioned sexual penetration and so declines the tourists' request. The spies in Gilead are called "The Eyes," whose main job is in fact to enforce blindness—to ensure that the handmaids themselves do not see and can never be seen.

In Bradbury's novel doubled language and the repression it attended were countered to some degree by the "truth" that Montag was to find in the language of the classics that could be burned to ash but never truly forgotten.

In Gilead, no such countervailing force is present, and both the actuality and deception contained in words shine forth in equal measure with each utterance, leaving Offred powerless and alone in her revolutionary thoughts for much of the story. She is allowed to walk with another handmaid during the course of her daily errands, but this interaction, like the interpreter's question, is another test. In an early scene Offred and Ofglen exchange the usual, required pleasantries, and Offred tries to read in her partner's gaze and intonation, in fibers of meaning so tiny even the Eyes cannot spy it, a spark of rebellion:

> During these walks she has never said anything that was not strictly orthodox, but then, neither have I. She may be a real believer, a Handmaid in more than name. I can't take the risk.
>
> "The war is going well, I hear," she says.
>
> "Praise be," I reply.
>
> "We've been sent good weather."
>
> "Which I receive with joy." . . .
>
> . . . Sometimes I wish she would just shut up and let me walk in peace. But I'm ravenous for news, any kind of news; even if it's false news, it must mean something. (26)

By novel's end our understanding of "false news" must include every utterance in the novel: the reports of war Offred hears on television, her clandestine meetings with Nick and finally Ofglen, even her own reportage is impossible to gauge for honesty and accountability. Is there a resistance movement, an "us" that Ofglen invites Offred to join? Or should Offred be wary when it "occurs to [her] that she may be a spy, a plant, set to trap [her]" (218)? Does it matter that "they only show us victories, never defeats" (106) on the news when the helicopters could be props, the prisoners of war actors? What does it mean when Nick, at novel's end, delivers Offred over to rescuers (who could just as easily be torturers) by using her real name when, if he were part of the spy network, even that kind of ultrasecret information could easily be uncovered? What is to be our response when, in the middle of Offred's reconstruction of a romantic liaison with Nick, she interrupts the narrative to warn us, "I made that up. It didn't happen that way. Here is what happened" (338)? Does her fantasizing ultimately undermine her project, weakening her ability to record and thus survive the horrors of her imprisonment and exploitation? Or is this entire narrative, maybe even these so-called horrors, nothing but fantasy—the ravings of a madwoman that scholars of such literature may many centuries later find intriguing but ultimately mystifying?

At one point in the story Offred is brought by her Commander to a house of prostitution for a night of costumed kinkiness, where Offred's loved and lost friend Moira serendipitously works as a "Jezebel." As does Anna Blume in her inner sancta, Offred finds here in this whorehouse cum liberation front the comforts and freedoms of an earlier time and draws deeply from Moira's wide-reaching and empowering wealth of information. She learns of her own mother's banishment to the Colonies—as in Auster's novel, an arrangement of forced labor camps on the outskirts of the central zone, again described here (but not really depicted) as a fate worse than death. She hears the story of Moira's harrowing, almost successful escape from Gilead on the Underground Femaleroad and her capture and relegation to this place that, while having its benefits (not the cigarettes so much as the freedom to sit and smoke them), has finally drained the life force from her. She is indifferent and careless in the telling of her story, and after their brief encounter Offred can only hope for her well-being, as Offred "never saw her again" (325).

While neither this venue of relative freedom nor the "black van" Offred finally surrenders to are revealed as sources of survival for the women, what little hope we may have for Offred's future lies in the structure of the novel's last sentence. She is led away from her commander's house by two guards whom, Nick says, are really conveyors of refugees for the Mayday Underground, and Offred, with no other choice than to follow and hope, "step[s] up, into the darkness within; or else the light" (378). These references to her final journey being a "step up" that is ultimately "light" rather than dark tip the scales of our uncertainty, at least to a tiny degree, in Offred's favor. Whatever hope we glean from this formulation, however, is irrevocably undercut by the "Historical Notes" that immediately follow the novel proper, a provocative epilogue that Atwood has set up as a "critical apparatus"—a lecture delivered by an inept and patronizing male scholar to a conference of like-minded scavengers of Offred's life and other artifacts from the now-defunct Republic of Gilead. The offstage constructed here is the final frontier, the last word that a mere narrator like Offred is powerless to defend herself against or, in many cases, even hear.

This otherworld to the territory Offred works so hard, and has maybe even given her life, to map out is revealed as ignorant of, mostly indifferent to, Offred's story, destroying her chance for textual survival. While the speaker and his collaborator are largely receivers of the lopsided history-as-usual that has come down to them, the gaps they cannot fill in the story make them impatient with Offred's very effort, and she is ultimately almost erased from her own story. There is, we learn, a wealth of information as to who the commander possibly was—a central figure in traditional histories yet in Offred's story only a menacing shadow. There is also, according to these "scholars," a little more information about "Luke" and "Nick," especially the Mayday Underground and The Eyes, male-run organizations of which Nick was a member. Yet there is finally nothing definite to be said of Offred, not even her name—and, most centrally, not her fate—and she herself is blamed for the scanty factual information surrounding herself: "many gaps remain. Some of them could have been filled by our anonymous author, had she had a different turn of mind. She could have told us much about the workings of the Gileadean empire, had she had the instincts of a reporter or spy" (392).

Thus Offred's emotional, sensual, intensely personal worldview is rejected by these hyperrational "reporters" for the enormous *lack* it represents in the fulfilling of their needs. They occupy a world so far offstage from that of Offred's that communication between the two is, we come to understand, all but impossible. Unfortunately, it is this other territory that is before us now, at novel's end, and that remains to remap the Republic of Gilead along its new rulers' own conventional, equally repressive lines. The magnitude of Offred's loss and tragedy is elided in Professor Pieixoto's barrage of speculations as to her outcome and in Offred's romanticization in his last remarks as "Eurydice," mythic and alluring in her mute transience. Unlike the otherworlds of Auster's and Bradbury's novels, this territory offers Atwood's protagonist no entrance and thus no escape, instead securing only for her oppressors a point of refuge and the silencing last word that attends such a position.

Likewise, George Orwell's *1984*, which was fairly obviously a model for Atwood's own project,[30] holds out a place of refuge only to snatch it cruelly away from the novel's heroes at the end of their story, leaving them stranded and doomed. As a founding example of the alterapocalyptic novel, it has in many ways been unequaled since,[31] and the nightmarish society Orwell depicts is the most repressive of all those discussed so far, its language most overburdened and paralyzed by false meaning. In the "critical apparatus" Orwell included at the end of his novel,[32] the intricacies and absurdities of "Newspeak" must be charted out, as no natural familiarity with "Oldspeak" (standard English) would suffice in understanding it. In Auster's country words disappear; in Bradbury's small town the classics are sent up in flames; and in Offred's Gilead even shop signs are merely pictorial, so high a crime is reading. But in Orwell's Oceania, the disappearance of all of these—stories, pictures, and history itself—is the dreaded ritual surrounding the disappearance of those whose lives these words shaped and documented. A disappeared "story" (word, news article, novel, or life) always is revealed to have posed a threat to the reigning political structure; thus, according to Orwell's appendix, a word like "free" maintains its "free from" implications but must sacrifice those elicited by "free to" to the notion of "service," so that in Newspeak "to serve" is also "to be free." The signifier "service" (really subservience) is now not only suited in its original meaning but saddled with its opposite as well, and one of the ultimate goals of Newspeak, implies the unnamed linguist of the appendix, is to halve all of language in just this respect, doubling—and thus disabling—meaning: "Newspeak was designed not to extend but to *diminish* the range of thought, and this purpose was indirectly assisted by cutting the choice of words down to a minimum" (247).

Each of three vocabularies works in a similar way, eliminating certain concepts through the grafting of them onto words with opposite meanings or hybrid words that are simply nonsense. The "A" vocabulary consists of the bulk of everyday speech, but the "debulking" process will eventually eliminate most root words, leaving just a few nouns or verbs and many repetitive and complicated suffixes and prefixes to drag them down. The fewer verbs available, the less agency or exercise a society enjoys; the fewer nouns and adjectives, the narrower the field of vision (recall Offred's huge blinders). In the "B" and "C" vocabularies political language and scientific jargon, respectively, hypertrophy and explode; the longer and more multipurpose a term, the less meaning it has and the less harm it can do: "doubleplusgood duckspeaker" (254). It is this meltdown of language into phantasmagoric hybrids that has sealed the fame of this novel, with concepts such as "doublespeak" and "thoughtcrime" defining "the Orwellian" and influencing our understanding of world politics ever since.

It is indeed a private, unspoken wish for a "space" (an offstage) to call his own that constitutes Winston's fateful "thoughtcrime." The buying of a diary in which to record his thoughts is a secondary and much less serious gesture; although it could be used as evidence against him, the nervous tics and premature aging produced by the lies he lives under (recall Montag's "fat") will undo him eventually anyway: "He thought of a man whom he had passed in the street. . . . They were a few meters apart when the left side of the man's face was suddenly contorted by a sort of spasm . . . : it was only a twitch, a quiver, rapid as the clicking of a camera. . . . He remembered thinking at the time: That poor devil is done for" (56). Stashing himself into an alcove in his cramped room, the one place unreachable by the roving eye of the telescreen, Winston scribbles into the blank pages of his diary the horrors of his censored life in an effort to communicate with the future. Although this offstage is certainly temporally situated, it is brought into immediate proximity, as if it were a neighboring, more neighborly country, by Winston's address to it: "*To the future or to the past, to a time when thought is free . . . : From the age of uniformity, from the age of solitude, from the age of Big Brother . . . —greetings*" (26–27). As did the "scholars" of Offred's story, Winston addresses this other time as a "second present," as a situation with as much immediacy and significance to him as his actual current moment.

Soon other offstages usurp the power and attraction these withouts, "the future" and his diary, initially hold for him: the wooded love nest he shares with Julia, the seedy bedroom in a proletarian section of the city they eventually find, the thrilling inner escape offered by Goldstein's *book,* which Winston pores over and gathers the strength necessary for revolution from. But like the ever-shifting battle lines that set Oceania against Eastasia one week and Eurasia the next, like the ominous and ultimately horrendous tortures waiting in Room 101, all these other secret territories are eventually revealed as government weapons, elaborate traps set for the likes of Winston and Julia, both of whom are captured and sentenced. Winston had taken a chance by reading the surreptitious glances of Julia as welcoming instead of threatening but longs to succeed once more in "reading" the equally cryptic yet promising O'Brien. It is this communication that Winston forces and ultimately misinterprets that results in the pair's downfall.

While the horrors of Room 101 seal Winston's capitulation to the powers of Big Brother, his understanding that no counterforce exists, that all rooms he enters from here on will be extensions of Room 101, broaches this capitulation in the first place and starts him irrevocably on the path to self-destruction. His revulsion by the revolting rat torture, his betrayal of Julia—these horrors have finally released him at novel's end, and he is left with only utter, drunken hopelessness and the perception of a world without end, without edges, that has driven him completely over his own brink, without hope of return:

> Winston, sitting in a blissful dream, paid no attention as his glass was filled up. He was back in the Ministry of Love, with everything forgiven, his soul white as snow. He was in the public dock, confessing everything, implicating everybody. . . .
>
> . . . O cruel, needless misunderstanding! O stubborn, self-willed exile from the loving breast! Two gin-scented tears trickled down the side of his nose. But it was all right. . . . He had won victory over himself. He loved Big Brother. (245)

In the pub or at the Ministry, drunk or doomed, crying tears of redemption or madness—all places and all states of mind fuse into one, as all language congeals into a suffocating and fatal mass. While Auster's and Atwood's stories offer at least a shred of hope for their protagonists' escape, no such possibility exists for Winston. Were he liberated by the armies of "Eastasia" the next hour, the sanity necessary to claim that freedom has been sealed off and bombed to oblivion.

In the ultimately downward trajectory characterizing Baudrillard's scheme of things, and in progressively alarming fashion, Auster, Bradbury, Atwood, and Orwell depict worlds getting roomier all the time—as airplanes, flowerpots, books, news, the past, friends, and lovers disappear one by one. But these otherworlds nevertheless make space for only an ever-amassing nothingness, pressing down on and paralyzing whatever and whoever remains. While there is probably still enough "stuff" occupying the spaces of Auster and Bradbury to enable optimistic conclusions, those lands of Atwood and especially Orwell are barren and bereft—of hidden treasures, last paths of escape, even (but most importantly) co-conspirators and the presence of mind to recognize them; the relentless opening up of the societies they describe will shortly close off life or freedom (if there is a difference) completely and permanently.

• • •

As in most any survey of postwar literature, the work of Thomas Pynchon requires incorporation here yet stands by itself in several respects.[33] In fact, Pynchon's most famous "rockets," those screaming across the sky of his epic *Gravity's Rainbow,* are painstaking reproductions of 1930s and 1940s Nazi weaponry and therefore only metaphorically related to the nuclear devices preoccupying Pynchon's contemporary audience so much more. Steven Weisenburger has carefully documented Pynchon's sources for the rocket construction scenes in *Gravity's Rainbow;* and multiple other critics have explored the historic, scientific, and mathematic verities behind Pynchon's seemingly fantastical story.[34] Thus, while it is tempting to substitute the more serious nuclear conflict for the now seemingly trite "romanticism of the blitz,"[35] Pynchon's dexterity with these archaic, dust-gathering historic minutiae is essential to the book's mind-bending impressiveness; also, the quaintness of a Second World War without blood, death, or concentration camps resonates with the musical-comedy veneer glistening ironically across the entire narrative. And while Pynchon's later *Vineland* recalls a 1960s counterculture that was certainly antinuclear in its original incarnation, Pynchon's heldover hippies are more interested in foiling the domestic plots of Reagan-era police and other operatives and have little in the way of a specifically nuclear message for readers.[36] Additionally, Pynchon's omnipresent apocalypticism does not describe a nuclear-delivered Armageddon but instead an eagerly awaited, Puritan-generated reckoning day, on which elect and preterite will be identified, divided from each other, and then sent to their separate destinies.

Thus Pynchon's work does not treat alterapocalyptic themes in any of the overt ways examined above but instead reflects an alterapocalyptic perspective so developed and ingrained as to influence and define its every movement. For the "alter," as several critics have already begun to observe, specifically the alternate and hidden universe as it touches on and inflames the paranoid suspicions of those in "this" world, is Pynchon's most accomplished narrative device. Richard Patteson has delineated the dual narratives of *V.* that eventually verge at the "base" of the novel to form their own "V" configuration, while V. herself inhabits two worlds—the empires of turn-of-the-century Europe and the wholly simulated landscape of a Baudrillardan postmodernism.[37] Susan Strehle has pointed out the multiple instances of doubling and duplicity in *Vineland,* observing that almost every character has a counterpart who eventually takes a separate path, "illuminat[ing] Pynchon's concern with choice and responsibility" (102). These many doublings among characters in *Vineland* reflect the larger narrative duality—1960s counterculture as it still challenges yet is all but vanquished by Reagan-era repression and control—while the smaller doublings in *V.* remind the reader of the war between two supervening worlds—the inanimate as it threatens and depletes the animate world. In Pynchon's own writing we find this theme encapsulated in the words of a Mexican anarchist in *The Crying of Lot 49:* "You know what a miracle is. . . . another world's intrusion into this one. Most of the time we coexist peacefully, but when we do touch, there's cataclysm" (88).

In *Gravity's Rainbow,* the key conflict is between a force of corrupt and dangerous government operatives and an increasingly aware and powerful counterforce that is ultimately unable to prevail. Chiefly, it is guileless but fortunate Lt. Tyrone Slothrop pitted against an invisible but powerful "They," who chase him about Europe in the late war and immediate postwar periods in an effort to learn the secret connecting multiple London bomb sites to the erections he has had and satisfied with various partners in each of these locales. Interestingly, Slothrop is lured toward the conspirators' clutches by being sent "on leave" in France, an idling, transitional plane between the opposite worlds of war (London) and peace (the reconstruction zone in Germany), which allows Pynchon to ease from one state of affairs into the next in mid-paragraph, without so much as a hat in the air. In many respects, the entire novel is "on leave" like this—in the lab instead of in battle, in London during the war instead of on front lines or in death camps, in Germany after reconstruction has begun, at the site of various bombings only after they have happened—always with time enough for a song-and-dance or banana frappé. Hiroshima, on the other side of the world from the beaches of France, is not even a blip on Slothrop's screen; finally, I find this sort of spatiotemporal game-playing consummately postmodern but strategically questionable in this novel of ostensible political import.

The contest between force and counterforce plays itself out on some smaller fields as well. The conspirators' initial interest in Slothrop's prescient physiology (itself the product of an old conspiracy) is led by the efforts of dog-behaviorist Edward Pointsman, whose determinist outlook is countered by that of the "Antipointsman," the statistician and semihero Roger Mexico: "in the domain of zero to one, not-something or something, Pointsman can only possess the zero and the one. He cannot, like Mexico, survive anyplace in between. Like his master I. P. Pavlov before him, he imagines the cortex of the brain as a mosaic of tiny on/off elements. . . . But to Mexico belongs the domain *between* zero and one—the middle Pointsman has excluded from his persuasion—the probabilities" (55). Mexico's postmodern uncertainty principles are thus pitted against the classical binarisms of the outdated Pointsman. Despite the philosophical mileage Pynchon gets from this debate, however, both men work to define and contain Slothrop—Pointsman as he plots to capture him for experimental purposes, Mexico as he plots the points of erections and bombings on matching Poisson distribution graphs.[38] Elsewhere in the novel, Vaslav Tchitcherine, a Russian operative inside the German zone, plots with almost no reason (Fowler 65) against his half-brother, the Herero hero Enzian; the rocket engineer Franz Pökler engages in a battle of wits with Weissmann/Blicero and, as the classic "cause-and-effects man," with his intuitive, dissatisfied wife, Leni. Between each pair, the conflict is less personal and idiosyncratic than abstract and philosophical, such that we may regard each contestant "in his own little world," which insulates each to a large degree but also engenders the volatility of the various encounters.

The twinned or intertwined relationship is essential to Pynchon's vision, as it takes two (at least) to form a conspiratorial plot that threatens unsuspecting victims and inspires the subversive thought and action of those who find conspiracies everywhere. Many critics have described Pynchon's "paranoid" characters and storylines, but in fact almost all are forced to confront not imaginary but actual threats to which they often respond with their own counterplots. The joining together that creates first the conspiring pair and then the conspiratorial network becomes an alternate world, an "invisible kingdom" intent on keeping its existence permanently behind the curtain. Its moments of slippage, as it reaches in to grab its next victim or as it inadvertently exposes itself, instigate and solidify the "counterforce" that will always have some success but never total victory. Pynchon himself notes, however, that conspiracy is also connection, perhaps the only means of connecting left in this contaminated, paranoid postnuclear age: "If there is something comforting—religious, if you want—about paranoia, there is still also anti-paranoia, where nothing is connected to anything, a condition not so many of us can bear for long" (*Gravity's Rainbow* 434).[39] While multiple critics have divided those occupying the hidden world (the masterminding conspirators aided by powerful technology) as elect against those struggling through the visible one as preterite (the passed over) in Pynchon's worldview,[40] in fact the elect includes not only the conspirators themselves but all those connected to them, and to the rest of the world, as targets and victims: only when Slothrop no longer serves the interests of "Them" does he decline to preterite status, becoming prey to the most powerful conspirators of all—the forces of entropy—and dissolving entirely into the narrative atmosphere.[41]

Yet the plot-counterplot narrative forms its own world against yet another, more radically other world widely and immediately familiar to any Pynchon reader—the chaotic plotlessness and linguistic confusion that are the hallmarks of his style. Again, *Gravity's Rainbow* best provides this frustrating, confusing, sometimes "grindingly dull" (from a blurb on the book's own back cover), sometimes hilarious and amazing experience of reading Pynchon; narrative digressions extending for pages, fantasies that were reality a moment ago, Ph.D.-level excursions into math and rocket science, anarchist lightbulbs, and impromptu musical numbers mounted by soldiers, bureaucrats, or laboratory mice are the matter that stretches this novel to its 760 pages and simply dares the reader to keep reading. Certainly the absurdity and confusion reigning in this other world to the novel proper reflect the alterapocalyptic tone and sentiment as I have defined it: before doing battle with Pynchon's first word, the reader understands from the novel's massive size that within is a realm governed consummately by doublespeak, if not quadruple- or quintuplespeak. Whereas in other alterapocalyptic novels characters speak in code so as to enlist, deceive, or betray each other, the author here is speaking in equally bloated and disorienting code *to us*, presenting a similar array of harrowing outcomes based on the various directions our response might take. Finally this alternarrative provides an enigmatic and treacherous yet potentially liberating realm of nonrule to counter the more strictly controlled frame of the traceable story; Pynchon's novels do not merely describe an elsewhere or offstage to a dystopic narrative landscape but instead create these two worlds around the reader and the reading experience. Here readers share with characters that glimpse of the alternate universe with all its threats and promises; here readers are carried or shoved from one world to the next and back again without reason or warning and sometimes forced to occupy both worlds at once. Pynchon's work settles consistently before and beyond (not alongside of) nuclear themes, yet his effective reliance on the alternate universe, the altered consciousness, and a markedly alternative prose style nevertheless partakes of and comments significantly on the alterapocalyptic.

Two Small, Deserted Islands: The Preapocalyptic and Extraepidemic

Among the protagonists of the alterapocalyptic narratives discussed here, it is finally only Bradbury's Montag who is depicted as successfully outwitting and outlasting his persecutors and flourishing in the place that is his refuge. Indeed, Montag outlasts much more than a few aggravated government censors; Bradbury treats us to a bona fide nuclear apocalypse that takes place, once more just offstage, but does enough damage to radically alter Montag's world and our estimation of his future. But since Bradbury assigns to such a war the bizarre and problematic role of ultimate global benefactor, necessary and purifying evil, his story helps define not so much a separate genre of apocalyptic literature as a difficult to sustain gesture within—the *preapocalyptic,* which genuinely *looks forward to* and longs for the bomb and all its "cleansing" devastation, as life in its current form has become intolerable.

What an author decides is an intolerable world will vary, but a preapocalyptic strain in narrative is dangerous to the degree that it envisions global conflagration as a viable and necessary lesser evil.[42] Bradbury's apocalypse is exhilarating, even beautiful, as it choreographs an explosive dance for Montag, who views in disbelief but relative safety: "He blinked once. And in that instant he saw the city, instead of bombs, in the air. They had displaced each other. For another of those impossible instants the city stood, rebuilt and unrecognizable, taller than it had ever hoped or strived to be, taller than man had built it, erected at last in gouts of shattered concrete and sparkles of torn metal into a mural hung like a reversed avalanche, a million colors, a million oddities . . . , and then the city rolled over and fell down dead" (143).

After the bomb, Montag's community of scholars dusts itself off and re-congregates at river's edge. After a campfire breakfast, the leader, Granger, reminds them of their mission to preserve the classics, and a hopeful light dawns: "The day was brightening all about them as if a pink lamp had been given more wick. In the trees, the birds that had flown away quickly now came back and settled down" (146–47). This depressingly naive view of the aftermath of nuclear war is only worsened by Bradbury's implicit definition of a "survivor" in this universe—a male, intellectual "rememberer" whose brain is big enough to contain the contents of entire books that may have been burned but are preserved intracranially for the benefit of future generations. Fortuitously, the unread masses (once again represented by Montag's wife Mildred) have been destroyed in the recent bombing; no one remains, Granger promises, except "lonely people" with interest and sympathy enough to "ask what we're doing" and hail the efforts of these philosopher-kings.

Erich Fromm, who has commented on *1984* and other dystopias in postmodern literature, discovers a mechanized dystopia in the text of existence itself in the 1950s and 1960s—a "technological nightmare" that had turned people into zombies and made the darkest alternative to "boring aliveness" seem attractive. In *The Revolution of Hope,* Fromm argues that "the rate of our automobile accidents and preparation for thermonuclear war are a testimony to this readiness to gamble with death" (43), and we note this readiness in Bradbury's acceptance of the bomb and its aftermath for the radical change it would produce.

Kurt Vonnegut's *Player Piano* depicts another such Frommian "technological nightmare" and, like Bradbury's text, supports the worst alternative to it. Vonnegut assembles at the end of his novel a collective of brilliant but rebellious manager/engineers (all male except for a token female "doctor" who serves mainly as the protagonist's secretary) who have decided to overthrow the machine-driven nightmare that is modern society. The debacle Vonnegut depicts at the novel's climax is hardly an apocalypse, but the author nevertheless produces a scene of significance and finality for the engineer-heroes' witnessing:

> Bodies lay everywhere, in grotesque attitudes of violent death, but manifesting the miracle of life in a snore, a mutter, the flight of a bubble from the lips.
>
> In the early light the town seemed an enormous jewel box, lined with the black and gray velvet of fly-ash, and filled with millions of twinkling treasures. . . .
>
> "All right, so we'll heat our water and cook our food and light and warm our homes with wood fires," said Lasher.
>
> "And walk wherever we're going," said Finnerty.
>
> "And read books instead of watching television," said von Neumann. (315–17)

Note that the destruction these men witness, as that witnessed by Montag in *Fahrenheit 451,* is of a fragmented, atomized quality and that these fragments, so uniform and patterned by the hand of chaos, are once again beautified, here as "millions of twinkling treasures." Note also the similarity between Bradbury's survivors and Vonnegut's, who, like Montag's commune, will live simply, walk for miles, and read all the great books. Much that is problematic in Bradbury's vision is softened or countered by the irony in

Vonnegut's, but in both the appeal to intellectual snobbery, and the snob's simple faith in an all-cleansing final fire, stand out. While the heroes are eventually captured and dragged back into their technological dystopia, the suggestion is strong that the leveling of the industrial town of Ilium was a good thing and that these heroes, or men much like them, will inevitably return to wreak similar havoc on a national or international scale.

A corresponding genre in AIDS literature, the extraepidemic, is exemplified, or so at least one queer theorist has argued, in the early writings of Peter Cameron. I argued early in this chapter that the "para-AIDS" novel—that written alongside of yet uninfected by this crisis—is as yet an impossibility. Still, in Cameron's *One Way or Another* and *Leap Year,* Myles Weber finds that AIDS is "not mentioned" in the earlier text and sees nothing "analogous to a life-threatening illness" (70). Cameron's work, says Weber, is extraepidemic in that it is "post-AIDS," "set during a time in which AIDS prevention techniques have become widely understood and generally practiced in this country, at least by sober adults" (72). Certainly such a reading is necessary to redeem for gay readers a depiction of themselves as healthy, sexual human beings, but Weber is revealingly defensive of the novelist's word choice and characterization;[43] likewise, he advances the following problematic argument: "the sexual histories of Cameron's gay characters predating the widespread acceptance of sexual precautions do not put them at risk of past exposure. During *that period of vulnerability* . . . each was involved in a long-term monogamous relationship if he was sexually active at all. . . . as long as Cameron's gay characters (and comparable men in real life) continue to act with care as a matter of course, none is at particularly high risk of exposure to HIV. . . . Cameron's fiction simply reflects this reality" (72; emphasis added).

In Weber's optimistic estimation, young men who were not sexually active during the early and mid-1980s only have to stick with condoms and limited promiscuity to consider themselves "safe." Statistics on gay men in their twenties reveal that the Weber formulation is an alarmingly popular assumption. AIDS is considered an old man's disease, a crisis that belongs to a "bygone" generation whose activism and years of behavior modification filtered the pool of HIV-positive partners, allowing young men unlimited sexual freedom.[44]

This disturbing redefinition of a widespread epidemic, with repercussions we have not begun to understand and no magic bullet in sight, as a mere "period of vulnerability" reveals Weber's utopic assumptions. He reads Cameron's work as pure metonym, as that which refers to nothing outside itself and, were this reading correct, condemns this text to removal from, irrelevance to, the world around it. As I have argued earlier in this study, the metonymic does not exist without always being part of that larger, opposing principle of the metaphoric; here the "reality" Weber describes is largely utopic fantasy.

To a lesser degree—though to a much more important one, because of these texts' huge following—Armistead Maupin's *Tales of the City* series (1978–89) partakes of this desire to treat the AIDS crisis in all of its overwhelming messiness as a series of isolated incidents. This gesture is understandable when the *Tales* are regarded as a single book—with multiple recurring characters and situations—divided into six volumes, which is divided again, sharply in half, by the advent of the AIDS crisis: an interesting study in temporal positioning, *Tales* is a story begun before gay San Francisco and the rest of the world had ever heard of AIDS and concludes intraepidemically at the height of this crisis as it affected the gay male population in the United States. The early "gay liberation" volumes are exactly that—liberating, light, and tremendously fun. Remarkable for their inclusion of gay and straight, male and female, youthful and middle-aged characters (if all of a liberal, colorful sort), the first three volumes feature long passages of dialogue, much white space, and a "readability ratio" of about 1:1 (one book per one afternoon at the beach). The feeling is much less of "serious literature" than a script for a long-running soap opera; surely these stories, appearing originally as snack-sized installments in the *San Francisco Chronicle,* must have been readers' favorites.

To watch this series "survive" the AIDS crisis in the way it does, however, presents interesting problems and questions. Language on the back cover of the early *More Tales of the City* (1980), describing this "divinely human comedy . . . roll[ing] recklessly along," belongs not at all to the darker, sadder, more cynical world configured in the final three books. *Babycakes* (1984), the first to regard AIDS in any way, is much longer and more dense than the earlier three; in the Harper and Row first edition, the type is small and the breezy dialogue and abundant white space are sacrificed for thick paragraphs of third-person narrative. In the fourth and fifth volumes, "me-decade" materialism and self-centeredness affect all the characters, especially the centrally placed, previously unspoiled Mary Ann Singleton. While Maupin manages to find humor in a villainous detective falling to his death, in cannibal rituals, and even in the Jonestown Massacre in the first three volumes, death is treated much more heavily in the final three; four characters die of AIDS, one of a heart attack, one of an infection after giving birth, one after a brutal bludgeoning; a central heterosexual marriage also ends in ruins.

But despite the perhaps inadvertent narrative elements marking these stories as "AIDS-infected," Maupin's intentional handling of the AIDS crisis is careful and controlled, and thus in some respects surprising: in the fourth volume AIDS is barely mentioned, while Jon, a central gay character, suffers the entire AIDS spectrum from diagnosis to death *between* books four and five and is thus separated from the reader and the reader's experience of his death by this intertextual gap. In the fifth book one minor character is introduced and then dies from AIDS-related causes, while in the sixth another character who was fairly important in the first two books is only a homophobically neutralized obituary. Michael, another central gay character, is HIV-positive and suffering minor symptoms but for the most part is alive and well. In fact, Maupin is wonderfully effective in treating HIV-positivity (Michael's faked orgasms during phone sex, his ever-sounding dosing beeper, and his panicked then groundless fears of a Kaposi's sarcoma lesion) and AIDS illness (in moving depictions of Geordie Davies, a straight woman, and Charlie Rubin, a gay man), but these "treatments" are most infrequently administered (for perhaps a paragraph or half a page every fifty to seventy pages) and interweave discordantly with the surrounding "foolishness"—Mona as the mistress of a grand Gloucestershire estate, hijinks at a lesbian summer camp, Mary Ann's selfish career preoccupations.

Maupin's most detailed descriptions of "AIDS-related illness" are indeed alarming—Brian, who once had a sexual relationship with Geordie, suffers the weight loss, flu-like symptoms, and drenching night sweats often accompanying early stage HIV infection—but end up as false alarms: the central straight male character is spared these trials. And while Maupin may be implying that during this period straights simply "could not know" what this illness was like, his efforts to wall off and minimize the actual incidents of HIV-positivity in the story do not help straight or gay readers to "know" the situation any better. Finally AIDS spoiled a good bit of the fun in Maupin's series—as it did in so many other elements of gay culture and gay life—and the author's efforts to keep the fun "roll[ing] recklessly along" nevertheless is a noble effort that in part succeeds, but in part fails, in disturbing ways.

• • •

To posit an unscathed world like the one inhabited by Bradbury's or Vonnegut's community of scholars, Cameron's twentysomethings, or Maupin's denizens of Barbary Lane in an epidemic- and plague-ridden time is to risk making "islands" not only out of infected characters but out of these utopic texts themselves. As they move from the mainstream, socially embedded genre of realism to the fantastic and purposely disconnected genre of escapism, these texts lose the chance to speak effectively to readers, to serve as guides to the past or the present. Texts recognized as preapocalyptic and extraepidemic represent dangerous illusions of the desert isle, heldover fantasies from the early modern period that in contemporary contexts are time bombs waiting to explode. Of course we cannot observe nuclear war over a copse of trees and dust ourselves off to continue a long day's journey in the way Bradbury's Montag does; of course young gay men who forget the lessons of their immediate past and secure themselves in the false hopes that *their* circles of society are untouched by disease are only setting themselves up for another wave of diagnosis and tragedy.

Texts infected to whatever degree by these generic tendencies are comparatively rare among the literature emerging from these two plague periods,[45] likely due to the difficulty in maintaining such false dreams. In each of the texts I have discussed here, other (even opposing) theses emerge that reveal them as examples of the more mainstream genres I discuss elsewhere in this chapter. While Bradbury's novel "anticipates" the bomb, it speaks emphatically against repression and censorship in ways I describe above; Vonnegut condemns the technological nightmares (including the bomb itself) he represents, providing beneficial social commentary in this way. Cameron's fiction in many ways acknowledges the very crisis Weber finds no mention of.[46] In depicting gay characters whose lives include AIDS-free issues as well, Cameron gives us an understanding of contemporary gay men that corresponds much more closely to reality in this age. That AIDS in Maupin's universe has become so universal that the most AIDS-symptomatic figure in the series is a heterosexual woman speaks effectively against the impulse to closet and forget this crisis, instead arguing in favor of a universal recognition of and response to it.

Deathbed Dictations: The Intraepidemic

In bold contrast to these "escapist"[47] genres, the intraepidemic and postapocalyptic texts I examine below acknowledge and explore fully the horrors of the crisis that shapes their respective eras. Where the escapist forms attempt and fail to inhabit a realm of safety, an island of metonymic detachment, the intraepidemic and postapocalyptic texts recognize correctly that the only purely metonymic state is that attached to the profound and permanent isolation of the grave. The characters of these stories fight bravely against this isolation and fragmentation, even though many are doomed to lose these battles. While the pre-epidemic attached great regenerative powers to texts and the alterapocalyptic presented words overloaded with multiple, debilitating meanings, the language of these last two genres simply explodes—off the page or off the stage in an aggressive, even threatening, but moving and irresistible, embrace of the reader or viewer.

In the intraepidemic, the *sexualized* body gives way to the thoroughly *technologized* body, which is forced to rely on gadgets and apparatuses to simulate sex, give it identity, save its life. Texts belonging to this genre describe the relationship between these two forms of embodiment, acknowledging the significant impact of low technology (telephones, latex) and high technology (e-mail, artificial respirators) on sexuality in this age. Here, homophobic and/or virophobic characters rely on technology to "metonymize" the threat of AIDS, to separate themselves from each other, or to build a wall around AIDS-infected characters. Turning once again to the generic marker for direction, we observe that the intraepidemic text has, theoretically speaking, nowhere to go. Unlike the "pre," the "alter," the "extra," or the "post" marking other genres of plague texts in this chapter, the language and characters of these novels, plays, and nonfiction accounts cannot go backward, forward, outside, or offstage. Shunned and quarantined by a fearful society, or terrified themselves of becoming infected or infecting others, these characters take the only direction left—inward to depression, illness, and isolation but also toward self-realization, acceptance, and inner strength.

Interestingly, the work of both gay and straight authors belongs to this genre, as AIDS is an issue powerful enough to influence the work, however indirectly, of thoughtful writers on both sides of this fence. The straight stories I examine here ask of technology a less-than-urgent question regarding sex today—"How do I stay 'safe' and still have fun?"—while gay-authored texts search for answers to much more vital inquiries—"How do I keep my T-cell count up?" "How do I stay alive?" Meanwhile, neither type of question is met very successfully by the state of the art, as vastly networked and exorbitantly expensive as all of it may be: the sex simulators in these texts are frustrated or frustrating (to characters and readers); the interpellated "patient" gets nothing for his patience except more and more symptomatic. The two technolove stories I am about to discuss both describe heterosexual desire, as it is mostly misdirected or thwarted by the hardware employed to express it. Neither story makes direct reference to AIDS or HIV, but they operate by new rules so thoroughly alien to traditional notions of sex and intercourse that only a thoroughly devastating sexually transmitted phenomenon such as HIV can account for this transformation.

Avodah Offit's *Virtual Love* tells the story of two sex therapists, an experienced female and her younger male protégé, who use their respective e-mailed musings on the erotic feelings they have for others to forge a platonic love relationship and ultimately to underscore the half-siblinghood between themselves that they discover at novel's end. Marc's sexual narrative revolves around a young and vulnerable patient, an especially inappropriate object choice, and his computer connections with a kindred spirit, instead of defusing or deflecting this "tainted" desire, only fuels it, serving as an aphrodisiac to his fantasies. Aphra, similarly misfiring in her communicative efforts, enters her thoughts on Marc's erotic emissions not in responses to him but in a private e-mail journal hidden by an anonymous ID she chooses for herself. These lengthy "do not send" files, which take up a healthy majority of the narrative, turn out to be genuinely revelatory, the stuff out of which true connections are formed, but Marc is not privy to this information for much of the story, and the "virtual" of the novel's title takes over and snuffs out the "love" the author may have expected us to find here. While the blurb on the book's cover describes the two analysts as "fall[ing]—almost wordlessly—in love," in fact they actually only *make* love—on the night before they attend their "fathers'" funeral(s) and discover that there is only one father between them and that they are half-siblings. This further weakens and pathologizes the notion of love in our current, technologized age. As one reviewer remarked, "Offit may have succeeded too well in her re-creation of the fragility of connections. The story itself seems vague and rootless, most of its various participants floating in and out of the reader's consciousness without really taking hold. In that sense, it is only partly reflective of a life 'lived' on line" (Bray 9).

This reviewer's frustration with the unaccounted for and misplaced "lust" and "rage" of the lead male character, Marc, mirrors my own irritation with Nicholson Baker's character Jim in the phone-sex erotic comedy (to use both terms loosely) *Vox.* As Offit's novel is epistolary, nothing but e-mail entries, Baker's *Vox* is one long phone conversation undertaken by two ordinary folks (no 900-number professionals cheapening this modern-day love story) who verbally turn each other on and get each other off over the course of this contemporary example of the world's oldest narrative structure. Jim and Abby are supposed to be equals: no *physical* power struggle can enter into a relationship in which either is free to hang up on the other at any time. They are supposed to be likable. They are supposed to be sexy. Their orgasms are probably supposed to accompany the reader's own. Yet Baker only proves that technology is no facilitator of, or improver upon, the traditional heterosexual relationship; if anything the same old gender roles reassert themselves, while in this new technologized (metonymized) context their many and various "hang-ups" will likely prevent their ringing each other again, once they have hung up on each other this time.

Once more sexiness and connectedness lose out to technology and isolation, a defeat crystallized in the idea of the way Jim and Abby "click." Early in their conversation Jim says he likes Abby's voice, acknowledging he watches a lot of "X-vid" and noting that with voices it is different: "At least with this, as opposed to pictures, at least there's the remote possibility of someone clicking. Perhaps it's presumptuous of me to say that we, you and I, click, but there is that possibility" (34). This "click," which is the aim and definition of all successful couplings, here reverberates both warm and hollow. Granted, there are sexy associations with "clicking": Jim and Abby click off their lamps to be in the dark with each other, Jim makes a "clk" sound in his throat when he gets too sexually excited to talk, and Baker is no doubt suggesting an association between this word found frequently here and the equally ubiquitous "clit" that Abby "dithers with" and Jim fantasizes about to fuel his own fire. However, the "click" between these two has a mechanized edge that competes with and overrides its erotic heart. At one point Jim describes the false darkness of a television setting, such as when the actress "turns out the bedside light, click," there is only "a high light level with the impression of darkness" (39). Technology's impressive but uncanny ability to create this false romance inspires a wave of anxiety in Jim, who does not want Abby to hang up and call him back to share expenses for their pricey call:

> "But then you'll have to turn your light on again to write my number down," he said. . . .
>
> "What if in this one isolated case the number slips your mind?"
>
> ". . . if you do call, but because of the break, even that one-minute break, when we aren't connected, what if fate shifts, and we're suddenly awkward with each other, and we're never able to resume the intimacy that we seemed to hit so easily the first time?" (40–41)

Obviously Baker's definition of intimacy, "so easily hit the first time" and so fragile it could not withstand a "one-minute break," reflects the tenuousness of all such connections in an intraepidemic age. Jim becomes sensitive, even oversensitive, to the sounds on Abby's line—the clink of ice cubes, the shifting of the phone ("What was that noise?" [56])—in an effort to distinguish these clicks from the click that will signal the end of their weakly forged relationship. While Abby claims to "*like* the sound of pauses in long-distance conversations—the cassette hiss sound" (25), her postorgasmic observation that "the hiss on the phone is very loud now, isn't it? . . . It's always louder at the end of conversations" (163) sounds much less "companionable" than menacing. Thus, while both of these novels argue that technology has succeeded over death by allowing "connection" and metaphorization where only metonymy (celibacy or death) threatened before, the cold, hard apparatuses employed as romance facilitators never fail to come between the two lovers or between the reader and her acceptance of the lovers' mechanized lives.

Variations on the phone-sex love story evident in Robert Chelsey's *Jerk-*

er; or, The Helping Hand denote the marked difference between straight and gay authors' stake in technology as defense against the AIDS crisis. Where the cut connections between Marc and Aphra and between Jim and Abby symbolize only anticlimax, the fizzling or resublimation of sexual desire, in *Jerker,* the ever-lengthening periods between Bert and J.R.'s phone-sex calls, and J.R.'s final inability to reach Bert at all, getting only his answering machine instead, signal sickness and ultimate death for one of the sex partners of this play. In the early scenes, the long-distance lovers are hot and horny; this "NC-17" production includes nudity, masturbation, and ejaculation. Inexorably, however, the AIDS threat infects and saddens the dramatic narrative—"J.R.: A friend was telling me yesterday: when he beats off? He fantasizes it's four or five years ago, before. . . . He can't even *fantasize* he's doing what he wants to do with another man unless it's before . . . all this" (476)—and the men talk less and less to turn each other on but more and more to verbally cuddle and comfort each other. At one point J.R. confesses, "I guess it was the *affection* I wanted. And you know? I think that's still basically it, still what I want the most" (484). The more realistic Bert challenges whether J.R. has always wanted to just be held or whether it is the epidemic that has forced this lesser, safer alternative on both of them. The play, under the virus's constricting pressure, shifts genres from porn to romance to tragedy: J.R. is left helplessly dialing and calling into Bert's unresponsive phone machine, with Bert silent and gone. Despite the marked difference in tone and message, in Chelsey's play, as with the two straight-authored technosex narratives above, this low-tech instrument sexually connects its users only momentarily but is finally no match for the separating, alienating ravages of AIDS.

Often the locus of isolation in the specifically AIDS-related and, significantly, gay-authored intraepidemic is the hospital bed, or the bed at home once devoted only to hot sex and warm bonding but now converted to the sickbed. In "Current Status 1/22/87," an especially concrete and technical survey of his own HIV status that appears in *Love Alone: 18 Elegies for Rog,* Paul Monette describes the coloring of his medicine: "the royal-and-white of the *ribavirin* rather / like the flag of an island nation which I am" (34). The image of the patient as island in a sea of technology also figures centrally in several important dramatic treatments of the issue, including Larry Kramer's *Normal Heart,* William Hoffman's *As Is,* and Tony Kushner's *Angels in America,* all of which depict various characters in bed, being attended to, comforted, but forsaken as well: in Kramer and Hoffman, the central lovers are reunited romantically—or even, in Hoffman's case, sexually—in the hospital bed after conflicts that disrupted their respective "marital" beds almost drove them apart. The same marital conflicts—resentment over diverging health statuses, fears of contamination—separate Louis and Prior in Kushner's play, but here Louis cannot overcome his motives for leaving Prior, while the sickbed becomes the site of an entirely different kind of "communion"—between Prior and the Angel.

The hospital bed is the catalyst for some of George Whitmore's most graphic accounts in his collection of essays *Someone Was Here*,[48] and Craig Rowland varies this theme in his essay "The Examination Table." The hospital or hospice bed or the bedroom turned into the hospital room are the settings for several of Adam Mars-Jones's more moving short fiction works. In "Slim," "Remission," and "The Changes of Those Terrible Years" (all from the collection *Monopolies of Loss*), major characters or the narrator himself suffer debilitating AIDS-related symptoms and illnesses, convalesce, and think about the beauty and sadness of their lives. In each story the home-based bed is the site not so much of high technology but the outreaching tentacles of the technocracy that supports it. Although human counterparts to the web of machinery and microchips they represent, the "home health industry" that descends on these men in the outpatient setting (in the form of volunteer-program "buddies" or social workers from hospice organizations) is no better comfort—even much less so for the promise of connection its humanity first offers.

In Peter Cameron's *Weekend*, Tony dies in the guest room of the perfectly appointed country estate of his half-brother and wife: "They had arranged to rent a hospital bed but it had not yet been delivered. So in the room were two twin beds, two antique wooden beds, a pair" (69); yet his death is "what is wrong with this picture" in more ways than one: "Tony lay on one bed with an arm hanging down over the edge, his head thrown back. His eyes were closed. The pillow lay on the floor" (69), while his lover, Lyle, attempts to cross over what now separates them irrevocably by assuming the position of peace he wishes for his beloved departed: "Lyle lay on the other bed, the way Marian imagined dead people should rest: flat on his back his hands crossed on his stomach, as if he were assuming Tony's death" (69). Lyle's metaphorization of Tony's death, a beautiful gesture as well as just a surrender to exhaustion and grief, has, of course, little effect: Tony is removed from the house and buried, while his memory causes discord among surviving family members. Cameron's own epigraph to the novel, from James Schuyler—"Violence gathers in a small place: a room, a bed, a glove"—warns the reader that these homelike images breed both love and tragedy, that the smaller space—that is, the bed within the country house—generates the suffering that spins outward and engulfs all present in its vortex.

James W. Jones has commented that the "gay space" identified by queer theorists over a decade ago[49] "requires a new definition because of AIDS. The division between interior and exterior has long been central to gay texts, but now its meanings vary" ("Refusing the Name" 238). This interior/exterior dichotomy of gay literature (and subjectivity itself) includes the "outed" existence as opposed to the closeted one, which has meant the difference between life and walking death to many gay men and lesbians. Jones argues that now interiors suggest positive associations with shelter and refuge from a harsh world (as in his reading of Robert Ferro's *Second Son*) yet recall the isolation of the closet by also signifying the quarantine (as in Edmund White's "Palace Days") that leaves the infected only each other to turn to. I would add that the hospital bed in these intraepidemic texts shares both the qualities of shelter and quarantine that Jones says the interiors of the intra-AIDS "gay space" are meant to suggest.

Where sexuality fails here to connect characters with each other or with readers or viewers, the language itself reaches out to and affects deeply all who hear the stories of these dying men. These narratives are among the most poignant, poetic, and moving in all the AIDS-related and queer canons, making contact with the reader powerfully and indelibly when contact within narrative boundaries is no longer possible. In the last moment of Adam Mars-Jones's "Slim," in his collection *Monopolies of Loss,* the narrator watches the inept and unfamiliar "buddy" assigned to him by a local AIDS service organization as he disappears after a visit, return to the world of the healthy and mobile: "There is something dogged about him that I resent as well as admire, a dull determination to go on and on, as if he was an ambulance chaser condemned always to follow on foot, watching as the blue lights fade in the distance" (18). In "Remission," Mars-Jones's narrator considers illness a "failure of . . . imagination. It seemed to me then, reeling as I was from the impact of the fruit in the yoghurt, that . . . with a little imagination, I could taste anything, take pleasure in anything. The yoghurt didn't stay down, of course; it wasn't such a new beginning as all that. But what it had to teach me it taught me on the way down; on the way up it had nothing to say. And even that was a lesson of sorts" (*Monopolies* 165).

In Edmund White's "Oracle," from his collection *The Beautiful Room Is Empty,* a young Greek prostitute returns the older Ray from grief to life by seeing him for several nights of reviving sex, then spurning him: "In pop song phrases [Ray] thought this guy had walked out on him, done him wrong, broken his heart—a heart he was happy to feel thumping again with sharp, wounded life. He . . . cried as he'd never yet allowed himself to cry over George, who'd just spoken to him once again through the least likely oracle" (209). In John Weir's *Irreversible Decline of Eddie Socket,* Polly discovers Eddie in his hospital room, fallen on the floor. Announcing she will call a nurse, Eddie responds,

> "Please don't. I'd rather lie here. Polly please don't leave. It's so good to see you. The only thing I was missing was company. I don't mind the floor. I got up to go to the john, it sort of leapt at me, you know, the tiles sort of hugged me, pulled me down, and it's cool down here, and anyway, I've never liked chairs, or beds, or—"
>
> "And what about the john?"
>
> "I got there anyway," he said, sourly. (245)

Despite (or perhaps because of) the graphic details of sickness and suffering offered here, these moving, fictionalized accounts reveal such deep sadness, sorrow, and loneliness that sympathy can be our only response.

In addition to these several literary examples, dramatic productions seek to reach out to audiences with equal effect. Marshall W. Mason's production note to Hoffman's *As Is* stipulates that "the audience must be kept from feeling 'safe' from this subject, so the actors of the 'chorus' must act as a bridge between the fictional characters and the real theater event" (xx). In this play, as well as in Kushner's, boundaries are broken down through the use of the split scene—the same setting used to stage different actions, sometimes even simultaneously—and the casting of the same actor in several roles. Larry Kramer also employs multicasting techniques to dissolve the boundary between stage and audience by directing that the walls of both stage and auditorium be covered with fields of the same startling information: death counts, government atrocities, comparisons with the Holocaust and the "Tylenol scare."

Shaun O'Connell posits that "the best literature on AIDS is found in the theater, for several reasons. Not only has the world of the theater been shaken by the disease, but the theater has long been the proper medium to bear bad tidings in artful design in times of crisis" (490). O'Connell cites Ireland's Abbey Theatre at the start of the twentieth century and New York's Group Theater a few decades later as examples of this powerful activist medium, and he adds to this list the gay theater that has developed throughout the AIDS crisis. Indeed, one of theater's primary strengths is its ability to metaphorize audience and actor, performance and "reality," and the plays, novels, and nonfiction that I examine here all partake of this same "dramatic" impulse to break down the "fourth wall" that perpetuates suffering and loneliness.

Forward Lunges: The Postapocalyptic

If the language of these intraepidemics fights successfully to whatever degree against the isolation and "metonymizing" depicted therein, the language of the postapocalyptics achieves this success (reaching out to and connecting with the indifferent reader) by surrendering to the explosive, fragmenting forces that threaten it. Derrick De Kerckhove has argued that it is the "phonetic alphabet that made the bomb possible" (73), meaning that the "Greek atomism" that broke language down into the isolated abstractions we know as alphabetic letters is a direct precursor to the atomism threatened in the nuclear age. As discussed in the last chapter, Derrida refers to a similar threat to the stability of language, insisting that "the archive" of "literature"—that body of discourse that "produces its referent as a fictive or fabulous referent" ("No Apocalypse" 26)—would not be able to reconstitute itself after a nuclear attack. To lose such an archive would be to wipe out our entire epoch, to lose the faculty of "literary memory" itself.

In the postapocalyptic novels that I examine below, language has been blown to bits—abbreviated, fragmented, fused into mystifying hybrids—and strikes and disables the inhabitants of these worlds with bomb-like force. We can identify a range of such linguistic manipulations across several texts: in the world according to Neville Shute language seems barely affected by the encroachment of a massive nuclear attack; in the works of Anthony Burgess, Russell Hoban, and Raymond Briggs traditional modes of expression are altered to near-unrecognizability. These radical changes force a reader into a process of constant metaphorizing, of attempting to graft new names onto old meanings and to force meaning out of an unyielding sea of word fragments and nonsense. Often these new formulations mark the very presence of illness—conditions menacing, urgent, and irreversible—in language and society; and the gap between our *sense* of what is happening and our actual *understanding* of it, a gap that is sometimes never crossed, makes these narratives as stressful to ingest as they seemingly are to live out. Thus these stories infect *us,* through our very reading of them, with the experience of chaos their characters face, turning reading into an almost painful experience. As with the alterapocalyptics, language here suffers to the degree that its respective society has. The more confounded and devastated the novelistic vision, the more ruined, howling, and violent the linguistic forms that describe it.

At the benign end of this scale, used here almost as a counterpoint to a definition of this genre, are novels like Shute's *On the Beach* and Denis

Johnson's *Fiskadoro;* despite the seriousness of their subject matter, both novels' sunny climates and calming ocean vistas shade their dystopic island landscapes toward prelapsarian paradise. Importantly, both novels' settings *are* islands, bounded on all sides by seemingly impervious boundaries in the manner of early modern utopias (and the purely metonymic). Both authors mean to depict and condemn the disastrous nuclear war that is visited on their settings, yet each has guided his reader into a pocket of tropical calm that, while ultimately succumbing to the inevitable storm, still fails to frighten and thus convince in a way we expect from this kind of narrative.

Shute's characters are paragons of stoic acceptance, even as they poison themselves and their children to avoid the ravages of radiation sickness, and their methodical, all-tucked-in existence is embodied in Shute's strictly controlled prose: "Peter left to catch the ferry truck back to the Navy Department; he picked up his letter of appointment and his [baby buggy] wheels, and took the tram to the station. He got back to Falmouth at about six o'clock, hung the wheels awkwardly on the handlebars of his bicycle, took off his jacket, and trudged the pedals heavily up the hill to his home. He got there half an hour later" (29). David Dowling has noted that "the trouble with Shute's world is that *everyone* seems to be as sensible and stiff-upper-lipped as his military heroes. . . . the characters, like Moira, are reduced to posturing rhetorical figures; even Holmes, administering fatal pills to his wife and child, is noble" (68). Dowling finds a "thinness at the heart of the novel" (68) that is a striking feature of both it and the 1959 film of the same name. Language here is calm and ordinary, and its juxtaposition with the chaos ensuing is at first startling but ultimately incongruous and disappointing.

Likewise Johnson's *Fiskadoro* depicts a postnuclear island paradise, inhabited by an ethnically varied yet harmonious enclave that again makes the post-apocalyptic seem edenic, a superior sociopolitical arrangement to even our own prenuclear society. Fiskadoro Hildago takes clarinet lessons from the gentle and gifted Anthony Cheung, whose 100-plus-year-old grandmother, half French and half Chinese, recalls memories of girlhood in Vietnam and watches over life with silent wisdom. Mr. Cheung's half-brother is a black Rastafarian, and Mr. Cheung enjoys the friendships of other black men on the island. Our first glimpse of the island is explicitly Club Med: "In the shallows the white of [the Key West sand] turns the water such an ideal sea-blue that looking at it you think you must be dead, and the rice paddies, in some seasons, are profoundly emerald. The people who inhabit these colors, thanked by the compassion and mercy of Allah, have nothing much to trouble them" (3). Even at the funeral of Fiskadoro's father (dead not because of nuclear poisoning but because he lost a romantic, Hemingwayesque battle with a fish), the setting is abundant and expressionistically beautiful: "the neighbors helplessly baked breads or cakes or artfully arranged slices of fruit on precious china platters and carried these offerings across a pink and blue landscape toward Belinda's house" (61).

Yet from the first a nuclear-based threat looms over and eventually undermines this fragile paradise, showcased vividly in the neologisms, the mutations in language, that radiate their hazardous history and eventually ruin the lives of their speakers: "Twicetown," formerly known as Key West, has been renamed because of two nuclear duds that landed there but did not explode; an old seer has a vision of "Colonel Overdoze," the atomic bomb pilot whose name suggests not only the "overdoes" that defines nuclear violence and the "overdose" of seemingly drug-induced insanity that inspires it but also the only worthwhile activity taken up in the nuclear aftermath—the "(bull)dozing" over of unlivable cities. The most frightening of these tainted words is "kill-me," an insidiously simple rendering of the cancers that appear as dreaded "durezas" (lumps) and afflict many on the island, especially Belinda, Fiskadoro's mother. While the islanders are powerless to understand or treat the "kill-me" that settles in Belinda's breast, they know what she has and, interestingly, treat it as a contagious disease. A visiting neighbor wipes the rim of a cup before accepting it from Belinda, and Fiskadoro, holding his mother's hand in her last hour, "didn't care if he caught it, and sometimes hoped he would" (199). As I argue in the early pages of this study, cancers in the aftermath of nuclear explosion would indeed spread throughout geographic regions like contagious diseases, and here is one of the more explicit depictions to be found of cancer as plague, of nuclear war as contagious disease.

The neologisms swirling through Kurt Vonnegut's apocalyptic texts always intensify their comic/absurd effects yet, despite their silly sounds, mark these worlds as drastically skewed by the occurrence of environmental disaster. In *Cat's Cradle,* Felix Hoenikker is the comically named counterpart to Robert Oppenheimer; on the day the bomb is dropped on Hiroshima, Hoenikker is home in his pajamas playing cat's cradle with a piece of string. The "bokononism" that so preoccupies the narrator is a religion based on "bittersweet lies," yet even though it draws diverse members of the human family together into a spiritually directed "karass," the "wampeter" (talisman or icon) for the narrator's karass is the deadly next invention of Hoenikker, *ice-nine.* Near the end of the story, the *ice-nine*d corpse of San Lorenzo's ridiculous dictator slides into the sea, bringing violent and instantaneous completion to this strangely named world:

> There was a sound like that of the gentle closing of a portal as big as the sky, the great door of heaven being closed softly. It was a grand AH-WHOOM.
>
> I opened my eyes—and all the sea was *ice-nine.*
>
> The moist green earth was a blue-white pearl.
>
> The sky darkened. *Borasisi,* the sun, became a sickly yellow ball, tiny and cruel.
>
> The sky was filled with worms. The worms were tornadoes. (211)

In "The Uncertain Messenger," Tony Tanner suggests that reading Vonnegut's novels causes us, like Billy Pilgrim of *Slaughterhouse-Five,* "to become unstuck in time" (127); certainly this sense of floating free, which easily resembles the escape of energy from matter and the disastrous "unstuckness" this escape can produce, is assisted by the strangeness of the language itself, which transports us so completely into absurd and menacing worlds.

In *Slapstick,* the world undergoes similarly silly but cataclysmic events—violent swings in the earth's gravitational pull, followed by a series of economic and epidemic aftershocks, these latter named the "Green Death" and the "Albanian flu." As a sort of emotional defense, U.S. president "Wilbur Daffodil-11 Swain" gathers his nation into 10,000-member artificial families (like the karasses of *Cat's Cradle*), based on a computer-generated middle name issued to every citizen, and the program is warmly received: Daffodil-11s flock to Indianapolis to form utopic societies of courtesy and support; "13" clubs spring up all over the country and do big business. In a paradigmatic scene, a young black girl leads a large gathering of the Daffodil clan with dignity and confidence; those contributing foolishly to the conversation are gently chided and redirected.

We are here at the heart of one of Vonnegut's favorite philosophic injunctions: that Americans, and people everywhere, leave off with falsely structured "clubs" such as nationalities and religious sects (lampooned as "granfalloons" in *Cat's Cradle*) and find unity with each other in large, loosely organized families of common interest or maybe even just common decency. While the challenge to nationalism works well in *Cat's Cradle,* the alternative suggested here seems equally artificial, comical, and socially detrimental: descriptions of these utopic families flirt shamelessly with sentimentalism; the "Chipmunk-5s" are a weakly excused "slave" colony. While I assume Vonnegut offers these false families as defense against the environmental and political disasters raining down on the narrative, my own sense of them is of more strangeness and craziness, one more aftershock from the gravitational upheaval and biological mayhem afflicting the story's inhabitants.

Significantly, *Deadeye Dick* is one of Vonnegut's most linguistically conservative experiments, offering little if anything in the way of the word invention or wordplay that marks his more apocalyptic stories; accordingly, the "neutron bomb" dropped on this story's Midland City is a much less satisfying, literal rendition of nuclear catastrophe than are the metaphorically suggestive environmental disasters to which Vonnegut treats us in earlier texts. Gary Giddins points out that "having destroyed the world in *Cat's Cradle* and the United States in *Slapstick,*" in *Deadeye Dick* "Vonnegut gives us his smallest and most painless holocaust to date" (251). In fact, Vonnegut's "actual" bomb is really just a metaphor for several other themes of importance to the author. In his preface to the novel, Vonnegut explains: "There is a neutron bomb explosion in a populated area. This is the disappearance of so many people I cared about in Indianapolis when I was starting out to be a writer. Indianapolis is there but the people are gone. . . . I also say that a neutron bomb is a sort of magic wand, which kills people instantly, but which leaves their property unharmed. This is a fantasy borrowed from enthusiasts for a Third World War" (xii, xiii). Later he links this bombing with the more generally understood notion of a "bombed out" city, one which has been abandoned for the strip malls and car culture of the suburbs and can no longer sustain itself or its remaining inhabitants.

Elsewhere Vonnegut metaphorizes radiation poisoning into just deserts for Rudy Waltz's philistine heartless mother. Because she is such a lazy, do-nothing presence in the home, she is exposed to radiation from a contaminated mantlepiece before which she spends endless hours hanging about. While she eventually dies from her exposure, the building contractors remove the contaminated piece and restore the Waltzes to their home within twenty-four hours. A Sheetrock wall and a paint job remove all trace of the nuclear threat, while "the whole beauty" of the neutron bomb that strikes Midland City is "that there was no lingering radiation afterwards" (226). Rudy informs us that "security is excellent" around the zone of disaster, that "the perimeter of the flash area is marked by a high fence topped with barbed wire, with a watchtower every three hundred yards or so. There is a minefield in front of that" (225). Throughout this study, I have been challenging such easy faith in the impermeable barrier between safety and something so dynamic and toxic as the effects of radiation; here Vonnegut comes curiously close to borrowing not only the language of World War III enthusiasts but their enthusiasm as well. Finally the novel's neutron bomb is doing the work of so many other disasters—governmental apathy and interference, American provincialism, white flight, and the curious "disappearance" of Indianapolis (when it is Vonnegut himself who "disappeared" from his native context)—that it cannot function as the bomb at all. Instead it is comic, contrived, and perfunctorily conclusive to the novel, as Giddins describes it, "a kind of howdy-do from the world of current events" (252) that fails to cohere with the larger narrative. Finally, it pales in comparison to the antinuclear, antiwar, proenvironmental statements made obliquely and metaphorically in Vonnegut's other, more authentically postapocalyptic texts.

Anthony Burgess's *Clockwork Orange* is an interesting combination of alter- and postapocalyptic elements, and, as with Vonnegut, it is the invented lexicon (no longer silly but strange and violent) that marks this literary world as devastated by some unnamed catastrophe in its past. As alterapocalyptic, the text divides between Alex's intensely dystopic Nadsat universe and the outside or offstage represented by the "Ludovico" scientist's laboratory—a repressive space that encroaches on and chokes off Alex's linguistically and physically violent realm: the scientists themselves, most of Alex's victims, even the "pre-pubes" Alex's gang encounters in a record store—none of these understand his outlandish, Russianized vocabulary, and by novel's end his world and the language he describes it with both seem profoundly threatened and shrinking fast. It is this casting of Alex and his language *as* threatened, as victim instead of victimizer, that emphasizes the alterapocalyptic strain in this novel. As threatened as it may be within the bounds of the story, however, Alex's vibrant and arresting Nadsat vocabulary certainly survives the comparatively pale Ludovico episodes (as Alex himself does) in the minds of readers: this text is marked deeply by its exploded, fragmented language and thus is marked primarily as a postapocalyptic text.

Certainly, it is Alex's language that constitutes his world, his apocalyptic setting that in many ways seems overarching and complete, that presents no point of return or escape. He is the only narrator of the story, and while he relates the voices of the establishment in standard English, he interprets and contextualizes these—and everything else he does and witnesses—in Nadsat, the mystifying dialect of his youth culture that borrows numerous Slavic (Soviet) and Germanic (Nazi) roots and diphthongs while also truncating, uglifying, and infantilizing much of its vocabulary that comes from English word forms. Alex addresses readers as "my brothers," a Westernization of the Soviet "comrade"; and the various examples of baby talk, "lubbilubbing" (for making love) and "eggiweg" (for egg), add to the frightfulness of their sound, suggesting either that it is children whom these thugs address (and thus violate) or that it is children themselves doing such violence to language. His words are threatening, then, to the others in the story for their subversive (political) emphases while also being threatening to them and to us for the violence they contain.

And foster in Alex and his "droogs" as well. We might almost wonder which came first: the unending flow of malevolence dealt out by these marauding, abusive punks or the language that seems to not only accessorize but inspire it. The words themselves—"devotchka" (girl), "pischcha" (food), "pyahnitsa" (drunk)—are disturbing to read, jawbreaking to pronounce, and headache-inducing to understand. Their foreignness and the consonant violence they carry with them seems to make an ugly scene even more unnerving. Alex watches a film of thugs robbing a store and beating up its owner: "it being only three or four malchicks crasting in a shop and filling their carmans with clutter, at the same time fillying about with the creeching starry ptitsa running the shop, tolchoking her and letting the red red krovvy flow" (107). That anxiety created between a sense of wrongdoing and our understanding of it is especially heightened here. It is as if we are witnessing one violent crime after another without the ability to "read" the situations properly, leaving us powerless to stop them or even to denounce and remove ourselves from them.[50]

Interestingly Alex's language and the violence it garnishes/produces is equated with a cancer, as the Ludovico method—an intravenous medication that causes vomiting and aversion to the violence with which it is associated—largely resembles a regimen of chemotherapy that kills the sickness while almost killing the patient. Burgess, through his "saving" of Alex, leaving him and his violent ways intact after many such experiments at novel's end, suggests that you cannot and thus should not try to cure social cancers this way, that the therapy always kills both the sickness and patient (Alex's "free spirit"). We might feel the urge to argue with such a proposition, as no one can finish Burgess's novel without great concern for the society into which this little Nadsat will eventually be rereleased.

In Russell Hoban's *Riddley Walker,* the violently altered language of this postnuclear "Inland" (England) produces a similar anxiety in reading as those novels I describe above. Peter Schwenger notes that the novel is an exercise in hermeneutics, the story of a boy's "unriddling" of the universe, and that "the text's language, the conjectured speech of a devastated society. . . . slows us to the pace of an oral culture, defamiliarizing the act of reading itself so that this process too becomes an unriddling" (*Letter Bomb* 31). Like Burgess's, Hoban's language is garbled and eviscerated. It too is childish, although while Burgess's baby talk multiplied unnecessary syllables, reproduced the hyperarticulations of a child's budding romance with language, Hoban's is the guttural ramblings of a inconsolable toddler: "parbly" and "barm" are "probably" and "bomb," "Arga warga" the onomatopoeia for a screamingly painful death.

Hoban's entire story is reproduced in this thickly mutated language; almost no standard English survives, nor do any of the standard markings of contemporary civilization. Both "Inland"—an interesting hybrid of the "island" England is and the "inland" that is the opposite of a utopic island paradise—and its national tongue have been transformed into something muddy, dangerous, and forever in darkness; the corruption of the words spoken by its isolated and contentious tribes reflects the ruin of their daily lives and the dishonesty of their thieving, itinerant "governors." This language reverts to an anaplastic state ("prime minister" significantly recast as "Pry Mincer"), explodes into its component syllables ("Inner G" for "energy"), and fuses into hybrids that are close to unrecognizable ("thatwl" for "that will"). Apostrophes, commas, and periods are crushed in these fusions—"The littl Man the Addom he begun tu com a part he cryd, I wan to go I wan to stay. Eusa sed, Tel mor" (30)—linguistically enacting the slippery slope: unable to stop themselves before the brink of total war centuries earlier, this civilization (if that term even applies) is incapable even now of cutting off a simple sentence in time. Hoban has stated that in *Riddley Walker* language itself is another of the story's protagonists,[51] and certainly words in this story perform a central, indeed heroic, function: their distinct form brings home the nightmarishness of the world they describe, and our need to avoid this world at all costs, in profoundly effective ways.

In Raymond Briggs's antinuclear "storybook" *When the Wind Blows,* "narrative" mutates into the most radical form to be considered here—a verbal/pictorial hybrid, with the "pictures" being the comic book drawing belonging in many Western cultures to a specifically juvenile realm. Briggs's comic strip is incongruous and disorienting, depicting plain folks doing ordinary things but whose lives are suddenly, graphically cut off by the "fabulous" war machinery more typical to the comics genre. The story is presented in oversized-book format, which brings its simple domesticity and the monstrous battle gear that destroys it disturbingly close. Interestingly, Briggs's mutant "literary" style has caused some confusion as to what exactly his work *is: When the Wind Blows* was assigned the Library of Congress call number UF767.B695, classifying this book under "Nuclear warfare—Popular works"—a category that applies not to "bomb" novels like Peter George's *Dr. Strangelove* or Burdick and Wheeler's *Failsafe* but instead to the oversized texts of more overactive imaginations—that is, "survivalist" guides to shelter-building, food preservation, weapons' construction, and the like—and also to sensationalized nuclear "almanacs" designed to shock readers with their detailed and harrowing predictions. In the library where I first found this text, the UFs are as far-out as UFOs: one must walk to the farthest aisle in the farthest back corner of the second floor, dig past the extra book trucks and desk chairs, and blow the dust off the call numbers to find them.

Interestingly, Briggs's anti-Thatcher fairy tale *The Tin-Pot Foreign General and the Old Iron Woman* has been similarly misread: a satiric condemnation of the British-Argentine war over (the heads and homes of) harmless, sheep-herding Falkland Islanders, this oversized book tells its story in a large-print, one-sentence-per-page format with nightmarishly caricatured cartoons, including a spread-eagled, red-headed female robot pulling large sums of money from huge breasts, and moving charcoal sketchworks of dead, falling, and wounded soldiers. The call number of this text begins with PZ7, a children's literature designation that places the book alongside titles such as *Nowhere to Play* and *The Singing Turtle and Other Tales from Haiti* in the Latin American collection.

Meanwhile, a dramatic version of Briggs's *When the Wind Blows,* adapted by the author in 1983, has been neither ghettoized nor misread, receiving the legitimizing "PR" designation of late twentieth-century British literature that both of his other works deserve as well. Ironically, the story-as-play suffers thoroughly, in my opinion, from the downsizing and mainstreaming it undergoes, stripped of its cartooned format and oversized presentation. What, we must ask, is so confusing if not downright threatening about the message Briggs sends and the way it has been sent to us? Peter Schwenger begins his own study of nuclear theory and literature with just this question, crediting Briggs's *When the Wind Blows* with producing in him his original impulse, indeed urgent need, to write: "there was an intense anxiety in me that I could not account for, assigning it first to one cause than to another. . . . Only a long walk allowed me to realize that a book so innocuous as to be first cousin to a comic book had invaded my unconscious and was still working there. How could this be?" (*Letter Bomb* xi). Schwenger finally answers this question by demonstrating how this anxiety in him (and us) emanates from the unconscious-invasiveness of all nuclear texts, never really returning to the specific mystery and undeniable power surrounding this "first cousin to a comic book." Here, then, we should examine the particulars of this text, its contribution to the post- (and thus anti-) apocalyptic genre, and the way it uses picture and language—indeed, pictures as language—to produce its vivid, unforgettable imprint.

The story centers on two aging, good-hearted Britons, James and Hilda Bloggs, recently retired from a bustling London life to a countryside more in keeping with their slowing, golden years. This move from the center of the metropolitan area is what allows them their few days of survival following a nuclear blast, even though this "grace period" is plagued by debilitating illness, fatigue, and fear. In the early frames of the story, the old couple prepare for a simple supper and ramble on about their own concerns in the interlocking, comfortable, but somewhat disconnected style of long-married couples. James studies the government pamphlets on bomb survival that he picked up at the library, Hilda mumbles to herself about what to serve for tea and how hard it is to keep the house clean. Sweetly, hopelessly, James gets up from his meal to construct a bomb shelter out of cushions from the sofa and forces his wife inside while radio-broadcasted announcements of approaching invaders grow more panicked and intense. An entire double page is devoted to a pink-rimmed whiteness representing the actual nuclear explosion, and the initial frames on the next page only fade into clarity as the two oldsters pull themselves from behind the makeshift shelter and examine the kingdom of fragments their cottage has become.

They are frightened and stunned but buck themselves up by assuring each other that the government has provided for such an attack and will restore power and water and milk delivery by the end of the week. They walk into their garden and observe the curious, world-blanketing silence. They trade idle bits of conversation back inside the shelter and bicker over whether it is safe to go upstairs and use the toilet. Soon, radiation sickness symptoms manifest themselves and multiply; Hilda is overcome by nausea and diarrhea, James bleeds from his mouth. Sores break out all over both of them. At last they are overtaken, rising in the morning to discuss breakfast and the lack of newspaper service, then settling down for an "afternoon nap" without even trying to execute the movements of normality. They crawl together into their shelter and Hilda suggests they pray. Their quiet, uncertain words to heaven trail out from behind their cushions in the final frames.

To an American or British reader, having to digest the subjects addressed here—fatal illness, world history, nuclear bombings—in a comic book format is disorienting and disturbing. The simple domestic routines depicted in the early frames are confusing to a viewer who is used to turning to comics for anything but. Comic books in this society cater to a particular, limited audience—action- or romance-loving, easily bored preteens or that aspect of all our personalities that resurfaces however briefly on Sunday mornings. Comics here warehouse the larger-than-life, the "Booms!" and "Zowies!," the garish colors, the dizzying angles of view; and this overbubbling zaniness is contained and thus understood by explicitly *not* referring to subjects that we perceive as domestic and mundane so that when the bad guys descend, trailing rainbows of violence and destruction, our own worlds remain intact.

Briggs, however, has violated this sacred boundary, opening the comic book genre to include (i.e., incorporate) *us*, drawing his characters in soft neutrals and realistic detail with apple cheeks and hauntingly expressive eyes. Even the mind-bending Wile E. Coyote–esque violence that can be visited on characters in the drawn genres has been downsized and simplified in an eerily disconcerting manner. Instead of watching these characters dramatically exploded, decapitated, or sliced in quarters, they are bent over with dry heaves and stomach cramps. Their cheeks turn a little greener with each passing hour, just the way *ours* would. Briggs thus forgoes the excesses that the comics genre allows in an effort to realize the situation for the reader/viewer, to metaphorize ordinary life and an other to it, the chaotic though previously contained universe of the comic strip.

The comic form also speaks to our conscious or unconscious fears surrounding the fragility of children[52]—the terror they produce within us by wandering so easily and suddenly into harm's way and our own childhood fears, which erupted from vivid imaginations, traumatic nightmares, and the horde of goblins that lurked under the bed, just waiting for us to fall asleep. How to take up the comic *book* (and I mean to distinguish this act from a browse through the Sunday funnies) to offer up the time and concentration that trips the mechanism for "getting lost" within, without reverting to the status of child? What more horrific position from which to view the end of the world and the slow but inexorable deaths of two elderly innocents (here "grandma and grandpa") than from that of the helpless and frightened child? Emerging from such an experience, adulthood—the ability to understand, reject, even militate against such destruction—returns to the reader as an enormous relief but also, as authors like Briggs no doubt hope, an enormous responsibility.

I have been careful to delineate a regionalized reading of the comics genre because this is "read" so very differently in other cultures. In France and Latin America comics are much more popular than they are here, and in Japan they have been a popular diversion for children, teens, and even young adults ever since the Hiroshima/Nagasaki bombings that ended the war. There, the best of comic book artists are as popular as movie stars are in the United States, and comics' subjects include the not only typical action-adventure stories of samurai, sumo wrestlers, and kamikaze pilots but also the more ordinary "adventures" of office workers and high school kids. These stories, Peter Duus notes in the introduction to one such book-length comic, can function as cultural pedagogy, offering lessons in the virtues of the Japanese company man, the intricacies of the Japanese auto industry, strategies for trade with the United States, theories of math or physics. Certain comics, Duus notes, actually serve as textbooks in Japan, helping children through the difficulties of math and science with their engaging characters and larger-than-life illustrations.

Interestingly, Duus argues that the postwar boom in comics in Japan was the result of a need for cheaply produced diversion, as the "Japanese population, living in the ruins of its old dreams, was hungry for new ones. . . . there was an audience ready for escape from dreary reality to a world of fantasy, adventure, romance" ("Introduction" n.p.). And yet the first strips immediately produced and popularly received in Japan (and even to some degree in America) seem full of war and conflict. The popular *Tetsuwan Atomu* lost its nuclear referent but probably little of its atomic "heat" in the Americanized *Astro Boy* strip and television series of the 1960s. Duus himself notes that an equally early *Shintakarajima* (*New Treasure Island*) was neither romantic nor escapist but instead humanized the cartoon figure with feelings "immediately recognizable to the [Japanese] child—sadness, fear, anger, self-sacrifice, as well as joy, courage, and triumph" ("Introduction" n.p.). At the same time that cartoon artists were turning cartoon strips into the human experience, was their wide acceptance in Japanese culture indicative of the way human experience had turned into a cartoon?

Certainly, the Japanese were subjected during the bombings to violence that was unprecedented, fantastic, and total in a way only dreamed (or drawn) about in the past. How can one suffer and survive so many thousands of deaths in such annihilating and mutilating versions if one were not made of pen and ink as was Wile E. Coyote or made of a resolve ("self-sacrifice") not understood or estimated by the rest of the world? We might argue that Japan was looking to this elastic resilience, these unnumbered chances for absolute regeneration, both fundamental components of the comic book mode, for a model of their own reconstruction.

In succession to but also in rewriting this tradition, then, Briggs depicts a violence not futuristic but historical, not "fantastic" but horrendous, yet trades in the rubber-made characters of traditional comics for flesh and blood, which does not bounce back but merely succumbs. Our faith in the immortality of the comic book figure is undercut, as should be our perception of "unbeatable" Western forces and the "inhumanity" of the "evil empire" or other global target of our weaponry. We watch what we hoped would never happen happen fully, and because we watch instead of simply read, Briggs's nightmare *vision* more effectively clarifies our own dreams of a denuclearized future.

• • •

In addition to being so striking an example of the postapocalyptic, Briggs's comic book novel is also an exceedingly postmodern experiment in the overlap of space and time. If *reading* is a largely temporal activity that offers us meaning over a period of time and *viewing* more spatial, a function of apprehending an image instantly ("in no time") but with much reliance on the spatial elements of light, angle, and composition, the comic strip fuses these divergent functions by making words into pictures—bold, jagged, tiny and punctuated, "framed" by the balloons that showcase and attribute them[53]—and by making pictures into language that does not "flow" cinematically or "freeze" photographically but progresses panel by panel the way sentences do word by word.

In various ways the spatiotemporal has helped us to organize and understand multiple texts from each of the four generic corners of the postmodern-plague configuration outlined in this chapter; its ever-shifting dynamic disrupts the binaries of "here and there," "now and never," "me and not-me" that presided over the geography of rule and oppression during modern periods. Those generic elements that would deny this destabilization, that claim to have moved writers and readers safely beyond it, have been shown, when they are determined to exist at all, as dangerous strains in literary production that serve only to diminish a text's relevance to contemporary experience. By proceeding in rather taxonomic, structured fashion, I have meant in this chapter only to outline and clarify some themes arising from these two widely scattered, complexly overlapping, intently conversant postmodern plague periods. I do not mean to suggest that the historic and cultural complications attending these periods can be "squared off" and neatly comprehended, that they can be "boxed out" of our everyday concerns and considered only during election periods and scare campaigns. As I hope the title to this chapter indicates, the notion of plotting the "corners of a crisis" is largely ironic and, finally, impossible to imagine. Yet delineating the edges of these issues to whatever degree possible is an essential initial movement in ultimately understanding, controlling, and alleviating their effects.

3

Three Points of Sight: Gender in Plague Texts

DANGER ZONES AND OTHER POSTMODERN MYTHS

In a small showing of art in the lobby of a bank on Chicago's near north side, Christmas 1993, vivid, engaging paintings by children of the now-ruined Belarus/Chernobyl region revealed a significant pattern: whether the scene depicted was a deserted country road, a snowy field, an ominous wire fence, or an abandoned town, each roadside or broadside that figured centrally was marked with a simple sign—a wordless, empty triangle surrounded by a circle: ⃤. This sign stems from a family of triangular figurations for nuclear hazard and for civil defense against these hazards in both the United States and the former Soviet Union since the inception of atomic energy. In later manifestations, in laboratories and medical centers across America, radioactive contaminants are stored in areas marked with a fragmented triangle, reminding one of the cold war air-raid siren: ☢. The atomic symbol itself, ⚛, is three rings (electron paths) overlain to form a double triangle; these surround the circular, a nucleus that centers and grounds the structure.

While the origins of this signage are not well documented, we nevertheless perceive an inherent triangularity in nuclearism itself, which inclines toward just this sort of pictorial representation. Indeed, the atomic formula is distinctly tripartite or pyramid-shaped, in that a nuclear chain reaction is generated, as Louis Szilard discovered in 1933, with a catalytic element "which would emit *two* neutrons when it absorbed only *one* neutron" (qtd. in Hilgartner et al. 15). Likewise uranium manifests itself in three isotopic forms—one that is abundant but nonfissionable, one that is so rare as to be useless, and one that is markedly fissionable yet relatively rare, making the generation of nuclear energy much more expensive than it was initially thought to be. Significantly Robert Oppenheimer named the first above-ground bomb test at Alamogordo "Trinity," from the reference to a "three-personed God" in the famous Donne sonnet he had recently read (Hilgartner et al. 30–31). The intensely (homo)erotic nature of this poem, as has been extensively investigated by queer theorists in recent years,[1] is of significance to our reading here, as the triangle is a figuration of critical mass—nuclear and sexual—itself: the chain reaction is initiated by the addition to a stable setting (the original equal pairing) of a third element—the last, least extra charge necessary to radically destabilize (i.e., drive) the chemical reaction over its edge and generate a sustained, uncontainable explosion.

Likewise the triangle, in its raucous, attention-grabbing shade of electric pink, has become a symbol for gay rights and AIDS activism in recent decades. A favorite design for gay rights buttons, banners, and black T-shirts for more than a decade, the pink triangle is sometimes accompanied by words but largely independent of them: the quickest glimpse of this sign's signature color and shape informs the viewer that AIDS activism of a decidedly creative, outlandish, and aggressive type is likely underway somewhere in the vicinity. The figuration has been converted, and thus effectively subverted, from its earlier function as a marker for homosexuals interred in Nazi concentration camps; appropriately, this conversion has been assisted by *in*version of the design, from downward-pointing in Nazi camps to upward-pointing for AIDS activism. As with the Chernobyl triangle, the wordless incarnation of the gay rights pink triangle carries a special, arresting power; as opposed to the nuclear triangle's message, however, the pink triangle's statement is not a pushing away but a welcoming in: not "beware" but "be aware."

The circle surrounding the atomic triangle must be read as the line of separation between the danger zone within and the outlying realm of safety where the sign's reader is exhorted to remain. Within this circle, the asymmetry and disorganization that governs the triangle preside, contaminating and debilitating all who enter there; without, stability, order, and safe resources are yet to be found. The circle, then, is a mark of control, an intact boundary that, if not crossed, will contain the danger housed within it. It is again a principle of metonymy, of separate entities and solid boundaries, that has been entrusted with definition and control of the metaphoric, a chaotic crushing together or fusion of elements and properties that will not crystallize (or carbonize) into stable meaning for eons. As I have demonstrated in previous chapters, however, the pure metonym is linguistically—and now geophysically—pure fantasy; the metaphoric principle always threatens and "contaminates" the purely metonymic in the same way a nuclear hazard eventually escapes from and thus demolishes the idea of a solidified danger zone. Thus, the nuclear *is* this triangular instability, the explosion itself; yet as Peter

Schwenger has argued in *Letter Bomb,* and as I will examine below, it is the circular, the series of ever-widening rings of destruction, as well.

Meanwhile, the pink triangle of gay rights and AIDS activism has never been and would never seek to be contained by a circling border the way the nuclear triangle would, as containment in this case is another word for "closet" and is therefore anathema to gay identity and gay rights; likewise the pink triangle as AIDS symbol acknowledges the difficulty (if not impossibility) of containing the AIDS virus, therefore asserting that those who have failed to "contain" themselves through spreading of the virus must not be shunned by society. Any sort of line in AIDS iconography seems suspect and delimiting, and Lee Edelman in "The Plague of Discourse" has called into question the solidifying and scientizing effect of the straight line, specifically the pseudomathematic certainty promised in the lines of the equal sign between "Silence" and "Death."

If, then, the previous chapter was primarily structured by four generic designations occupying corners of a square, the governing figuration in this part of my study—which moves from the question of *genre* to the question of *gender* in plague texts—is the equilateral triangle, as it inevitably bursts the barriers of its circular containment zone. Specifically, this triangular configuration will signify the three-way relationships among characters in stories (and among characters, authors, and readers) that unify, polarize, and triangulate because of gender-based positionings. Relative to the equilibrium of the square, an explosive tension defines the triangle, an unevenness that leaves a question hanging, that closes off the possibility of closure: if the pair, the "couple," is a fundamental sign of stability, completion, and the private, protected union, the triad connotes open-endedness (with all its narrative and sexual connotations), volatility, and an inherent oddness that allows, even sanctions, voyeuristic intrusion. Of course the trio being intruded upon is marginalized by its triadic configuration and is thus powerless to close its doors and secure its privacy in the way that the societally supported couple always can. Narratively, the triangle is open-ended in that the characters involved cannot or will not pair off and thus close off the narrative trajectory of "happily ever after," as the third member is left "stranded"—more rejected than accepted and forever struggling to reverse this situation. Thus, position is of vital importance when reading gendered bodies in plague texts: who is in the middle of, or has come between, the other two? Who is in the position to choose between? Who is fighting to be chosen? Finally, the triangle is a sign of discord, even danger, in both postmodern periods considered here; yet it has been likewise used to disrupt the very systems of abuse and oppression that once structured them. Finally, it stands as both warning and invitation, as a zone of danger but also one of healing, pleasure, and peace.

Specifically, traditionally drawn battle lines between suitors in the love triangles of plague texts are disrupted, since the classic scenario of two (presumably straight) males challenging each other for the hand of an elusive (though presumably not lesbian) female has been radically altered. Again it is the triangulation principle itself, that figure which contains and yet cannot contain the free agent or "third wheel," that intervenes in and subverts the traditional heterosexual coupling. Steven F. Kruger observes that even gendered figurations assigned to cellular components by the biases of modern science—a male nucleus surrounded by soft, impregnable, feminized cytoplasm—*triangulate* at the moment of viral infection: "The cell, after all, itself already represents a 'marriage' of male and female, nucleus and cytoplasm, the 'ideas' of DNA and the material products 'coded' in those 'ideas.' 'Take-over' of the cell by HIV involves not just the phallic 'invasion' of the (feminized) cytoplasm . . . but an 'attack' on the (masculinized) nucleus and 'usurpation' of the central, governing position of cellular DNA" (37). As typical as this configuration may seem, Kruger finds here a "male homosociality, with two differently 'armed' male opponents battling for dominance" (37); and likely he borrows his concept of the homosocial from Eve Kosofsky Sedgwick, who argues in *Between Men* that the traditional romantic triangle must not be viewed so much as a contest *for* the favors of a woman as *over* the body of a women by which the two contending male lovers demonstrate their desires and desirability for each other.

Interestingly, if not fully explored by Sedgwick, the growing strength of the feminist movement has had much to do with the queering of the love triangles in plague texts, since the stronger and more interesting their female characters are revisioned by feminist readings to be, the stranger or "queerer" a (presumably straight) male character's preoccupation with another male character becomes: when Orwell depicted the characterological triangle of *1984* in 1949 it was "natural" that Winston would seek and find passionate communion with his alter ego, O'Brien. "Naturally" Julia, the female lover, would be sexually available but mentally and emotionally disappointing, and Winston's turn to O'Brien as his new sphere of meaning at novel's end would seem nothing out of the ordinary, even only proper, as demanded by the literary conventions of those times. I will argue below, however, that it is a powerful feminist reseeing of Julia's role as not natural and appropriate but distinctly unnatural—indeed, nearly fatal—to women that resulted in the simultaneous denaturalization of the male characters' relationship with each other. Feminism thus romanticized fully (i.e., *equilaterally*) the triangle that had been distinctly isosceles in early postmodern sensibility, paving the way for a fuller enunciation of those male-male relationships to be done by queer theorists a generation later.

In the AIDS texts I examine here the triangle outlines a figure—male or female, straight or gay—divided between and strengthened by access to competing sensibilities (traditional and nontraditional versions of masculinity and femininity) and bearing an orientation-based double consciousness that entangles inextricably societal assumptions with personal truths. The "straight" (at least married) characters triangulated thus realize in themselves an awakening homosexual or bisexual orientation, inspired by the presence of an erotic object of their own sex; they face the choice between not only contending suitors but dramatically different lifestyles. The gay and lesbian characters presented as these new object choices triangulate and dissolve formerly stable, though obviously unfulfilling, heterosexual couplings by introducing their "straight" lovers to heightened sexual *and* social awareness. Characters in these texts of any sex-gender combination lean toward a traditionally, even stereotypically, feminine side when they demonstrate strong affinities for caretaking and nurturing, especially toward those dying of AIDS or grieving for those who have died. Stereotypically masculine traits (of aggression, self-interest) win out in the moments these characters look away from the suffering caused by AIDS and, I contend, in the failure to accurately position female characters alongside male ones in this depicted struggle, when so many real-life women have indeed made an important difference. This stereotypically male tendency manifests itself surprisingly often in texts authored by and featuring centrally gay men, whose "atypically" masculine ways of being seem to coincide not at all with the dishearteningly typical disregard for women on display as well. Finally the (hetero)sexist elements of these otherwise radical texts return the destabilized, energized "third term" (gay sensibility) to the larger *half* (mainstream masculinity) that would subsume it *whole*—slowing and solidifying these texts' potential to allay fears, change hearts, and save lives.

PLAGUE TEXTS AND THE FEMININE

Presence and Absence in Nuclear Literature

I would begin delineation of these plague triangles by examining over the course of several texts the two points, the original opposition between masculine and feminine, that the third point inevitably interrupts. As the disruption of the heterosexual status quo is one of the triangulating figure's chief strengths in these plague texts, it is important to describe this traditional pairing in terms specific to this study. While this masculine/feminine (and by extension straight/gay) binary is by no means exclusive to postmodern plague texts, we find that the damage done in these cases by such binarization pertains specifically to postmodern plague themes: ultimately, heterosexist ideologies based on opposition and difference lead to an absenting of women (as both characters and readers) that weakens and narrows the specifically antiplague effects these texts all originally sought to produce.

Interestingly, several male critics assessing Thomas Pynchon's work have praised its seemingly universal appeal and boundless range, contending that it describes "all existence . . . the thermodynamics of life itself" (Friedman and Puetz 346), that it "reveals the destructive powers of all systematic enterprise" (Poirier, "Importance" 156), that *Gravity's Rainbow* "envisions a global whole" (LeClair 37), and that Pynchon himself owns an "astonishing knowledge of what appears to be everything (Levine and Leverenz iv). Certainly, the range of subject matter that Pynchon "masters" as a writer has the simultaneous effect of "mastering" readers themselves, while the sheer size of the novels he produces (about which more will be said below) promises a world of some sort or other opened before us before even hefting one of them from the shelf. Yet surely each reader defines the "whole world" along lines as diverse and specific as readers themselves. Certainly some women readers might be less easily seduced by "army stories" populated by ironically drawn military authorities, large noisy guns, and boyish soldiers on leave and would be downright repelled by the overly sexualized, fetishized presence of Pynchon's every female character, with the male characters inhabiting mentally interesting, philosophically provocative, politically affecting roles. This imbalance has the effect of absenting women characters to a large degree—and perhaps women readers to an even greater one. Pynchon scholarship is overwhelmingly male-authored, few feminist responses to Pynchon exist, and male critics, even those publishing in recent years, revert to the universalizing "man" and "he" in their writings.[2]

The contrasting authorial decisions made with respect to depicting male and female characters are readily observed in Roger Mexico and Jessica Swanlake, a primary romantic couple in *Gravity's Rainbow*. Roger is defined by his role as a patriot, loyal subordinate, and all-around swell whose philosophy of life as random and uncontrollable, as opposed to determined and quantifiable, we are invited by the author to embrace. Additionally he "loves" Jessica, though readers must assume it is only her "pale nape" (31), "breasts bobbing marvelously" (31), "black slip and clear pearl thighs above" (38), and "marvelous round bottom" (39) that have won his lofty regard, as she is defined by and remembered for her physical attributes alone. Yet the sexualized anatomy reeled off in the preceding list does not even cohere into a *unified,* completely sexual depiction of her but is scattered over the course of several pages so that the (male) reader may linger over and invest erotically in each part. In later episodes, she continues as embedded in her physical state—shivering, suffering from a bad cold, crying, and sleeping; when late in the novel she betrays Roger's "love" by returning to her bourgeois fiancé, her presentation is no less physical but only mannish and off-putting: "hair much shorter, wearing a darker mouth of different outline, harder lipstick. . . . Her voice is perfectly hard" (708–9). Roger, who continues in his passionate obsession despite the harshness of her rebuke and appearance, ends their story as an innocent victim, with Jessica seeming heartless and mercenary.

Jessica's rather simple and naïve sexuality is contrasted to the high-powered eroticism emanating from blond and mysterious Katje Borgesius, a Dutch double agent who uses her sexuality to control and extract secrets from powerful men. Another of Pynchon's "exploded" female figurations, she too comes across as a package of parts—"very blonde hair" (92), "high heels instead of wooden shoes" (93), "dimples countersunk each side of her mouth" (93). Although we are promised an "intellect behind the fair-lashed eyes" (93), Katje still presents primarily as a talented consort, offering various sexual services to the powerful and perverted Captain Blicero and Brigadier Pudding and highly charged (with seltzer water even) yet still-traditional sexual refuge to the beleaguered Slothrop. Slothrop is the most embodied of any male character in the novel—his frequent costume changes, pendulous gut, boyish appearance, and bomb-dowsing erections call frequent attention to his physical self but do not reductively slant the picture in this way; rather, they complement the range of his mental and verbal elements and round him into a believable, involving "figure."[3]

In *V.* and in *Vineland* Pynchon's female characters are allowed larger roles yet play these in typically deceitful, sexually treacherous fashion, thus deserving their respective unfavorable ends. "V." is classically, canonically feminine in multiple respects, "V" turning out to be perhaps the most female letter ("O" notwithstanding) in the whole English alphabet. Not only do iconic female figures—the Virgin Mary, Veronica (with her veil), Queen Victoria—lend their names and emanations to the list of V.'s various incarnations, but "vortex" (of narrative, of history, of spreading legs), "veracity," "verge," "venereal," and of course "vulva" and "vagina" are easily associated with this enigmatic female character and reinforce her allegorical, inhuman ("inanimate") state.[4] Even the punctuation mark forever following her through the pages of the novel itself and the reams of critical response that have followed add to the classically, discouragingly, feminine picture that emerges: *no wonder this heartless, colonizing ice queen hasn't cracked a smile in centuries. She's always right before her period!* As with the female figures from *Gravity's Rainbow,* "V." is largely the sum of her parts—this time not sexualized but artificialized—her false eye, her bejeweled navel, her golden feet. Her dismemberment by avenging subaltern children at the novel's end only completes V.'s transformation into inanimate, exploded matter that she herself had initiated. Despite the presence of sympathetic female characters such as Rachel Owlglass elsewhere in the novel, V.'s overarching presence—as icon, as allegory, as hideous *thing*—controls and defines the reader's response to the role of the feminine in this novel.

Molly Hite's interesting assertion that *Vineland,* "informed by a meditation on power and gender" (136), is therefore Pynchon's "feminist" novel draws its support from rather questionable evidence. Hite cites the lesbian relationship between Frenesi Gates and D. L. Chastain, as well as D.L.'s martial arts skills and self-possessed attitude, as feminist elements in the story. Additionally Sister Rochelle, head of a large, all-woman commune of martial arts practitioners/Eastern philosophers, is allowed to articulate a feminist version of an edenic past ruined by "phallic spoilers." Yet the fact that these feminist commune dwellers go by the condescending diminutive "Ninjettes" and that D.L. is "bought" by Ralph Wayvone to do away with Brock Vond, then inadvertently poisons Brock's Japanese "double" while in bed with him, does much to undermine any feminist strides these characters may begin to make.

More curiously, Hite also finds a feminist statement in the "self-abasement that appears to define feminine sexuality in the character of Frenesi Gates" (140) and adds that Frenesi is Pynchon's "most fully feminine character" since she combines Leni Pökler's political idealism but also Katje Borgesius's "turncoat mentality" and Gerta Erdmann's "submission and abasement" as they were presented throughout *Gravity's Rainbow* (140). Like D.L., Frenesi is a traitor to the men she sleeps with, selling out her liberal-idealist lover Weed Altman during trysts with his (and, we would think, her own) archnemesis, Brock Vond. Again, Hite would turn this negative female behavior into grounds for her feminist reading (141) but to do so must rely on obfuscating jargon ("extreme submission provides a paradoxical route away from the merely temporal" [141]) *and* on our implicit understanding that Pynchon's ironic tone through all of this signals an actual condemnation of the action he sets forth. When Hite points out that "underlying Vond's cocksure posturing is a secret terror of female sexuality as predatory and violating" (139), the ironic distancing Hite (and perhaps Pynchon) hopes we derive from Brock's outrageously misogynist attitude is undercut by the fact that both D.L. and Frenesi *are* "predatory and violating," treacherous and destructive to their male lovers.

Hite sees profeminist "entanglement" in "Brock's fantasy of putting a pistol to Frenesi's head and forcing her to go down on him in front of all the other countercultural detainees at the PREP camp" (135), yet the language Hite uses to enlarge upon this reading is impossible to differentiate from the kind of remarks feminist critics have used for decades against standard-issue sexism in literature: "the operations of oppression become synonymous with the operations of masculinity. The masculine becomes by definition that which oppresses, that which creates its own subject class, thereby constructing the feminine" (138). Perhaps sensing the shakiness of her argument at this point, Hite makes the unexplained leap to the assertion that "this account of the construction of masculinity in turn indicates how relations between men, and ultimately masculinity itself, are thereby depending on the woman" (138). Finally, Hite's connection between Pynchon and feminism is weakly defended and unconvincing; *Vineland*'s women *are* sexual predators and political sellouts; its male characters, even the worst of them, are correct in their negative assessments.

In fact Pynchon's use of male-sadistic *fantasy* is, for me, the most offensive and troubling of his many sexist authorial gestures. Often these fantasies involve young girls forced violently into intergenerational, even incestuous, sex acts with the fantasizer in question. In *Vineland,* in addition to the fantasy described above, Frenesi's daughter Prairie mentally consents to sexual initiation at the hands of Brock Vond, who only refrains from capturing her for his own purposes because the helicopter he is suspended from suddenly whisks him back into the atmosphere. In *Gravity's Rainbow,* Slothrop's relationship to Greta Erdmann's young daughter Bianca is first sexual fantasy, then sexual exploitation, then a sexualized death—"Icy little thighs in wet silk[. . . .] cold nipples . . . the deep cleft of her buttocks, perfume and shit" (531)—that haunts him throughout the remainder of the novel. Bianca's status as sexualized child is furthered by the role Greta forces her to play—bad girl being spanked by her mother—before a crowd of masturbating onlookers.

Most disturbing of all are Franz Pökler's fantasies regarding "Ilse," a young girl, presumably his daughter yet appearing mysteriously with little to say about their shared past, perhaps an impostor deserving punishment:

> He hit her upside the head with his open hand, a loud and terrible blow. That took care of his anger. Then, before she could cry or speak, he dragged her up on the bed next to him, dazed little hands already at the buttons of his

> trousers, her white frock already pulled above her waist. She had been wearing nothing at all underneath, nothing all day . . . *how I've wanted you,* she whispered as paternal plow found its way into filial furrow . . . and after hours of amazing incest, they dressed in silence, and [. . .] down at last to the water and the fishing boats, to a fatherly old sea-dog in a braided captain's hat, who welcomed them aboard and stashed them below decks, where she snuggled down in the bunk as they got under way and sucked him hours while the engine pounded, till the Captain called, "Come up and take a look at your new home!" [. . .] The three of them, there on the deck, stood hugging. . . .
> No. (420–21)

How much strength to reverse and condemn the atrocious little yarn preceding it can a feminist readership expect from that absurd little "No"? Returning us to the "reality" of the unfolding story, from a fantasy we had been led to believe *was* reality a moment earlier, the "No" attempts to undo Franz's incest by restoring it to its "proper" plane—considered and wished for but not acted upon—and to elicit the reader's admiration for this heroically self-restraining character: "What Pökler did was choose to believe she wanted comfort that night, wanted not to be alone. Despite Their game, Their palpable evil, . . . by an act not of faith, not of courage but of conservation, he chose to believe that" (421). Of course distinctions between fantasy and reality in literary representation are ludicrous: a fantasy—about killing, raping, or beating—is a "fact" of novelistic presentation, as is a bit of action or a moment of truth that "really" happens to characters therein. As Hite seemed to be arguing with *Vineland* above, Pynchon here asks his readers to disregard the prosecutor's last remarks: because the most heinous crimes against women and children happen in these novels only *as fantasies,* the decency of these fantasizers in their waking moments is to guide our response to them. Of course even in a real courtroom it is as difficult to disregard a prosecutor's last remarks as it is to "run three times around the building without thinking of a fox" (*Gravity's Rainbow* 47). In a novelistic universe, where distinctions between fantasy and reality are entirely spurious, it is important, for reasons I have delineated above, to not even try.

• • •

Lesser-known authors, perhaps overly influenced by the male-dominant style that shapes and defines the canon yet, continue in this vein of separating and/or absenting female characters, reducing by half the reach and relevance of their respective worldviews. In Russell Hoban's *Riddley Walker,* traditional gender-based dichotomies control both character and action throughout, as the novel is heavily populated by male characters, who perform heroic or villainous actions, and is almost empty of female characters, who tend to hang about the blighted postnuclear village—when they appear at all. The male characters, especially the boy-hero Riddley himself, tell stories, find answers, and walk paths of ancient mystery that hint of a technologized, civilized past. Most often female characters are replaced by female figurations ("icons," in Peter Schwenger's terminology) that are defined by rounded, hollowed-out shapes connoting the presence of *absence*—whether it be the circular path that Riddley "walks," the "woom of Cambry" (a crypt buried where the Canterbury cathedral used to stand), or quite simply and quite offensively—and as will be the case in several bomb novels here—the *hole,* the ground zero that has been created and simultaneously blasted to oblivion by the bomb's contact. In *Gravity's Rainbow,* the sites of Slothrop's many sexual conquests correspond perfectly to the sites of subsequent bombings, while throughout *Riddley Walker,* and especially throughout Schwenger's reading of it in *Letter Bomb,* the masculine is identified with Hoban's every central theme. But as I will show below, such singular engendering is, while not completely false, decidedly only half the story.

Twelve-year-old Riddley's middle-aged lover and mentor, Lorna Elswint, the only major female character, gazes tellingly at "the full moon, all col and wite and oansome" (32) while delivering words of insight and inspiration to Riddley. Her message, about the mysterious origins of "the idear of us" and the equally mysterious origins of narrative itself, causes Riddley to wonder which came first: us or the story of us that we (only think we) produce—and it sets him off in search of an answer. Since, as Schwenger points out, "Lorna's words produce Riddley's journey" (*Letter Bomb* 33), and the novel works to erase the distinction between journey and journeyer, we might argue that "Lorna's words produce" not just Riddley's journey but Riddley himself. In a philosophical birth-giving Lorna is thus defined not only as bearer of life but also as sender on its way: she who stays home and waits or, rather, she who *is* home, which in Hoban's novel is also the path of the journey.

Throughout the novel Riddley goes, in ever-widening circles, in search of answers, treading on the circular that is also a treading on the feminine, being buoyed along invisibly by it and absorbing its energy for his own use. Schwenger describes the Power Ring as a seductive, circular (again, feminized) source of knowledge for Riddley, "an image of narrative" (*Letter Bomb* 39) that *is* the reading of the story, the apprehension of vital knowledge. Yet Schwenger then inscribes a distinction he has been applying elsewhere in his essay—that between the Ring and the ringer of Rings, the circle and the "Walker" who treads it: "the power of narrative comes not from individual words [the Stonehenge-like 'stannings' or 'broakin teef' of the ring figure] . . . [but] from *motion,* motion that is circular, repetitive, and cumulative" (*Letter Bomb* 39)—that is, Riddley's approach to and movement around this static, receptive, female figuration. Elsewhere Schwenger correctly reads the image of a green and "blipful" light sweeping over the darkened towns as "a radically ungoverned idea of the circle that here represents narrative" (*Letter Bomb* 40). This image indeed disrupts the relationship among circularity, the static, and the strictly feminine, as it creates a circle that is not moved upon but itself moves, that combines principles that had heretofore been separated falsely (sometimes by Schwenger and sometimes by Hoban) into gendered categories. Again, however, Schwenger recoups this potentially subversive "blend" to the realm of the strictly masculine, as he describes the green sweep of light as Hoban's icon for "the 1 what goes thru chaynjis" (144), a "1" who is explicitly defined not only as Eusa (the god-figure of this society's myth) but also as the exploding, mushrooming, "Littl Shynin Man."

The Eusa myth of Riddley's society contains several stories of Eusa's attempt to control and split open this "Littl Man"—the Addom (atom/Adam)—during an intense embrace or wrestling match between them. This and other homoerotic elements in the story, while doing much to disrupt the hetero-dynamics and restrictive definitions of masculinity in the novel, continue nevertheless to define primarily figurations of *men.* The all-boy's club that is formed by Riddley and his travel companions, the Ardship and Pry Mincer, and presided over by the passionate adversaries Eusa and the Addom is rife with queer associations. At one point Riddley is captured by the Pry Mincer's henchman, who grabs him "from behynt" and hauls him before the Pry Mincer's gang who, like Riddley, search hungrily after the secret of power: gunpowder, if not atomic weaponry. The scene is menacingly suggestive of gang rape as the Pry Mincer threatens to "tern [Riddley's] up side down weare going to empty your pockits" (118); and Riddley resists Goodparley's "going thru my pockits" to find the phallic "blackent . . . figger" (118), an old wooden Punch puppet that Riddley hides there.

Later in the novel Riddley speaks more benignly, and much more explicitly, of his seizure by and rapture in a masculinized "Power":

> Fealt like it were the han of Power clampt on the back of my neck fealt the Big Old Father spread me and take me. Fealt the Power in me I fealt strong with it and weak with it boath.
>
> . . . I begun to feel all juicy with it. Juicy for a woman. Longing for it hard and heavvy and stanning ready. Not just my cock but all of me it were like all of me were cock and all the worl a cunt and open to me. . . . I tryd to hold it like that but I los it I wernt man a nuff right then. I cud boy for the other but I cudn't man for her what has her woom in Cambry. (159)

Here Riddley admits to and revels in a vibrant bisexuality that for the moment is more successfully consummated with the male object of his desire, and we understand that at this point in the story Hoban equates the apprehension of knowledge explicitly with the male-male sex act. None of this overt queerness makes its way into Schwenger's reading, however; his argument, as structured by the binary oppositions walker and path, teller and tale, male and female, forecloses such an inquiry. Hoban himself reheterosexualizes any suggestion of queerness between the male-male couplings in his story with his recurring insistence, "the two shall become one." The biblical reference to the wedding ritual makes explicit the male-female opposition and leaves intact the primacy of the male Eusa figure, "the 1 what goes through chaynjis. If hes chemistery or if hes a man" (139).

That this "1 what goes through chaynjis" is male, even if "hes che*mistery*," is a novelistic assertion resting this time not on the reinforcement of gender dichotomies but on their antifeminist manipulation, on a usurpation of an almost solely feminine attribute to the domain of the strictly masculine. For while male characters lay aggressive claim to the dynamism and creative power of constant change, who but women spend their lives "going through chaynjis"—often to the horror and scandalizing of men? Whose "chaynjis" besides women's have been blamed for everything from madness to chronic illness to the inability to hold public office, yet whose "chaynjis" are responsible not only for Riddley's journey itself but what meager creation of life there is in his ruined universe? Significantly, it is the moon that inspires Lorna to inspire Riddley on his way. It is her earlier going through changes (menstrual cycles) that endowed her with reproductive ability in the first place and her final change (she is probably postmenopausal) that mark the years of her wisdom, the source of her probing questions and Riddley's subsequent search for answers.

Once again this productive force that so naturally emanates from the feminine is borrowed upon but then quickly extracted from it, as Lorna fades into an inspiring memory that Riddley only calls up periodically throughout the rest of novel. Schwenger notes, "'Always on the road' walking has no beginning or determinable end" (*Letter Bomb* 34), yet it is definitely the case that Lorna neither walks nor maintains her significance for us without "determinable end." Replacing her, and countering the seductive but productive forces of the "woom of Cambry," is the luring and lurid gynophobe's nightmare, "Auntie," a vicious and revolting vagina with teeth, whose every visitation brings certain, protracted, agonizing death to men. Thus the feminine in Hoban's novel is nowhere near "always on the road," progresses not circularly but in a steadily linear, increasingly negative fashion. Schwenger's silence on this issue allows for a sustained and consistent examination of his "essay's icon," the circling of ground zero, in Hoban's novel but fails to point out that the feminine, as far as it is less than fully incorporated into this post-modern postapocalyptic vision, diminishes the power of this vision, calling into question its ultimate meaning for the "idear of [all of] us."

In contrast, in Tim O'Brien's *Nuclear Age,* the hole that protagonist William Cowling digs feverishly throughout the novel is an entirely masculinized "presence." Even though this hole, similar to those in Hoban's novel and to the circle of the supplement analyzed in Schwenger's attendant reading, is described as "the absence of presence . . . the presence of absence" (198), O'Brien nevertheless endows this absence with a "thereness" not found in these other texts—due, I would argue, to the very maleness that is also one of its attributes. Indeed, its ever-increasing girth; its complex function as security and threat, home insurance and homewrecker, monument to the madness of the cold war and justification for insane reactions to it; and its riveting, commanding, distinctly masculine voice make this hole neither a setting nor a symbol but a fully realized character, surpassed in complexity and impact only by the heavily felt presence of the narrator himself.

Significantly, the hole is far more compelling than any of the female characters O'Brien has to offer us here. William loves all three of them—his wife, Bobbi, his daughter, Melinda, and his girlfriend/co-insurrectionist from his draft-dodging past, Sarah Strouch—madly. Yet each of their presences is so shallow, so clichéd and mechanical—in short, so frustratingly *absent*—that they must be seen simply and reductively as "holes" once more, no more than hazy images if not absolute blanks in the reader's apprehension of the story. Late in the novel William recalls a time he missed his wife, who had "disappeared . . . two weeks; her diaphragm went with her" (287), revealing the (w)hole of his estimation of her and the limited significance of the feminine that follows from it: "I'd go to the medicine cabinet and open it and just stand there. It was like watching a hole. The diaphragm, I came to realize, was one of those objects whose absence reveals so much more than its presence" (287).

The hole William digs in the backyard is witty and engaging, as Schwenger puts it, "ironic and hip" (107),[5] addressing William with *"Hey Man," "brother,"* and *"tiger"* and throwing out one-liners that are not jokes but vital, irresistible imperatives:

> *Dig,* it says. At times I'm actually cowed by its majesty. It has a kind of stature—those steep walls plunging to shadow, the purity of line and purpose, its intangible holeness. There it *is,* you can't dismiss it. It's real.
>
> *Be safe,* it says.
>
> It says, *Survive.* (197–98)

In marked contrast the language emanating from O'Brien's female characters is ineffectual and bothersome. Bobbi writes childishly simple poems with titles like "The Mole in His Hole" and "Martian Travel," Donna-Reedly pinning them to pajama tops and cereal boxes as if they were any Saturday's "honey-do" list. While William fell in love with Bobbi (in the course of about ten minutes) because of a poem she pinned to his lapel, the verse is now an irritant, a constant plea to stop his crazy digging, his obsessing over the nuclear threat. Yet the poetry is so obscure—

> Here, now, is the long thin wire
> from Sun to Bedlam,
> as the drumbeat ends
> and families pray:
> Be quick! Be agile!
> The balance of power,
> our own,
> the world's,
> grows ever fragile. . . . (65)

—that William is undeflected in his madness and rightly informs his daughter in defense of his bizarre actions that "mommy's a fruitcake" (63).

Daughter Melinda is a typical novelistic "kid" in that she is a repository of backtalk, precocious allusions, and contraband swear-words, yet she is too often guilty of tossing off clichéd expressions, belonging more to William's own era, like "Simple Simon" and "I'm a goner." This archaic diction is symptomatic of Melinda's dislikability and profound "typicality"—in fact she is not a kid at all but a smaller prototype of William (and, no doubt, O'Brien) himself, sporting a fluency with argument, logical sophistication, and nonchalance during real crisis that marks her as entirely too grown up. Finally, she is two-dimensional and trite; and this "review" is only significant in light of my larger, gender-related concern: as female character she is, again, more absent than present.

Sarah, the most visibly drawn and most fully felt female character (functions, no doubt, of her marked sex appeal), fails to engage the reader as fully human either, due once more to the maddeningly inhuman pattern of her speech. She talks, even when not relaying guerrilla war tactics over the shortwave, in staccato, half-baked headlines that are meant, no doubt, to attract and seduce but only mystify and annoy:

> "Naive Sarah. All that time I kept thinking, Hang in there, baby—he'll be back. Wanted to be wanted. Not a peep."

"... Anyway, it's still politics as usual. Key West, the old Committee. Not quite the same, I'm afraid—mostly just dreams. Super Bowl, remember? Never made it." (289)[6]

Thus William and his hole emerge shortly as the novel's main characters, as those whose all-important message—that the nuclear threat is at the heart of all manner of postmodern psychoses—must contend with and defeat multiple persistent, nearly successful, feminine incursions if it is to be fully heard.

In fact, this hole is the latest manifestation of the bomb shelter William has been trying to secure himself within all his life. As a boy he built a fortress against the traumas of frightening radio announcements and air-raid drills at school by layering his family's Ping-Pong table with pencils (lead to keep out the radiation), cushions, blankets, and other absorbent matter in an effort to feel completely safe. O'Brien resists depicting this move as a "return to the womb," as the author would argue this is not some universal, unconscious impulse in all of us but a distinctly neurotic manifestation of the nuclear age. Instead, then, it is not William's mother but his father who is associated with these nightly forays into the basement and with the effort to reassure him that the world is not after all as close as all that to total destruction. Aside from his father, another early male influence and William's first friend is Chuck Adamson, hired as William's analyst but soon more or less transforming into his patient. Chuck talks constantly, suffering from a diarrhea of the mouth distinctly counter to the role of the analyst yet demonstrating the uninhibited flow of expression that William himself longs for, that will also attract and subordinate him to the smooth-talking hole. For while William surrounds himself with an array of intriguing, freely expressing male "holes," we learn early on that an additional neurosis derived from his cold war traumatization is a lifelong battle with constipation that accompanies emotional and sexual inhibitions as well.

Thus the masculinized hole found throughout O'Brien's story is a verbose, sometimes articulate speaking mouth but also a seductive, compelling anus.[7] We find in such holes not only O'Brien's implied thesis that both the cold war and, finally, crazy, kidnapping William himself are both full of shit but also a homoerotics of the nuclear age, manifested obviously in the all-male activities of bomb-shelter building, draft dodging, and Vietnam vet rap groups that so richly represent the middle period of the cold war. In this light, Bobbi's indignation and Melinda's confusion at William's growing obsession with the hole are made more complex, even justified: what wife would not rail against the realization that her husband is "getting his" from some other "hole," this time demonstrably male, and, to her added mortification, carrying out the affair right in the backyard? Bobbi protests that the ever-widening dimensions of the hole are threatening the foundation of the house, but we all know the institution this "little homewrecker" threatens is not so much concrete as abstraction, not the value of the real estate but the value of the "nuclear" family that is about to cave in to it.

The romantic triangle formed by William, Bobbi, and the masculinized hole is ultimately expanded to include a fourth member—daughter Melinda—immediately defusing its homoerotic potential. When William drugs both Bobbi and Melinda and constrains them within the hole for "safekeeping," he enacts the kind of male-to-male trafficking in women that has been described by feminist theorists as early as Emma Goldman.[8] In a ritualistic suburban sacrifice cum self-fulfilling prophecy, William likewise literalizes Lacan's seminal depiction of woman as Other, as she who *is* the phallus, the affirmation and extension of him who *has* it: depositing his precious "parts" within the masculinized hole, William constructs a double date that hopefully will appease the hole (actually his own tormented psyche) and ease the homoerotic tensions created by the triangulation—Bobbi for himself in her "rightful" role as his wife, and Melinda for the hole, for the facing and fixing of the nuclear mess that is her and all her generation's legacy.[9]

With everyone now paired off, the story ends shortly thereafter. William learns that the hole he digs—both the security it offers and the threat to home and stability it portends—is actually within, and he battles successfully against the internal despair, the nihilism that is driving him toward murder and suicide. He puts down the dynamite he is about to activate, in an effort to beat the nuclear blast to the punch, releases his family, who begin to forgive and reaccept him, and dismantles the hole by exploding it with the dynamite intended for his family. The novel's message, "to live is to lose everything, which is crazy, but I choose it anyway, which is sane" (310), is supportable, even admirable, but is only advanced here at the expense of adequate treatment of and thus meaning for women suffering this same nuclear experience: the novel's women characters revert to their typical, two-sided dimensions; its interesting, feminized male hole is blasted out of existence.

Philip Wylie's *Disappearance*, predating these other texts by several decades, reveals that this impulse to "absent" women from the postwar scene, let alone from the nuclear debate, is no recent derivative of the Vietnam War or the Reagan era in the United States. Wylie's problematic attitude toward women—whom, with his theories of "momism," he blamed for a weakened, effeminate U.S. society—manifests itself readily in *The Disappearance*, a nuclear/science fiction "fable" that was one of his most widely read productions.

In the story Dr. William Gaunt and his wife, Paula, suffer a simultaneous, postbomb "disappearance" from each other's lives into thoroughly separated but temporally identical dimensions. Each is left in a world with only his or her respective sexual kind, and the novel grants us the double perspective of both the men and women; that is, both seemed to have "disappeared," and thus both genders maintain a claim to hereness, to the presence necessary to narrate and thus analyze the crises and rebuild from them. Not surprisingly, the women flounder with government and commerce, while the men eventually restore order, yet Wylie argues that it is *men* who have so disarmed women in this way and are thus to blame for this demeaning of women that simultaneously demeans themselves. Wylie's overarching thesis—that, thanks to the "attitudes of men," both genders have always lived in debilitating, if unacknowledged segregation anyway—is surprisingly progressive, given his misogynist pronouncements elsewhere. Perhaps even more surprisingly, the anticommunist Wiley holds up Soviet women in the story as skillful, industrious, yet nonaggressive counterparts to the flighty, fashion-obsessed American women: "they didn't know how to fire naval guns or launch the torpedoes they brought. Just how to run the ships" (190). Russian productivity and industry are analogous to the reproductive capability that all of the disappeared women of this dual world took with them. By novel's end it is obvious that the women will have eventual success with the parthenogenesis that will enable their species to continue, while the men struggle much more desperately with a similar proposition.

Yet for all his pretending to an enlightened mindset, Wylie ultimately reinstates the divisions between masculine and feminine worlds, specifically the dichotomy of presence versus absence—or, more specifically, action and inaction during the time of political and metaphysical crisis. While the men almost immediately call a congress, circulate position papers, travel the world surveying atomic blast damage, and aid in the reconstruction project, the women in their separate world stay at home (the suburbs of Miami), store up rations, sew and cook, and "degenerate" into lesbian activities that "threaten" to seduce Paula more than once. The men do not even seem to eat; the women do not appear to have noticed that there has been a nuclear war. Theirs is the realm in which minority characters (women, of course) are allowed to remain, where children (girls, of course) have pivotal roles in the plot. They are threatened not with war or labor strikes but with a force of nature, a hurricane that damages the Gaunt house and indirectly causes the death of Paula's granddaughter. The narrative of the men's sections is abstract, theoretical, and sweeping, while the women's passages are homey, intricate, and tending toward overdramatic revelations. Overall, the women seemed removed from the heart of the larger conflicts, spinning their wheels in undersized local actions and lacking the ability to restore their cities to full power.[10]

We find in Margaret Atwood's *Handmaid's Tale* and in Marge Piercy's *He, She, and It* helpful responses to this marking of the feminine as absence and the masculine as singularly present in these cold war and nuclear texts. In both, the feminine is not only permitted but assumed as the controlling perspective and shaper of events. Issues of reproductivity and domesticity are interrogated and problematized to challenge the co-optation of women's abilities to reproduce and nurture life that the "fathers" of nuclear capability would claim belong solely to them.[11] In these views we find not only the more informative analogy to the "spark" of nuclear energy but likewise the impulse toward the preservation of life that is its harnessing for peaceful means.

In Atwood's universe, a worldwide breakdown in reproductive capabilities caused by male-engineered environmental manipulation and limited nuclear war forces a desperate association between women and their reproductive potential. Saddled with the nearly impossible responsibility of restoring human life when men have nearly wiped it out, the few remaining "handmaids" (those possibly capable of giving birth) of Gilead are "honored" with constricting uniforms more appropriate to nuns, rigorous scrutiny of their every word and movement, and weekly sexual assaults by "generals" desperate to father children "on them." Now that the powers inherent in reproduction are all but demolished, successful childbearing and the multiple barriers to it are returned forcefully to the feminine realm. It is never questioned whether the generals involved in these trials with the handmaids are in fact physiologically able to reproduce; it is always assumed that a failed attempt at impregnation rests with the women: it is they who are eventually punished, cast out of their houses or sentenced to death, if "their" infertility does not correct itself soon enough.

Atwood harshly criticizes the sanctioned sexual activity in this devastated, depopulated society, depicting all of it as brutal rape. She re-empowers the feminine by depicting the handmaids' reproductive capabilities, however threatened they may be, as essential to the future of Gilead. Offred's flight at the novel's conclusion, whether into the arms of loved ones or captors, nevertheless "castrates" the general she left behind. As one of an ever-diminishing endangered species, Offred's own choice to absent herself causes the general—at least, though most importantly, the generations that were to have followed from him—to simultaneously disappear.

In contrast, the enclosed and stringently corporate "multis" of Piercy's universe offer women and their partners multiple high-tech methods of reproduction. Here it is considered backward, and thus subversive, for Piercy's Shira to have carried her son Ari a full nine months and to have borne him in the traditional way. Piercy suggests that low-tech, old-fashioned birth produces a mother-child bond so strong that it causes a child to "belong" to its mother (and, more controversially, to its mother's mother and grandmother) as it can never belong to a father and his line: "Malkah told her that . . . men came, men went, but she should remember that her first baby belonged to her mother and to her but never to the father" (40). The story supports this philosophy too easily perhaps, as Shira's ex-husband Josh is a lazy and indifferent father, ultimately using his son as a pawn to lure Shira back to the Y-S multi. Yet Piercy's overall charge against men in this postholocaust world is in fact correctly placed, in light of the enormous damage they have done: through wars and industrial exploitation, men have ruined the livable environment and can offer relative though strictly monitored security only to the "techies"—the middle-class corporate employees and technically skilled workers—who have survived. Thus, Piercy's children are as endangered as Atwood's in the postnuclear nightmare, and in both novels men battle women not only for claim to their reproductive power but for the commodification of children that will ensure their respective futures.

One such "child" successfully ends this battle, freeing children and the mothers who love them through the ultimate self-sacrifice. This is Yod, the cyborg-with-the-heart-of-gold (or maybe titanium) who, having been programmed by both a man and a woman, is not only intellectual, executive, and physically unstoppable but also patient, thoughtful, and highly in tune with a woman's needs, specifically Shira's and her grandmother/his "mother" Malkah's, both of whom become his lover at some point in the novel. À la Arnold Schwarzenegger in his second Terminator incarnation, Yod is a better father to Shira's son than the boy's natural father ever was; and Piercy credits both his male/female hybridity and his cyborg (human/machine) qualities as the proper formula for world survival: "we're all unnatural now. I have retinal implants. I have a plug in my skull to interface with a computer. I read time by a corneal implant. Malkah has a subcutaneous unit that monitors her blood pressure and her teeth are half regrown. . . . Avram has an artificial heart and Gadi a kidney. . . . We're all cyborgs, Yod. You're just a purer form of what we're all tending toward" (155–56). Meanwhile, Yod is prevented from assuming the full status of "citizen" (i.e., person) in the utopic Tikva where he was born,[12] preventing him likewise from continuing in his role as Shira's lover and Ari's father. He is sent, as he was created to be, to Shira's former multi to destroy her persecutors and, through his self-destruction, their plots to learn his technology and take over her free town. As is Shira's son Ari, he is the child/possession, this time sold into slavery and sacrificed to his family's wishes.

Finally, while Yod might be what "we're all tending toward," he is still a cyborg and not a human, thus expendable because readily reproducible, thanks to technological advances. As with the intraepidemic stories discussed in the previous chapter, technology infuses this story with a utopic quality, an element of optimism that coincides with several others—the multiple childbearing options, the matrilineal communities suffused with Jewish spirituality, the "romance" novelistic structure spinning off countless romantic triangles[13]—but clashes with Piercy's supposed overarching thesis about the preciousness of children's lives. Technology enables Shira and her community to "wall off" Yod from themselves, to send him to his doom in the Y-S multi; meanwhile, regardless of Tikva's somewhat "robotic" response to his plight, certainly technology is positioned here as both giver of life and bringer of death (for cyborgs), a source of utopic and dystopic outcomes in the story.

Thus both Atwood and Piercy emphasize the fragility of humanity's reproductive capability and the ultimate failure of technology to perpetuate our race for us when our hypertechnologized bodies have failed. In response to the power-usurping fantasies of some male nuclear novelists,[14] specifically the untenable claims of Hoban, O'Brien, and Wylie discussed above, these feminist authors remind readers that women's views and abilities must be included integrally if not primarily in the decisions we make regarding the progress and future of life on earth. In several respects in both of these novels the "children" of the female protagonists are not so much their flesh-and-blood (or flesh-and-silicone) offspring as their peace-loving perspectives and the individual narratives that they leave as records of suffering and loss but that as records are triumphs as well—over hostile ages that cannot outlast or destroy them. This new form, then, of "writing from the body" emphasizes communication and record-keeping and opposes itself to (by inserting itself in place of) "domestic" terrorism and nuclear warmongering that would be writing's, and all our other offsprings', deathblow.

Positivity and Negativity in AIDS Literature

Despite assumptions to the contrary, women suffer the same absenting in several gay-authored texts directly and indirectly treating the AIDS issue that they do in the nuclear texts;[15] and although I would argue that these absences ultimately weaken a text's significance (if for no other reason than their conformity to the straight male authorial standard), the reason for women's diminished presence here is in part explainable. In the gay male context, in fact, AIDS has simply been much more of an issue than it has for either the lesbian or straight female communities that intersect it. Indeed lesbians have consistently comprised the lowest risk group since the disease's appearance; and while the incidence among straight women, especially in minority communities, is on a drastic incline,[16] these groups were not a significant factor at the time most of the current AIDS canon was produced.

The masculine-identified "presence" in the nuclear texts examined above translates here into a mostly male "positivity," with women both suffering (and, let's face it, enjoying) a relative "negativity"—that is, separation from the worst that HIV and AIDS means for its victims. But to be negative (female or male) in many of these stories is also to not understand, often to not care enough, and sometimes to simply not exist. Even "negatives" who make appearances in these texts are "absent" in the way the women in several of the above novels are, appearing as ultraminor characters verging on two-dimensionality who form unlikable impressions in our minds if they manage to leave an imprint at all. In Paul Monette's *Afterlife,* Steven ponders the status of negativity, which strikes him as prehistoric, a relic from a forgotten age: "Steven was thinking about his roommate: negative. Was anyone he knew negative? He couldn't imagine such a thing. For years, it seemed, ever since Spot appeared on Victor's ankle, he had assumed the worst scenario, that all gay men would die. . . . And though he heard now and then about somebody testing negative, he put no faith in it. The test was bullshit like everything else" (149). In Monette's *Borrowed Time,* a friend declares he will have nothing more to do with negatives, as the mundanity and blatant eternality of their lives relative to his own bore and infuriate him. Monette himself insists that all those "negatives" out there who are really only positives in denial should be forced to be tested "so I will have people to talk to" and mount an activist movement alongside (165). Note that in the long quotation above, negativity has a self-canceling property that prevents Steven from even considering it. A negative test, removing the "patient" from the realm of tests, hospitals, and patienthood itself before the needle is withdrawn from the vein, is either an ontological impossibility or just "bullshit"—a false negative that will soon be corrected with a follow-up test and positive diagnosis.

In addition, then, to negativity constituting a sort of political limbo within the gay community, it also presents a linguistic and philosophical aporia—the "other" half of a binary opposition that simultaneously does not exist.[17] While I am excited by this structure of a binary opposition that dissolves simultaneously into a half that is whole, I note that the secondary problem that always follows binarizing—subordinating one member of the pair to the other—persists, as the negative voice, most often the voice of women, is consistently diminished if not silenced in these male-authored AIDS texts.[18]

Alan Hollinghurst's *Swimming-Pool Library,* for instance, a "pre-AIDS" novel that I examined in chapter 2 for its multiple AIDS-related implications, houses a large and engaging cast, sprung from multiple races, classes, orientations, age groups, centuries, and media-produced representations, yet all from the same sex category. The equivalent of a half page scattered throughout the novel is devoted to Will's sister; beyond that, we may as well have returned to Philip Wylie's all-male universe from *The Disappearance.* Interestingly, more than one critic[19] has advanced the notion that there are plenty of women in this novel—all just happening to come to us in the form of disempowered or effeminate men; I am intent here, of course, to reserve the category of women for those who actually "body" as such and find it in Hollinghurst's novel to remain objectionably empty. Likewise, Peter McGehee's *Boys Like Us* and *Sweetheart* contain several female characters, though none of them rise above caricature and hackneyed, however loving, stereotypes drawn from his native American South. In the hip and urbane North of these novels (Toronto to be exact), Zero MacNoo and his lovers and friends enjoy a satisfying sexual lifestyle and simultaneously confront the horrors of AIDS in a manner consistent with the erotic noir atmosphere promised by the Stonewall Inn editions' cover art for both novels. Interestingly, tone and even genre shift markedly when Zero makes his way in each story to his home in Arkansas. Here, broadly comic female characters predominate—Mom sprawled across the hood of a fast-moving car or plowing into a lobster-shaped butter sculpture, Doll with her "enormous haystack" of hair fretting another birthday, and the magical-realist Stellrita, impervious to death, grief, and weather conditions, sitting in the rocking chair on her front porch for well over a century. Closing the book in the middle of one of these Arkansas episodes, the reader is caught off guard by the sexy, New Age cover art that reflects so well the stories' prevailing but completely unrelated agenda—a contrast underscoring men's and women's stark separation in this novelistic world.

Perhaps even more problematic are texts that treat women centrally but in ways still closely resembling the troubling depictions of canonical (straight) male authors. Armistead Maupin's tremendously popular *Tales of the City* series features three female characters among the denizens of San Francisco's Barbary Lane—the loving and "grandmotherly" Anna Madrigal (who is in fact the benefactress of a sex-change operation), her confused and abrasive lesbian daughter, Mona, and Mary Ann Singleton, a wide-eyed ingenue from Cleveland (at the start of the series) who is transformed into a steely and self-serving "career girl," who by the end of the series leaves San Francisco to host a syndicated talk show in New York. It is remarkable to observe the ways in which these three characters diminish in presence, interest, and/or reader sympathy as AIDS manifests itself in *Babycakes* (the fourth volume), claims the life of a central gay male character in *Significant Others* (the fifth), and threatens the life of yet another central gay male character in *Sure of You* (the sixth and final installment). Mrs. Madrigal—even in early volumes a janie-one-note ensconced in the rooms and gardens of her dear old house, a warming smile ever on her lips, a bowl of homemade joints blooming perennially on the coffee table—is a marginalized presence in the fourth and fifth volumes and a character played out a world away (in sapphic Greece) in the sixth. Mona is also removed (to Seattle, London, and Greece) from plots related to AIDS diagnosis and death in the fourth and sixth volumes and barely mentioned in the fifth; a scene in which Michael informs her of his lover's death while she has been away from San Francisco is the harsh medicine she needs to reclaim her family and re-establish herself, to a certain degree, in their lives.

Mary Ann's transformation—from a sweet, naïve young woman who spends much quality time in the company of gay men into a frigid, materialistic grump who forsakes her colorful family at 28 Barbary Lane for the career fast track—coincides so closely with the introduction of AIDS into the *Tales* that it may be regarded as partially the source of her physical and emotional flight. In *Sure of You,* Mary Ann seeks out Michael after a long break in their relationship but only when she wants support and comfort while deciding to dissolve her marriage. As Michael correctly points out, the focus is primarily on herself and her career gains (221); she is hopelessly obtuse on the issues of gay identity (219) and Michael's own HIV-positivity:

> "I wish there was some way to convince you I'm not dead yet."
>
> She gazed at him, blinking.
>
> "That's the way you've acted," he added. "Ever since I told you I was positive."
>
> She pretended not to understand. "What do you mean? Acted how?"
>
> "I don't know. Careful and distant and overpolite. It's not the same between us anymore. You talk to me now like I'm Shawna [Mary Ann's five-year-old daughter] or something." (220)

The plot synopsis found on the back of *Sure of You* likewise does much to separate issues related to AIDS from the female characters of this story, Maupin's most AIDS-focused number in the series. The dust jacket of the Harper and Row first edition makes no mention whatever of the way this story will address the crisis. Significantly, the focus is on the non-AIDS elements instead: Mary Ann, her troubled marriage, and her career ambitions. Michael, the only HIV-positive character remaining, is "used" (late and briefly) in the précis the way Mary Ann herself uses him: as a mediator between the dissolving heterosexual couple who "spill out their hearts to him," with Michael described as only "contentedly gay and newly entrenched in a marriage of his own." I noted in the previous chapter that one of the few characters in the series to be visibly sick with AIDS is a straight woman who is movingly depicted in her suffering; she is, nevertheless, only briefly treated, quickly walled off from reader contact and sympathy by the author's overriding concern to keep the story (and its enjoyability) rolling along. While Maupin, a gay author writing widely received gay fiction, offers several engaging portraits of women and some touching scenes detailing the fears and sadness born of AIDS-related illness and death, it is disappointing that his series concludes without ever combining these narrative strengths in a successful manner.

In Monette's novel *Afterlife,* Margaret is certainly closer to this crisis than any of the female characters discussed thus far, yet the author allocates to her the traditionally feminized role of caring for her dying male friends, once again well away from center stage, where the emerging love relationship between Steven and Mark constitutes the main plot. Early in the story Margaret, though supported by the text for her good intentions and her continued and upbeat presence in this community of symptomatic men, is derided for her germophobia with a subtle, biting choice of words: "'Well, if I knew *you* were going to be here,' said Margaret, sweeping into the vestibule, 'I would have brought your tickets.' She nuzzled the air beside Mark's cheek, then turned and held out a hand to Ted" (9). This distance that Margaret maintains from the men of her community works ultimately to justify their distancing themselves from her. At a climactic Thanksgiving party near the end of the novel, Margaret is ghettoized alongside the other minority figure in the story, Ray Lee, whose Charlie Chan English—"Pie—lookit pie. . . . Margaret help. She did crust" (209–10)—coincides not at all with Monette's otherwise enlightened, progressive perspective. Ray is referred to by the omniscient narrator more often as "the Korean" than by his own name, and Steven notes earlier in the story, with only the slightest embarrassment about such stereotypic attitudes, that "Ray Lee wasn't sexual. He seemed somehow above all that, androgynous and rarefied" (122).[20] Margaret arrives at the dinner accompanying Ray Lee, whose condition is now so frail that he must be hauled upstairs in a wheelchair she unpacks from the trunk, fed his dinner by other (female) guests, and taken home immediately after pumpkin pie by Margaret, whose recently failed (heterosexual) romance leaves her evenings free for such ministrations.

From the beginning of the scene Margaret is embedded in traditional domestic roles, bearing a covered dish up the steps to Steven's apartment, taking credit for having "instructed Victor in the sin of over-roasting" turkeys (212). Her heavy-handed nursing of Ray Lee—she hovers around him, strokes his hair, and massages his head—verges on a sexual attachment to him. None of the theses emerging here—that men this sick are as unattractive to gay men as are straight women, that men this sick should go "home to mama" and leave the healthy men alone, that Ray Lee's "sickness" is manifested now by his attraction to and reliance on Margaret—reveal Monette as appropriately attuned to the reality of sick (ethnic) men and the women who would be present in his community.

While several female characters in Tony Kushner's *Angels in America: A Gay Fantasia on National Themes* are tragic, dramatically central figures in this AIDS-related story, the pattern discerned in the preceding texts is somewhat reinforced here: the closer a female character gets to the crisis itself, the more minor her role is (e.g., the doctor); the more necessary she becomes to the story as a whole, the more removed she is—by ignorance, selfishness, prejudice, madness—from the reality it represents (e.g., Harper and her mother-in-law, Hannah). Especially, the female angel concluding this play functions in disappointingly traditional ways, and I distinguish this "concluding" angel from the "beginning" and "middle" angels who contribute so memorably to Kushner's play.[21] The distinction is once again gender-based, as both the angel pictured on all the posters, T-shirts, and covers of the Sarabande Press 1993 edition of *Part One: Millennium Approaches* and the angel wrestling with Jacob in Joe Pitt's telling boyhood fantasy are decidedly male, while the angel that descends in redemptive glory on the dying Prior Walter in the final moments of part 1 and hovers above his doings throughout *Part Two: Perestroika* is female.

Early in act 2 of *Millennium Approaches,* Joe recalls his early fascination with "Bible stories when [he] was a kid": "There was a picture I'd look at twenty times every day: Jacob wrestles with the angel. I don't really remember the story, or why the wrestling—just the picture. Jacob is young and very strong. The angel is . . . a beautiful man, with golden hair and wings, of course. I still dream about it. Many nights. I'm . . . It's me. I'm that struggle. Fierce, and unfair" (49). Only inches below the surface of what is a parable of Christian fortitude for this Mormon outcast is the longing he feels to surrender to this angel in ways never sanctioned by the Old Testament, in ways inspired and fueled by graphic pictures in the Bible itself. Kushner's smart depiction of Joe's ambivalence in part explains his choice of theme and title: in America the thrust of Christian fundamentalism only incites the "debauchery" that each Sunday it condemns to hell.

This "middle angel" is somewhat countered by the other male angels in the text: neither the "cover-angel" of *Millennium Approaches*' salable iconography nor the "angel of death" referred to by Prior Walter early in the play are "beautiful" or "golden" but are instead laden with associations of sickness and death. The angel on the cover is emaciated and enshadowed, crouched in a fetal position with his head thrust mournfully in his hands. His wings are lit with a softly colored spot, representing a redemption that aligns itself with the most traditional of Christian visions. Significantly, this angel figure is alone, likening him to Prior (dying of AIDS) and Harper (losing touch with reality), both of whom are abandoned at the conclusion of the play. Likewise the "wine-dark kiss of the angel of death" (21) is Prior's name for the first Kaposi's sarcoma lesion he discovers on his body, the first in a series of crises that prove ultimately too much for his lover, Louis.

With all of these moving and evocative male angels swirling through the early pages of Kushner's play, his choice of the feminine representation that descends on Prior's sickbed—"*Very* Steven Spielberg!" (118)—at drama's end is something of a surprise. It is interesting that Kushner describes this character in the cast list as "four divine emanations . . . manifest in One: the Continental Principality of America" (3), when Kushner's feelings toward America as demonstrated in the play are profoundly ambivalent. Certainly he is fascinated by the comminglings of race, sex, politics, and gender that make for such intriguing (if unlikely) bedfellows; certainly he has hope enough for our otherwise dismal civil rights history that "angels" (activists, including playwrights like himself) will one day be not only discovered but heard.

Yet his disgust with almost every "national theme" to have mattered to U.S. society in the last forty years is certainly even more evident throughout. Republicans and religious fundamentalists, red-baiters, racists, homophobes, and closet cases all come frequently and effectively under fire, and we cannot ignore the obvious connection between the angel—especially the *female* angel, with her secondary figuring as the Lady Columbia—and much of what infuriates Kushner about America. Appropriately, Kushner finds the redemption that defines part 2 not in the religious realm but in the political "emanations" of America's worst enemy throughout much of the twentieth century, the Soviet Union. Interestingly, however, one issue that should be equally anathema to this Walter Benjamin–styled marxist—the undeserved wealth and attending elitism of the upper classes[22]—is less thoroughly redressed and ultimately, I will contend, reinscribed in the playing out of Kushner's gender-based, angel-related thesis.

Prior Walter, whose fussy name suggests old-family origins, is indeed a blue blood whose family name is "stitched into the Bayeux tapestry" (51). In fact it is his own name stitched there, as there have been "Prior Walters"—that is, there were Priors prior to this one, spanning back through so many generations that our Prior is thirty-second in line, without even "including the bastards" (86). Interestingly, our Prior, the first to subscribe (exclusively) to a lifestyle uniquely indisposed to sexual reproduction, will conclude this family's illustrious tradition—tragically, prematurely so—as he is dying of AIDS. His moneyed status aligns him with Harper, who also came from and partly relinquished a social position when she married Joe, as well as with the female angel, whose regal dress and occupation of the upper planes of the theater space establish her as royalty, the play's highest represented social class. Likewise the angel, with her high-tech flying capabilities, is obviously the show's crowd-pleasing draw, a Broadway-style moneymaker who has been compared by one displeased critic with "the chandelier in *Phantom* or the helicopter in *Miss Saigon*" (Lyons 57).

The alliance among these three characters is strengthened through the ultrafeminization of Prior's character: he is by far the "nelliest" of the three leading gay men and the only one of all the cast to appear both in full Nora Desmond drag and stark naked during the course of the play. This alliance verges onto the unlikeliest of romantic triangles, as Prior and Harper "come together" in an intense emotional discovery that certainly outshines any interaction Harper has with her husband, Joe. Late in the play Prior confesses to his ex-lover Belize that he hears the early murmurings of this female angelic voice and, unexplainably, "gets hard." As with the character Ray Lee in Monette's *Afterlife,* the dying gay male is authorially consigned to the province of women in what can only strike the reader as the most bizarre of budding romances.

Prior's oddly occurring erections aside, the angel as high-tech, ultimately asexual commodity represents an "eternal life" that is highly problematic because in Kushner's play it is evidently available only to a few—specifically, those whose names can be traced back to the Bayeux tapestry. As with many of the texts discussed in chapter 2, once again it is the past, the backward glance, that is the saving and significant repository of a gay male culture that faces such an uncertain future. Yet as opposed to, say, the nineteenth-century Wildean past unearthed by Neil Bartlett—generic and anonymous, derived from dime tours and newspaper clippings, and thus belonging to everyone who would share in it—Prior is granted "eternal life" (i.e., is the one singled out for visitation by the angel), not because he will go forward forever but because he can go *backward* forever—in an unbroken, fully documented family line.

A few nights before the angel's first visitation, Prior is visited by some Priors before him, a medieval Yorkshire farmer and an eighteenth-century London fop, who surprise but finally hearten him with the news that "pestilence in my time was much worse than now" (86). These prior Priors describe "the spotty monster . . . Black Jack" as leaving "whole villages of empty houses" (86) and carrying off half of London in a deadly onslaught. To be sure, there is little comfort in the fact that only 10 or 30 percent, as opposed to 50 percent, of a population will suffer this postmodern plague, but Prior is given hope in the fact that there even *were* such similar plagues in the past, in his very own past, and that, as he puts it, "I'm not alone" (86). This is, of course, an important and redeeming discovery for him to make, but it is true, nevertheless, that Prior finds his deathbed community mainly through his "country-club affiliations," that the poor in similar circumstances are rarely so familiar with their ancestry.

Prior's contact with the salvific angel, then, is the crowning perk of having descended from a "good family,"[23] and, as perk, the angel inhabits the traditional feminine role of ornament in the treasury of wealthy men. Additionally, and despite her "hardening" effect on Prior, she is asexual herself; her voice is "incredibly beautiful" but ethereal, and she speaks mainly in biblical quotes and allusions. She is "saved" for the end of the play in a way representative of other texts that "spare" their female characters the worst occurrences and deepest emotional upheavals attached to the AIDS crisis, or that "spare" the reader from observing these characters' involvement with them (as in Monette). Finally this "angelizing" of women in these texts elevates them to mythic and irrelevant heights, at the same time removing them from the plane of real events where they might instead offer their own forms of comfort and healing.

• • •

Jill Dolan has compared lesbian playwright Paula Vogel with Broadway successes like Kushner and Terrence McNally, noting that in particular "Kushner's [writing] shares the depth of Vogel's political vision, and its hugely theatrical, non-realist imagination" (440). She voices frustration that lesbian writers with equal talent and skill have yet to cross from off-Broadway to Broadway environs and the wide audience acceptance that fosters and follows from such a move. In an interview with Michael Lowenthal, Kushner hoped that "the success of *Angels* has made a slight foot in the door for lesbian writers, because there has not been nearly enough of that" (11); but in fact Vogel's AIDS-related play *The Baltimore Waltz*, a 1992 Obie Award winner that has been staged in New York City and in regional theaters nationwide, remains a relatively obscure and unheard voice on this vital national issue.

In Vogel's play a young woman, Anna, and her brother, Carl, tour Europe while never leaving the cold, glaring setting of a hospital waiting area and adjoining patient's room. We understand at the beginning that Anna has been diagnosed with something terminal, Acquired Toilet Disease (ATD)—a device that injects humor and ironic social commentary into the proceedings but also suggests impending tragedy by so clearly referring to a real-life, gravely serious illness. In fact Vogel's brother Carl, to whom the play is dedicated, died of AIDS in 1988 and had once proposed a trip to Europe for the two of them that Vogel at the time was unable to agree to. Vogel has insisted that her writing, while certainly autobiographical, is not solely so (Savran, "Introduction" xiii), and in fact the character Anna is hardly a stand-in for the playwright herself, as she is quite ravenously heterosexual throughout the play. In addition to Vogel's curious decision to mainstream the story in this way, we must question her description of ATD, while terminal and toilet-acquired (i.e., accessing the body through private parts), as *not* sexually transmissible: a doctor reassures her early on that "taking precautions" is all she has to do, and Anna's travels through Europe include a roll in the hay with a male representative of each country visited.[24] Thus, regardless of Anna's sexual orientation, her no-questions-asked, fly-by-night contact with multiple anonymous partners in a story clearly meant to chronicle the pain and loss so consummately associated with AIDS is unexplained and largely unexplainable.

To the degree that this theme of sexual freedom and immunity is employed, Vogel's play resembles in disappointing ways Rita Mae Brown's contemporaneous novel *Venus Envy*, in which Frazier Armstrong, a beautiful and successful lesbian with a large, conservative Southern family, is delivered from a deathbed diagnosis when her lung and spine cancer turns out to be nothing more than a bronchial infection. Brown's "cancer" is potentially an AIDS analog in that it threatens the life of a gay person who is entirely too young to die and compels Frazier to send letters to each of her family members, informing them of her terminal diagnosis and gay orientation at once—a hello-and-good-bye episode reminiscent of those that countless HIV-positive gay men have had to undergo themselves.

However, the eleventh-hour reprieve that spares Frazier entirely, and reclassifies this novel from tragic social commentary to lesbian comedy, sharply severs Brown's analogy to, her dialogue with, the AIDS-related texts of gay men who have known the loss of many loved ones and in some cases face death themselves, who are clearly without the luxury of building such redemptive moments into any text they may write today. Brown's lesbian love story is suffused with the fantasy that interestingly characterizes so much of the second part of Kushner's *Angels in America*—the angel-graced earth scenes and the almost as equally miraculous reprieve granted to Prior, who not only did not die at the end of part 1, as we thought he would, but moves into part 2 as a central figure and immortalized prophet, raining blessings on the audience at the play's conclusion. In contrast, however, to Kushner's use of fantasy and magic, Brown's recourse to a deus ex machina is unnecessary, even ironic, since gay women, we must admit, need so many fewer miracles to ensure long natural lives for themselves, at least relative to their contemporary gay male counterparts.

Meanwhile, Vogel's reprieve of one of her characters is the least problematic of the three considered here. While in both *Angels in America* and *Venus Envy* once-dying characters spring from their sickbeds at a magic hour and in important respects never look back,[25] in *The Baltimore Waltz,* Anna is dying, very realistically and sadly:

> The Third Man: Anna has a difficult time sleeping. She is afflicted with night thoughts [an AIDS analog for night sweats]. . . .
> Anna: I feel so alone. The ceiling is pressing down on me. I can't believe I am dying. Only at night. . . . In the morning I feel absolutely well—without a body. And then the thought comes crashing to my mind. This is the last spring I may see. This is the last summer. (27)

This suffering continues throughout the course of the play, which concludes grimly and with finality in the death this story is really about, that of the brother, Carl. As the loving sister Anna (and no doubt Vogel) is, she literally dreams of taking her brother's suffering and infirmities onto herself in an effort to trade her life for his and in some way atone for the missed opportunities for sharing and togetherness (in Vogel's case perhaps the foregone trip to Europe) that the routine of life too easily forgives. In marked contrast, then, to authors like Kushner and Brown, who employ magic and miracles to secure "eternal" (for dying people, this means natural) life, Vogel acknowledges and even describes a dream of dying that offers no reprieve, suffusing her story with the weight and sadness appropriate to stories about AIDS and, more importantly, to women's involvement with it. As reality warms into the final scenes, Carl collapses into his hospital bed and Anna leaves the hospital carrying his memories and his favorite stuffed rabbit into the world that goes on without him. Although Carl comes back to life to waltz Anna offstage in the play's last moment, the audience is fully aware that this, too, is only a dream, that reality has fully taken its toll.

In line with this helpful response to the absenting of women from AIDS texts are two recent lesbian novels that include more fully not only a significant masculine presence but also a detailed treatment of illness and the fragility of bodies that is ultimately an issue for all of us. Sarah Schulman's *People in Trouble* depicts a romantic triangle positioning Kate between her husband, Peter, and her lover, Molly, who helps initiate Kate into her lesbian identity. Schulman plots Kate's sexual self-discovery to coincide with her discovery of gay male culture as well, of AIDS and the need for AIDS activism, of the many privileges she has always taken for granted and the magnitude of the suffering outside her door. Schulman, then, equates a lesbian consciousness with a politically enlightened, empowered state; once Kate accepts her lesbianism (which happens shortly into the novel), she is freed to act (to ACT UP) in ways that, while without immediate effect on the prognosis of many of her gay male associates, strikes a blow against harmful political ideologies that threaten the lives of those affected by AIDS.

The setting is New York City, with its large gay population and large contingent of wealthy, indifferent landlords and city planners who make life difficult, if not miserable, for its citizens living with AIDS. The Gay Men's Health Crisis is featured here, as several of Kate and Molly's friends are hotliners; ACT UP is likewise refigured in a black-and-pink-shirted group called Justice, whose members, like those of ACT UP, pass out flyers, protest at City Hall, and demonstrate during Catholic services. Donald Trump (though more accurately a composite of millionaires like him) is pilloried for his indifference to human suffering in the figure of "Ronald Horne" (a "Trumpette"), who, if not aggravating enough to Kate's community as he is, decides to run for public office, inciting a violent protest against the anti-AIDS policies he stands ready to enforce. Finally it is Kate's own work of art, self-reflexively titled *People in Trouble,* that catches fire at an anti-Horne rally, engulfing the greedy mogul in flames. Kate, of course, is never caught for "accidentally" setting the highly flammable piece aflame in the vicinity of the millionaire, and Schulman concludes the novel by savoring this sweet, envisioned revenge.

As Molly and Kate establish their relationship, they explore the gay and AIDS subcultures together; the novel is in one respect an inquiry into and celebration of "famous fag/dyke teams like the Catholic Church, Hollywood, and the Olympics" (157), as well as the AIDS activist community of New York. Schulman's estimation of the bond these two communities shares may sound a bit cold, but it also strikes a note of truth. In an early scene Molly's friend Pearl says it was AIDS itself that drove the two groups together—or, to put it more accurately, drove gay men to seek out lesbians for support: "I remember when the Saint wouldn't let women in. It was gross. But when AIDS happened men needed more friends. The back rooms got shut down and the bars needed more cash and started going coed" (76). In a later scene Kate realizes that her bond with a gay man has nothing to do with her "loving men, too,"—that is, with any semblance of a heterosexual dynamic between them: "*It was our gayness that connected us,* she realized later. *Not our love of men. It is the danger that brings you together, makes you need each other and feel so close*" (162). While the novel's conclusion (the assassination of Horne, revolutionary and unpunished) smacks of utopic fantasy, Schulman here finds a realistic plane of understanding between gay men and lesbians, identifying the trials they in fact undergo together: the "danger" Kate describes is not the threat of AIDS and AIDS-related death but that of homophobic and AIDS-phobic individual sentiment and city policies so stringent and hostile as to be life-threatening. In this universe, if an impoverished gay man or lesbian is turned out of an apartment in the midst of a New York winter, if a gay person is beaten during a hate crime and homophobic/virophobic police do nothing to intervene, these lives are threatened or extinguished. This threat, as defended against throughout the novel, becomes a workable if smaller-scale analog for AIDS itself, for the ways in which lesbians have indeed made the effort to share the burden and alleviate the suffering of AIDS-infected gay men. Thus the bond formed between these formerly diverging groups is drawn here as one of the few benefits to have emerged from the AIDS crisis, which, now beneficial and empowering to all concerned, must not be forgotten at the supposed dawn of the "post-AIDS" era.

Jeanette Winterson's poetic and moving *Written on the Body* features centrally a radically bigendered narrative voice whose character falls in love with a beautiful woman who is married to a successful doctor yet, ironically, is dying of a terminal illness. The novel is suffused with both the joyful rumination on and execution of a passionate love affair and the debilitating world-weariness brought on by chronic and profound illness as well. The narrative looks out, in its early moments, on a world already weakened, near death, that longs for an earlier, more vibrant time: "The grapes have withered on the vine. What should be plump and firm, resisting the touch to give itself in the mouth, is spongy and blistered. Not this year the pleasure of rolling blue grapes between finger and thumb juicing my palm with musk. Even the wasps avoid the thin brown dribble. Even the wasps this year. It was not always so" (9). The world is colored thus because the narrator has lost the woman s/he cared madly for—beautiful, fair-skinned Louise, whose hair is "mane-wide and the color of blood" (190). We do not know, by novel's end, whether Louise is "lost" because she has finally succumbed to a struggle with cancer or whether she simply remains, removed permanently from the nameless narrator, with her surgeon husband in her traditional and well-appointed marriage. Though the narrator is driven to distraction with the determining of Louise's outcome, both her death and survival are forms of the same tragedy: even if Louise is alive, she is removed from the impassioned narrator, who is little more than walking dead without her.

Throughout the story, this narrator is less ungendered than alternately gendered, as s/he rapidly and completely switches back and forth between masculine and feminine modes with delightfully perverse abandon. At times this narrative voice is active and masculine, boasting of many previous affairs with married women, stealing into their houses after their various relationships have ended to retrieve the belongings these spurned women try to horde. Even more masculine, I would argue, is this narrator's history of sexually transmitted diseases obtained from certain of these dalliances, as such diseases are most often transmitted when the penetration involved is of a type that lesbian sex relations can (in this case, fortunately) only simulate. The narrator's visit to the "Clap Clinic" not only momentarily determines a masculine gendering but also reinforces Winterson's underlying theme of universal suffering from illness, here a specifically sexual one: "plastic flowers in a plastic vase and all over the walls, top to bottom, posters for every wart and discolored emission. It's impressive what a few inches of flesh can catch" (47).

Yet this narrative "manning" is immediately undermined as the narrator is informed during the same scene that s/he is in fact not infected, suggesting to us that the type of sex the narrator had with the infected partner was "safe enough" (nonpenetrating) after all; earlier, remembering another affair, the narrator admits that this time infection is only a metaphor, is ultimately all in the head: "I had bought a new flat to start again from a nasty love affair that had given me the clap. Nothing wrong with my organs, this was emotional clap. I had to keep my heart to myself in case I infected somebody" (25).

Likewise the narrator is feminized, that is, lesbianized, by her estimation that Louise's traditional (heterosexual) marriage is a lie she is living, a "shell" to hide in, and that most marriages are abominations. At a high point in their affair Louise and the narrator have a mock ceremony that takes place significantly "outdoors" (i.e., it is an "outing" for both of them); likewise the figuration is of two brides plighting troths as the narrator notes that "our bouquets were Ragged Robin from the side of the canal" (19). The themes of outing and of outness, the thrilling outlandishness of gay life, are wryly suggested in the following lengthy passage in which the narrator again assumes the role of accommodating, facilitating male figure (but perhaps only the "butch" half of this kinky pair) yet also presents a lesbian profile through certain pointed double entendres:

> I had a girlfriend once who was addicted to starlit nights. She thought beds belonged in hospitals. Anywhere she could do it that wasn't pre-sprung was sexy. Show her a duvet and she switched on the television. I coped with this on campsites and in canoes, British Rail and Aeroflot. I bought a futon, eventually a gym mat. I had to lay extra-thick carpet on the floor. I took to carrying a tartan rug wherever I went, like a far-out member of the Scottish Nationalist Party. Eventually, back at the doctor's for a fifth time having a thistle removed [once again this pathologizing and endangering of the sex act] he said to me, "You know, love is a very beautiful thing but there are clinics for people like you." Now it's a serious matter to have "PERVERT" written on your NHS file and some indignities are just a romance too far. We had to say goodbye and although there were some things about her that I missed it was pleasant to walk in the country again without seeing every bush and shrub as a potential assailant. (20)

To be "out" while you're doing it, to prefer a sex that distinctly avers attachment to the traditional (i.e., marital) bed, to get your kicks (but also your licks) among the ever-overgrowing "bushes and shrubs"—all of these will get you a "pervert" sticker slapped on your file at the NHS. Ultimately it is just easier to call the romance off.

Even while the narrator, running so rakishly through all these women, is read as male, his "pervert" status is left intact by a history of previous "boyfriends," themselves with bisexual histories that keep the mystery of the narrator's gender spinning. "Crazy Frank," for instance, "didn't want to settle down. His ambition was to find a hole in every port. He wasn't fussy about the precise location" (93). Another boyfriend was Carlo, who eventually takes up with another man. This profile of the narrator-as-pervert, then—as not so much gay man or gay woman but thoroughly impervious to a determination of either—is consistently, even rigorously enforced, revealing perversion not as the pit of laxity and indifference it has been depicted as throughout the ages but as that which verges on an artistic achievement, an exhilarating tightrope act that is as thrilling to watch as it is to live.

Yet perversion, and the debilitating instance of having your "file at the NHS" stamped with any denomination, much less one so fraught with controversy, is linked throughout the novel with serious, even terminal illness that, as stated above, makes this novel so relevant as an AIDS text. In addition to a generally deteriorated natural world surrounding the narrator and narrative, and the multiple references to STDs and their nightmarish treatments, Louise contracts a deadly illness—chronic lymphocytic leukemia—that significantly resembles HIV. The narrator and Louise's husband discuss her condition in a terse dialogue that Winterson cordons off from the surrounding narrative with extra spaces, attempting to cordon off Louise's hideous diagnosis and the permanent separation for the lovers it implies:

> She looks well.
> The patient may have no symptoms for some time. . . .
> She's not ill.
> Her lymph nodes are enlarged. . . . She has too many white T-cells.
> Will she die?
> That depends.
> On what?
> On you.
> You mean can I look after her?
> I mean I can. (101–2)

Triangulated between these two competing lovers, Louise has a chance of survival (i.e., is dealing with a treatable form of cancer after all) if she returns to her heterosexual contract and makes use of the multiple facilities and technologies her surgeon/husband can provide for her. Contrarily, she will face almost certain death (i.e., an illness much more closely resembling AIDS) if she chooses the life of perversion, of continued relationship with her illicit lover—who finally capitulates to this brutal dichotomy and loses her, that is, *looses* her, so that she can live. No matter which outcome we might have, the cancer is clearly an AIDS analog, with its lengthy and confusing latency period, its reliance on T-cells (in this case too many instead of too few) as a measure of health, and its tendency toward easy bruising that presents in pale Louise as "burst figs . . . the livid purple of your skin," strongly resembling Kaposi's sarcoma.

Moments before the novel's end, the narrator is alone and bereft without her, then has a sudden "vision" of her: "paler, thinner, but her hair still mane-wide and the color of blood. . . . Am I mad? She's warm" (190). The story concludes "where the story starts, in this threadbare room," yet "the walls are exploding. The windows have turned to telescopes" (190), and the unknowability that is this novel's largest theme limits our view until the very end: "We can take the world with us when we go and sling the sun under your arm. . . . I don't know if this is a happy ending but here we are let loose in the open fields" (190). Separated by death or reunited blissfully on one side or the other of the great divide, the lovers are nevertheless running wild and "out" again, reinstating the certainty of uncertainty, that is, the perversion that defines them, a final time.

Vogel, Schulman, and Winterson, then, have written AIDS stories that successfully incorporate the feminine *through its very incorporation* of the masculine as well—Vogel through Anna's literal assuming of Carl's physical crisis and Schulman and Winterson through their sexual "perverts," a full depiction of whose sexuality is not possible without an analysis of the masculine within and around them as it coincides with the feminine and the feminist (that is, activist) within and around them as well. As AIDS writers, they also recognize the need to include the male, especially the gay male, perspective in their depictions of sexuality and sickness in this postmodern era. Finally, neither gender is "angelized," spared or removed from crisis, but is instead anchored firmly on earth, where all hands get dirtied, even bloodied, but offer healing as well. As opposed to Brown's comic novel, which removes the AIDS-analogous crisis from the women's story she tells, and the male-authored AIDS novels and plays discussed above, which examine less than the total effect of, less than a total response to, the ravages of this epidemic, these women-authored AIDS texts work to include both perspectives, offering women committed to this cause a position from which to speak.

TEXTUAL TRIANGLES

Even in the course of analyzing gender opposition in these plague texts, multiple traditionally masculine and feminine narrative components have begun to break away from their original, static roles into dynamic triangular relationships: in Tim O'Brien's *Nuclear Age,* Bobbi contends for her husband's loyalty with a masculinized hole; at the same time she fights alternately with this hole and with her husband over the possession and safety of her daughter. In Kushner's play, Joe triangulates himself between his wife and his lover, Louis, while also contending with a (feminized) Prior for the ability to reach and thus "cure" his mentally disabled wife. Kate must choose between her husband, Peter, and her lover, Molly, in *People in Trouble,* and Louise must choose between a husband she barely loves and a bigendered narrator in *Written on the Body.* Significantly, all of these triangles contain a "perversion"—either an explicitly gay relationship that forces the triangulated to choose not only between different partners but radically alternative lifestyles, or a more broadly perverted romance like that between Louise and her unidentifiable narrator or between the very gay Prior Walter and his two "girlfriends," Harper and the Angel—that keeps them humming with multidirected desire and keeps the reader guessing as to their final outcomes.

William, Joe, Kate, and Louise all must choose between a traditional heterosexual marriage that can give safety and stability (and in William's and Louise's cases, life itself) and a "mad" or "perverse," sometimes ill-inducing, sometimes deadly relationship with a queer or perverted counterpart. Yet as fraught with danger as these "alternative" relationships may be, an inner, strengthening truth is found each time, effectively countering the physical threats they may produce. Certainly O'Brien's William returns most enthusiastically to the married, suburban mainstream, while the other three characters take up a "perverted" but rejuvenating lifestyle, reveling in the multiple personal freedoms emerging from it, choosing perhaps even death (as do Joe and Louise) over a stifling continued existence within a traditional marriage bond. Schulman's Kate seems most enlivened by her alternative lifestyle, as Schulman's explicit equation between a lesbian relationship and the vitality and power attached to political activism makes Kate's choice clear. In all of these plague text triangles, however, the introduction of a radical alternative (instead of, say, the traditional heroine's "momentous" decision between straight male A and straight male B) not only invites (or forces) the text's characters (and those who read their stories) through markedly varied lifestyle changes but also introduces the possibility of other "radical alternatives" in our waking lives—peace instead of hostility, treatment and prevention of illness instead of red tape and false promises.

In fact these several triangles are among the most disrupted, disruptive, dynamic and promising of those to be observed in plague literature from these two periods. All of them are fairly recent productions (O'Brien's *Nuclear Age* [1985] being the first published), and all but one of them treat the AIDS crisis implicitly or explicitly and introduce actually queer characters into the story (again, O'Brien's text stands alone), so it is perhaps not surprising that here we would find the instability of the triangular figuration, described in the early pages of this chapter, at its boiling point. Perhaps equally unsurprising, in the older, male-authored, primarily cold war–themed novels and nonfiction to be discussed in the remainder of this section, dynamic and subversive triangulation—between lovers, lifestyles, and readerships—ostensibly does not exist: it is *only* a feminist and/or queer reading of these texts that sees or produces their three-way relationships—a reading that, while certainly applied to the texts instead of springing organically from them, is necessary to a full understanding of them nevertheless. In the earliest of these stories, from the immediate postwar period, a characterological threesome receives from a feminist/queer interpretation a new twist: instead of the coveted female choosing between male suitors, the male protagonist must choose between his "woman" and his "buddy," who both covet him in ways never observed (or acknowledged) by original readers. In later, more canonical texts, triangulation is denied through the exclusion of actual women (characters and readers) from the boys' club constituted by these texts' male authors and critical readers. Only the forced insertion of a feminist presence in this discussion pulls this two-way street into triangular shape; and this disruption, which would seem to "heterosexualize" the situation, also retroactively queers it, interrupting a lovefest with curiously queer shadings between multiple powerful men.

The discussion that follows is fundamentally informed by the theories developed by Eve Kosofsky Sedgwick in *Between Men.* There Sedgwick describes the homosocial triangle, which requires the presence of a third term (women) at the same time that this term is completely banished, sometimes by an exclusionary homoerotic desire but more often by heterosexual misogynist tendencies. The homosocial depends, then, on a triangular configuration to shield or sustain the primary pairing between the men involved yet also requires the removal or destruction of this third term, which interrupts and obstructs this very relationship. While homosociality is often considered to describe some mode of gay lifestyling, in fact the queering of the men's relations described by Sedgwick is only a secondary, sometimes even illusory, effect of the intense antiwoman sentiment found among straight men. Nevertheless, the equally intense "passions" between male characters or between male authors and their critics to be explored here cannot help but strike modern readers as distinctly homoerotic; if the AIDS crisis itself is not a primary theme of concern in the discussion to follow, certainly the sort of queer theorizing that was in part born from this epidemic and has in turn done much to alleviate its negative effects will be essential here.

• • •

Three early postmodern triangles position a male protagonist at the vortex of sex and the intellect, forcing his choice between the life of the body, promised by the female love interest, and the life of the mind, represented by the supporting male character. In Orwell's *1984,* Bradbury's *Fahrenheit 451,* and Vonnegut's *Player Piano,* all three of the lead male figures turn from female partners, whose functions range from disappointing to debilitating, to a male "equal" whose free mind and daring actions attract the male lead in ways his female partner never can. The two men in each novel forge a bond that queers more with each passing decade of (feminist and queer) readership.[26] All three male protagonists—Winston, Montag, and Proteus—attach themselves to women who are the beautiful and desirable reward of their accomplishments; all three of the(ir) women finish the story in greatly diminished roles, if they survive it at all.

By far the most positive female portrait is found in Orwell's Julia, who, as opposed to Bradbury's Mildred or Vonnegut's Anita, is an actual revolutionary with political agency and clever schemes for subverting the oppressive system controlling her world. Unlike Mildred and Anita, who are the "prizes" received by their husbands for conforming to a suffocating social order, Julia begins a friendship with and love for Winston only after he begins his own experiments in subversion. Thus, she is part of what he works toward, while Montag and Proteus run from what Mildred and Anita represent. Likewise Julia is still a vital presence near the novel's end, even if she is recast as a profound disappointment, a traitor to Winston's aspirations. Her confession of surrender in the face of torture by her captors is a moving and dramatic testament to the horrors of life under authoritarian rule.

Yet like Mildred and especially Anita, Julia[27] is ultimately condemned and discarded for an overt sexuality that is deemed irrelevant to the political struggle undertaken by the lead male figure. Winston accuses her of being a revolutionary "from the waist downwards" (129) (as if her brave disregard for Oceania's antisexual policy were of no subversive merit). Shortly after this statement is leveled against her, she is captured by thought police (i.e., removed from a position of consequence in the storyline) and does not reappear until very near the novel's end. Likewise Anita's drive to push her husband, Proteus, through an overmechanized career that he despises is attached to her aggressive sexuality—and similarly discarded—when Paul witnesses her seducing his much more corporate-minded rival and realizes, along with the novel's readers, that he is better off without her.

Only Montag's wife, Mildred, suffers actual death during the novel. Of the three women she is the weakest, most dependent, and therefore most dangerous to her partner's revolutionary plots. Whereas Julia and Anita betray their partners well after or well before each is pursued and captured by the governing regime, Mildred is a chief instigator of Montag's implication, turning in the books he has stolen (instead of burning) to the supervening authorities. Bradbury invites us to enjoy her fiery death as just deserts for her disloyalty: she, like the rest of Montag's ignorant and doomed society, perishes in a pseudonuclear scene of destruction, her final moment of horrid self-discovery no means of salvation for her: "she saw her own face reflected there . . . and it was such a wildly empty face . . . touching nothing, starved and eating of itself, that at last she recognized it as her own . . . and the entire structure of the hotel blasted down upon her" (142).

As with the women themselves, their (male) rivals are all ultimately incidental if not disabling to the male leads' respective searches for political freedom and personal growth. Each is finally unable to deliver on his promise of total fulfillment and freedom of movement with which they initially entice the male leads to join them. Yet, although these male-male relationships all fail to some degree, it does not mean that each was not "consummated" during some moment presented as intellectual communion but suffused with the homoerotic as well: Winston perceives in O'Brien a "flash of intelligence" that alerts him to O'Brien's shared hatred for Big Brother and the police state. Montag feels that he is almost turning into his intellectual mentor, Faber, and indeed the two men enjoy a physical union when Montag carries Faber's instructive and inspiring voice in his ear via a small transmitter that Faber has developed. Likewise, Proteus and Finnerty, after many years of separation, reunite when Proteus has left his managerial post at the Ilium Works, and they plot their antirobot revolution together.

If, as argued above, Orwell's text provides the most positive portrayal of women's contributions to social change, it simultaneously provides the most negative male-male relationship of the three texts examined as well. Finally, O'Brien is not only ineffective in aiding Winston's fight; he is the chief cause of Winston's downfall, the torturer who will drive him and Julia to betray each other and Winston to the brink of madness. Winston begins intensely interested in and enamored of O'Brien, admitting to himself that he writes his life-giving diary "for O'Brien—*to* O'Brien" and that the very thought of him keeps Winston's writing project going. Their moment of meeting verges on the sexual and sublime at once: "At last they were face to face. . . . [Winston's] heart bounded violently. He would have been incapable of speaking" (130). Yet the romance is quickly exposed as fraudulent on O'Brien's part; he has lured Winston into his confidence only to trap and imprison him.[28] His betrayal has the effect of reauthorizing not only Julia's presence in Winston's life but her version of revolution—"from the [heterosexual] waist down"—which still constitutes her and Winston's most effective subversion of Oceania's stifling regime.

Conversely, the women of Bradbury's and Vonnegut's novels are not reinstated as forceful presences in the social upheavals depicted there; instead the male-male relationships endure, succeed against an oppressive social structure to some degree, and foster all-male communes of intellectuals who are also "drinking buddies," a boys-only utopia that markedly queers these authors' prescriptions for a better way of life. Although "Montag-plus-Faber" do not make it out of the burning city together, Montag has inspired the aging genius with a burst of youthful vigor for which he effusively thanks the young fireman in suggestive terms: "I must admit that your blind raging has invigorated me. How young I felt! But now—I want you to feel old, I want a little of my cowardice to be distilled in you tonight. The next few hours, when you see Captain Beatty, tiptoe 'round him, let *me* hear him for you, let *me* feel the situation out. Survival is our ticket. Forget the poor, silly women" (93). Faber's plea to forget the women and join him (and Captain Beatty) in an invigorating game of cat and mouse leads to a confrontation (and secondary triangulation) among the three men that eventually results in Montag killing Beatty to protect Faber.[29] While this effort cannot save the aging Faber from perishing in the ensuing firestorms, their relationship prepares Montag for the community of (male) scholars he finds by the river at novel's end, with whom he witnesses the conflagration of his society and with whom he will share a life in the new postcensorship order of things. The explosion and purging witnessed by the men is orgasmic and cleansing; each moves on from the experience renewed and refreshed—reborn into intellectual integrity and into a close-knit community of men.

The scenario is almost identical at the end of Vonnegut's novel, but because the holocaust created in Ilium is not nearly so complete, Proteus's Finnerty is able to survive it with him. Yet a system of oppression remains in place that will quickly engulf the revolutionaries and punish them for their misdeeds. Instead of walking along the river reciting Bible passages to each other, Vonnegut's postlapsarian heroes drive over to meet their captors on the outskirts of town, sharing a bottle of whiskey as they go. Long ago they have each forgotten "the poor silly women" who tried to bog them down in their own selfish dreams, and the free thinkers—Proteus and Finnerty, Lasher and von Neumann—will face their judgment and excommunication stronger because they will face them together.

We note, of course, that in current-day assessments of these triangles, a new triangle is formed between (straight) feminism and queer theory, which each vie for the hand of "meaning" in these texts in a self-canceling fashion I am as yet unable to reconcile: Orwell has either produced a relatively encouraging portrait of the female revolutionary or has failed to capitalize on a homoerotics of social upheaval in his engaging but finally conservative treatment of the Winston/O'Brien compact. Conversely, Bradbury and Vonnegut's texts are problematic and regressive because of their withering attitudes toward women or are enlightening and subversive due to a newly asserted primacy of male homoerotic couplings, even groupings. Ultimately we may understand the feminist-queer theorist relationship as generational, though less Oedipal (i.e., matricidal) than dialectical, with early feminism inspiring and influencing the first wave of gay theory but now with new cycles of feminist and queer theories presenting constantly, sprung from the gender-based work of *all* their predecessors. Finally, both share in the project of enunciating and elevating interpretations of the "feminine," the "pervert," or the "activist" as they confront the threat of stricture and silencing in the Symbolic realm; and here a combination of approaches—a feminist application of queer theories—is what discovers the triangulating dynamism of these plague texts.

• • •

In a long and prolific career that began in the era of the above three novels and continues into the current day, Norman Mailer senses the queerness endangering the straightest and most canonical of literary relationships and devotes much of his own work to eradicating the dreadful threat. Like that of the classic "homosocialite" described in Sedgwick's work, Mailer's intense interest in men springs certainly from his equally intense dislike of women, especially women authors and critics. Meanwhile, and also in typical homosocial form, Mailer sees the "homosexual" everywhere in life, art, and politics, and the role this marginal figure has played in American culture clearly obsesses him. The male-male couplings between Mailer and the manly authors and characters he champions, between himself and the homosexual figures he despises, between the hipster and the homosexual in American society, and between Mailer and his many admiring male critics—all of these have been helpfully triangulated by the interventions of feminist readers of the 1960s and 1970s,[30] to whose complete and necessarily scathing replies I have little to add. Instead, I will focus here on multiple other gender-based triangles informing Mailer's work: specifically, how his view of the homosexual in his bizarrely conceived universe, as well as how his understanding of sexuality ("genitality") in general, forms the apex of his own triangular worldview—whose two opposite angles, politics and literature, affect every other aspect of life.[31]

In an introductory moment in *Cannibals and Christians,* Mailer blames "hypercivilization" for the fact that "the world is entering a time of plague. And the continuing metaphor for th[is writer's] obsession [with plague]—a most disagreeable metaphor—has been cancer" (2). The cancerous condition for Mailer is a buildup or backup of poisonous matter that a hypercivilized (i.e., sexually repressed) society is unable to clear from its system. Both the sexual conformity of the 1950s *and,* contradictorily, the sexual radicalism of the homosexual cause this cancerous condition, this constipation and hesitation that ruin the vigor and integrity of American letters as well as the quality of the men Americans vote into high public office. Mailer's favorite nonfiction modes—the political journal, the literary review, and the free-form "rant" (speeches, columns, interviews with himself)—enable him to define and develop the connections among these themes with the unrestricted, self-generated abandon that characterizes this "healthy" sexuality as well.

Commercialism aided by technology is the primary cause of this psychobiologic coitus interruptus; Mailer complains that modern man is doomed from his earliest days, and he borrows the cure from the philosophies of Wilhelm Reich, whose theories of orgasm-as-therapy he has readily accepted. In "The White Negro" (1957) Mailer defines the "hipster" as one who is driven, undistracted, and entirely motivated by self-interest, that is the incredible, "apocalyptic" orgasm—and then the next one and the next. The hipster code allows for violent confrontations of any sort on the way to achieving the ultimate orgasm(s), and in the course of the essay violence becomes a worthy substitute for or diverting alternative to the hipster's lifelong succession of orgasmic moments. Elsewhere violence is his ludicrous prescription for even serious illness: "If one were to take the patients in a hospital, give them guns and let them shoot on pedestrians down from the hospital windows, you may be sure you would find a few miraculous cures" (*Cannibals and Christians* 91). Andrew Gordon points out, however, that Mailer went well beyond Reich in his advocation of violence; "Reich . . . never talked very much about violence, except as another instance of the perverse behavior into which a sex-denying civilization drove individuals" (41). Thus for Reich violence between individuals in society is part of the pathology of "hypercivilization," while for his renegade student Mailer it is part of the cure.

Philip H. Bufithis explains this proviolence bent in Mailer (who profiles himself explicitly and volubly as an antiwar activist in multiple other instances) thus: "Mailer's radical assumption is, however, that each act of individual violence, no matter how heinous it may be, subtracts from the collective violence of the state. . . . He was later to suggest in his writings of the late 1960s for example, that the war in Vietnam was partly the result of our inhibitive lives" (58). Note the sexism that invades Bufithis's paraphrase of Mailer's continuing argument, providing its own base of assenting support: "Mailer is saying that if violence alone will overcome an enfeebling fear, let violence be. We might be better off closer to death than hag-ridden by the dictates of a conformist society or emasculated by an anesthetic modular world" (59). To be "enfeebled," "hag-ridden," or "emasculated" is the central crisis of Mailer's American under siege—the president, the author, or the average Joe—all figures male, of course, and all of them in desperate need of outlets for violent heterosexual expression.

In *Norman Mailer*, Richard Poirier reminds us that for Mailer sex is not only explosive but "creative"—a positive force pitted relentlessly against the general destruction and "formlessness" of modern life. Sex as creative act symbolizes and inspires brilliant, even revolutionary, writing, a product Mailer frequently laments as having all but disappeared from the stage of late twentieth-century America. Likewise it enables a fairer, more peaceful nation and improves international relations worldwide. Conversely, the noncreative sex of homosexuality gives rise to and can be blamed for dull, derivative writing and hysterical international relations, an assertion that nicely rationalizes Mailer's gut-felt homophobia as disseminated throughout his early career. In *The Presidential Papers* Mailer castigates the "faggotry" of Jean Genet (206) and locates "the lethal defamation of homosexuality" (Kate Millett's formulation [333]) at the root of the necessary violence of men. In *Cannibals and Christians* Mailer blames a perceived recent rise in the homosexual population on "a general loss of faith in the country, faith in the meaning of one's work, faith in the notion of oneself as a man" (201).

His fictional characters exhibiting queer tendencies—General Cummings (*The Naked and the Dead*), Leroy Hollingsworth (*The Barbary Shore*), and Marion Faye and Teddy Pope (*The Deer Park*)—all labor under, in Mailer's own words, "unpleasant, ridiculous, or sinister connotations" (*Advertisements* 206) that reinforce what he felt at the time was a widely held belief in the "intrinsic relationship between homosexuality and 'evil'" (207). The essay including these remarks, "The Homosexual Villain," was originally developed at the request of the editors of *One,* a "serious" homosexual magazine founded in Los Angeles in the early 1950s. Although it is largely a reconsideration of and apology for his homophobic attitudes, Mailer reprinted the essay in *Advertisements for Myself* with the disclaimer that it is "beyond a doubt the worst article I had ever written, conventional, empty, pious, the quintessence of the Square" (205). My assumption is that it is not so much the newly enlightened attitude about homosexuals but the apology itself—the admission of guilt that no doubt seemed to Mailer a bending-over before his readership—that led to the insistent and defensive retraction. My assumption derives from the new and central "function" granted to homosexuality in Mailer's later *Why Are We in Vietnam?* A dubious promotion to be sure, Mailer positions this form of "bad sex" (and the bad living that follows from it) not on an opposite plane from ideal, creative sex and the creative life it supposedly inspires but as the fundamental *precursor to* and *inspiration for* the vital and violent "brotherhood" that is a creative force. Mailer himself admits in "The Homosexual Villain" that his readings on homosexual subject matter and meetings with homosexual neighbors, inspired in part by the request to write the piece for *One* in the first place, led him to revise the galleys for *The Deer Park* to improve the profile of the gay Teddy Pope;[32] in *Why Are We in*

Vietnam? ♻ the explicit homosexual fantasizing of the boys D.J. and Tex is a narrative device that the "naturalizing," electrifying force[33] of the aurora borealis interrupts and redirects into a healthy, rejuvenating zest for "life": "the radiance of the North went into them, and owned their fear, . . . and they were twins, never to be near as lovers again, but killer brothers, owned by something, prince of darkness, lord of light" (204).

Mailer's rambling, complicated narrative makes the answer to the question "Why are we in Vietnam?" most unclear; and some readers (certainly this one) may construe the text to blame our involvement in Southeast Asia on the stupid bloodlust exhibited by Tex, D.J., and the host of "medium assholes" accompanying them on a hunting expedition through the Alaskan wilderness. Indeed, the boys' break from the older men leads to an episode of communion with nature and the experience of essential manhood for them, so that the return to the group hunt for defenseless creatures at the novel's end becomes sinister in comparison, resembling too closely America's persecution of native peoples in Vietnam.[34] Recalling, however, Mailer's distinction between violence among individuals as it "subtracts from" the organized, technologized violence of a national collective, we should instead consider the hunting/wilderness experience a valid and healing expression of violence and the "descent" (from Fairbanks to Dallas) to life in the lowlands itself the real reason "why we are in Vietnam." The novel's final, "hypercivilized" moment is a dinner party to send off D.J. and Tex to Vietnam. It stands in sharp contrast to the episode of the boys' "getaway" to the Brooks Range, "stripped" (of weapons and protective gear) and clinging together for warmth and enlightenment after an icy, life-threatening night. As is obvious, the queer shadings intertwine thickly with (and are finally indistinguishable from) the macho storyline of escape from conformity to a violent encounter with nature. Poirier argues that, finally, "this whole book is about buggery" (150), and Kate Millett concurs that in *Why Are We in Vietnam?* and throughout Mailer's work, "cruelty and violence spring out of the repressed homosexuality of men's-house culture" (332).

Thus Mailer's triangle of sexuality, politics, and literature is either a harmful or helpful force in society, depending on whether the sexuality in question is "creative" (heterosexual) or "destructive" (homosexual). In Mailer's early cold war writing, these two sexualities war over the identity and quality of this triangular force, while in his later cold war writing they interdepend and define each other. I picture the ubiquitous stamp on recyclable materials ♻ and see sexuality at the top of this triangle, feeding the creativity and/or perversity of political and social life, which in turn feeds the triumphs (Hemingway, Lawrence, Henry Miller), and crises (most contemporary male writers and *all* women writers) of the twentieth-century novelistic tradition. Quickly, however, this image dissolves as the arrows move forward and back, then in all directions at once. While I appreciate Mailer's attention to the societal crises of his era and the resonant language he uses ("sickness," "cancer," "plague") to define these ills, his insistence on narrowly defined sexualities as cause and cure is not postmodernism but puritanism and thus impossible to apply or even understand.

• • •

Arguing that Thomas Pynchon was himself influenced by Sedgwick's *Between Men* and by the theories espoused in Sandra M. Gilbert and Susan Gubar's *Madwoman in the Attic* as he composed *Vineland,* Molly Hite reads an admittedly resonant speech by Brock to Frenesi—"You're the medium Weed and I use to communicate, that's all, this set of holes, pleasantly framed, this little femme scampering back and forth with scented messages tucked in her little secret places" (214)—and counts this as evidence of Pynchon's feminist project. I argued above that it is difficult to find a truly feminist statement among the dense and dissolving layers of Pynchon's irony and inference, and here the echo of Sedgwick's feminist-critical voice is much easier to miss than the ridiculous misogyny of the male authors and characters she targets. Certainly, the homosocial is in play here, though acceptance of its detrimental effects is just as likely as rejection.

Such homosociality is reproduced in the curiously intense relationship between Pynchon and his many admiring male critics, some of whom have vigorously "explained" (i.e., justified) and supported the problematic writings of Mailer. In the introduction to an early and influential special Pynchon issue in *Twentieth Century Literature,* George Levine and David Leverenz cannot get down low enough to salaam before the great one: "One of the conditions of [Pynchon's] staying with his publishers, we've learned, is that they not publish books about his work. So as editors of this special number dedicated to Pynchon, we know there's not much we can do to please him. Wherever you are, Thomas Pynchon, we apologize" (iii–iv). Later the editors hope "the essays here don't look too silly" and sign off "with gestures of respect to an unwelcoming Pynchon himself" (iv). In the first essay of that issue, "The Importance of Thomas Pynchon," Richard Poirier blames only readers if Pynchon's work fails to please: "Tepid, condescending, unwilling or unable to submit to the intense pressure of Pynchon's work, they admire (when they manage to admire him at all) only what is separably cute or charming or what is compact or economical, like *The Crying of Lot 49*" (153). Later Poirier depicts Pynchon as some sort of higher being, simply incomprehensible to the rest of us: "it is nearly impossible to feel about our cultural (even, sometimes, about our biological) inheritance the way he does. We don't know *enough* to feel as he wants us to feel" (155).

Certainly, it is the sheer *enormity* of Pynchon's subject range and of the books themselves that impresses so many of these readers, that demands a response equal in size and significance, as if Pynchon had thrown down a huge gauntlet or, more likely, unzipped his pants and released a huge phallus, challenging all to a literary pissing contest. But Pynchon's "size" here is less a challenge that male readers can accept or reject than a compelling demand to which many have submitted in terrifically suggestive terms. Levine and Leverenz claim that Pynchon's "forte is to seduce us into grail-hunting postures that he then parodies" (iv); Poirier's insistence that we "submit to the intense pressure" of Pynchon's work is coupled with a later remark about Pynchon's "masterful and feeling" (156) revelations. Mastery is also an overarching concern for Tom LeClair, who exhorts readers to submit to the skillful hand of Pynchon and other postmodern "masters." Scott Simmon, speechless over *Gravity's Rainbow*'s incredible bigness, makes interesting Freudian word choices when he at last finds his tongue: "The theme of *Gravity's Rainbow* is so huge that to confine it in a sentence makes it sound ridiculous, but it might be called an historical and cultural synthesis of Western actions and fantasies. A mouthful all right" (55). Richard Pearce speaks not for himself but "the reader, whom Pynchon compels to join in the search" ("Introduction" 6) for order and meaning in Pynchon's first three novels, and Lawrence Wolfley claims that "we" will "invent [connections] equally adequate to our needs" when we lose the trail set down by "the director" of *Gravity's Rainbow* (101). Quite simply, "we perforce read on" (101).

"Sez" who? In their rush to contend with the multiple psychosexual issues that Pynchon's work no doubt presents to them, Pynchon's cohort of admiring "size queens" makes overextended assumptions about readers' responses that, I argue, vary markedly depending on the race, social class, and perhaps especially gender of the reader in question. I freely admit that it is only Pynchon's entrenched canonical status—derived as all canonical placements are, not by the merit of the work itself, but by the amount and kind of response to it—that has caused *me* to include readings of Pynchon here. Overall, I find his work tiresome and repellent, his jokes childish and unsuited to the novel as a genre, his snide attitude inappropriate to effective political statement. I am among the negative respondents to Pynchon's work[35] who would find fault specifically with the *narrowness* of his vision, with the way he in fact aimed for "everything in the world" but fell short by a wide margin. While others have offered realistic assessments of the failed humor, the frail characters, even the botched German in *Gravity's Rainbow* and his other works, my critique of Pynchon regards how poorly he has always handled *me*—my experience and my perspective, my presence as a female receiver of his work.[36] Thus it is these words themselves, perhaps those of any feminist response to Pynchon's work, that open the close coupling between male author and male critics into the dynamic and inclusive triangular figure I have been examining throughout. Of course this structure is weak and temporary, poised to snap back into solid duality as soon as this discussion breaks; I look to other feminist voices engaged in this discussion to open the conversation more fully and permanently.

BOMBSHELLS AND BASKET CASES: GENDERED BOMB/ GENDERED ILLNESS IN NUCLEAR TEXTS

The readings that conclude this chapter speak to the triangular—or, more specifically, *triangulating*—dynamic between the plague periods examined here. Because of the rich historic and discursive relationship between these periods, a solid distinction, much less opposition, between "this plague" and "that plague" (the nuclear and the AIDS crises) is, as I hope I have shown all along, impossible. Thus while both bomb and illness imagery have been enlisted to heighten the gendered depictions, oppositions, and triangulations in these and other postmodern plague texts, neither of these image groups is exclusive to cold war– or AIDS-related texts, respectively: the issue of illness, particularly psychological forms such as paranoia, depression, and psychosis, has done much gender figuration in nuclear and especially cold war novels, while the bomb continues as a pointed and haunting presence in many AIDS texts. The images from these differing crises, then, *triangulate* each plague period between them, in equilateral (i.e., equally productive and provocative) fashion. Thus, analysis of these images illuminates not only gender's essential relationship to issues of cultural and planetary survival but also the deep significance these two plague periods continue to have for each other. If I may be permitted one more diagrammatic aid, the triangular relationship among the issues considered here comes to light:

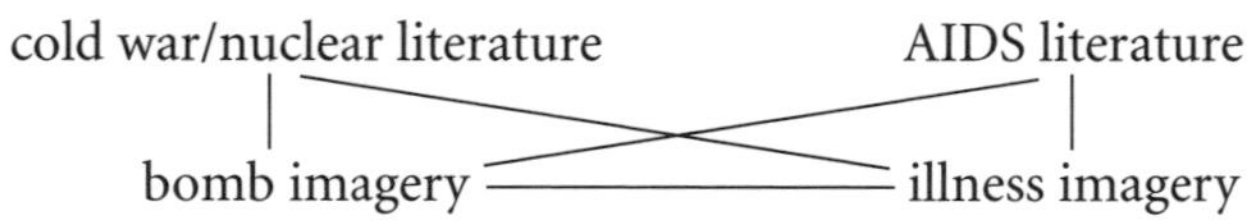

• • •

The connection between an exploding bomb and an explosive female sexuality has been informatively analyzed by Elaine Tyler May,[37] who discovers a connection between fear of the bomb and fear of women's newly gained liberation as productive members of the industrial war effort. With the return of American soldiers to the workforce, women's resistance to return to the role of homemaker/mother caused a panic in their male counterparts that elicited an equation between the bomb and unleashed feminine freedoms. As May notes, "It was not just nuclear energy that had to be contained, but the social and sexual fallout of the cold war itself" (94). Yet May also notes an explicitly sexual and thus more traditionally "feminine" association with the bomb that coincided with the more aggressive and threatening one outlined above. She describes a civil defense pamphlet that personifies radioactive rays as sexy women, noting that the implication here is that both women and nuclear energy "were potentially destructive creatures who might be tamed and domesticated for the benefit of society" (110). Likewise May points out the decision to name revealing women's swimwear the "bikini four days after the bomb was dropped [during underwater tests at Bikini atoll] to suggest the swimwear's explosive potential" (111).

Thus Philip Wylie condemns a "momist" character such as Netta Bailey in his novel *Tomorrow!* and offers in contrast his "bombshell," Lenore, who is both sexually attractive and effective in the civil defense of her city against a Russian air strike. She is a "geigerman" who dons a bright yellow suit and searches out "hot" material during drills, then during an actual attack forges into hot zones when the men around her hang back. While her aggressive behavior recalls the negative equation between the bomb and women's rights, her overt sexuality is almost immediately associated with the bomb-as-orgasm and thus recontained as traditional and nonthreatening. Interestingly, Wylie's mixed presentation of Lenore as both seductive and dangerous ("crazy" for wanting a man's job) is product and instigator of his own mixed perception of the bomb's ramifications: after multiple vivid depictions of the destruction brought by such an attack, Wylie fails to incorporate the added dimension of radioactive contamination to an accurate degree:

> He could see, in the heaving fire-light, that the dials on her gadget were jumping. But that didn't make her back away from the big slag heap, so he didn't back away.
>
> "It's hot," she said. "Plenty."
>
> . . . "Is it killing the men?" he asked.
>
> Lenore chuckled and shook her hooded head. "No. They'd be safe even sitting on it, for a matter of a few hours. But I wouldn't want it in my dining room for good."
>
> "Cigarette?" Lacey asked.
>
> Lenore unzipped her transparent face protector. "I'd love one!" (302)

It is interesting that Wylie was instrumental in founding the Atomic Energy Commission, advised the chairman of the Special Committee on Atomic Energy, and acted as consultant to the Federal Civil Defense Administration from the late 1940s to mid-1950s, and yet he still delivers this naïve estimation of the bomb's contaminating effects in his effort to support the feasibility of civil defense planning but also to recontain Lenore as nonthreatening and attractive, as receptive to the jumping dials of her Geiger counter as to a flirtatious remark.

While the bomb's terrifying yet exhilarating explosion has been associated almost exclusively with figurations of feminine sexuality, the bomb itself, with its obviously suggestive shape, has often been depicted as a phallic symbol, notably in Pynchon's *Gravity's Rainbow* and in Stanley Kubrick's film *Dr. Strangelove* (along with Peter George's novelization by the same name), where the bomb ridden by Major Kong to his (and the planet's) doom projects between his legs like an enormous phallus of destruction. Yet to determine the bomb as phallic symbol is in no way to balance the objectification of women-as-bomb with a similar objectification of men. As Lacan has persuasively argued, both the masculine and the feminine are enthralled by the phallic presence and both maintain an intimate—indeed, physical—attachment to it. Yet women, because they do not *have* the phallus, must console themselves with forever *being* the phallus and thus must contend with the *more* intimate relationship to the phallus and the added objectification it entails. Thus, even though a woman rides the phallicized bomb in Pynchon's novel[38] and a man rides it (significantly named "Lolita" despite, but also due to, its phallic suggestiveness) in George's, in both cases the bomb is being "ridden" (sexually subjugated) in traditionally oppressive fashion: as a sexual *object,* even (or especially) as a phallic *object,* the feminization of the bomb and the objectification of the feminine remain primary gender associations.

I noted earlier in this chapter that the bomb and its explosion, whether perceived as come-on or threat, feminine or phallic, are suffused with the notions of charged sexuality and high energy, of vigorous life and explosive potential and are thus contrasted to the opposite of explosion—cold war and espionage, the strain of normalcy during an age of lunacy—that are instead pathologized as "sickness" in nuclear texts. Much in medicine pertaining to the register of the "cure" requires a painful but necessary explosive moment—the broken fever, the lanced boil, the evacuated gastrointestinal tract—after which, and only after which, the wound begins to heal. In contrast, to put off such a necessary physical contortion may ease the condition of the sick in the short run but can worsen a medical prognosis overall. Interestingly, both anti- and pronuclear arguments are served by this set of analogies from the discursive fields of medicine and illness: a military hawk would defend the bombing of Hiroshima as the necessary "bad medicine" that ended the war, while a pacifist would insist that the only cure lies in the absolute elimination of nuclear weapons from the earth.

I have also argued in this study that the cold war, as originary postmodern plague, constituted a period of dissolving boundaries between "us" and "them" that transformed all acts of *violence* into epidemics of social and biological *illness*. Likewise the distance separating enemy camps, and the attendant ability to do violence "over there," without its having immediate and equally damaging repercussions "over here," disappeared: a strategic attack on any Soviet-allied territory would have brought immediate retaliation against U.S. interests and vice versa; there was no immunity from nuclear destruction, nor for that matter was there any safe haven from the contagion of cold war hysteria. Thus the *basket cases* found throughout nuclear texts are much more definitive of, yet much less often considered for their significance to, the cold war era than are the bombshell figures so commonly referred to by feminist commentators in this period.[39] However, as we locate many associations with the exploding bomb among stock figurations of women, I likewise find this condition of sickness brought to life by a return to this rich and generative trove. Here the equations between communists and sickness flourishes not only through depictions of female characters but almost as often with the aid of an intervening third term, "perversion"—that is, a homosexual lifestyle whose suspected inherent "weakness" produced a "limp-wristed" patriotism especially disruptive of national security. May observes a "sexual paranoia" that led McCarthyites (and the nation as a whole) to "link 'perversion' to national weakness" (96) and to persecute homosexuals as those most likely to succumb to the machinations of Soviet spies. In his study of cold war culture, Stephen J. Whitfield cites pundits of the 1940s and 1950s who described communism as "'something secret, sweaty, and furtive like . . . homosexuals in a boys' school'" (Arthur Schlesinger) and "susceptible to seduction" by Soviet spies, thus "'lack[ing] the emotional stability of normal persons'" (a 1950 Senate report). Likewise, Allan Bérubé documents a sharply escalating homophobia within the military in the postwar period that coincided with and exacerbated fears of communist infiltration.[40]

It must be noted that both female and queer male characters are "blamed" by probomb (anticommunist) nuclear texts when cited as a cause for cold war trouble—as perpetrator of espionage or treachery, as having weak constitutions in a time of nuclear crisis. Examples of these include the female spies/villains tortured and murdered by the heroic Mike Hammer in the novels of Mickey Spillane[41] and Pat Frank's character Helen in the popular thriller *Alas, Babylon.* In Frank's novel, Helen goes temporarily insane after a massive nuclear war, threatening the utopic stability of her family's structure. Stanley Kubrick's film version of *Dr. Strangelove* is crawling with perversions of "normal" masculinity, from the rarified Dr. Strangelove, to the effeminate President Muffley, to the hysterically silly General Turgidson. The villain of the piece, General Jack T. Ripper, perverts "normal" manhood through a hypermasculine obsession with war toys and war games that produces a patriotism spun out of control but also a decidedly queer attachment to other men. He suffers a mental breakdown, originating in a history of sexual dysfunction, an aversion to women that causes him to refuse to "share his essences" with them. In an uncomfortable scene, Ripper traps Colonel Mandrake in his office, drawing him close on a leather couch and whispering in his ear his plans to take over the army base he commands so as to initiate World War III. With phallic suggestiveness, Ripper wields a large gun during a shoot-out with his own soldiers, and Mandrake helps him through multiple orgasmic volleys by feeding him the necessary ammunition. Patriotism, pathology, and queerness also coalesce in the feminized Donald Pleasance character in Twentieth-Century Fox's *Fantastic Voyage.* His army scientist is a complex weave of villain (he is a spy for the "other side") and victim (he is also a shell-shocked veteran of World War II) of midcentury political upheaval. And in Wylie's *Tomorrow!* the eventual destruction of his "momist" nightmare, Netta Bailey, serves as a fitting end to the social ills (nuclear war included) for which she and her ilk are deemed almost entirely responsible.

According to Wylie, the dreaded "moms" of his era thought nothing of the welfare of their overworked, understimulated husbands or neglected children, pushed their nuclear families to attain and conform to middle-class status, and allowed their husbands to work themselves into early graves so as to surround themselves with fur coats and modern appliances. Momists were hyper-capitalistic and -individualistic; they thought little of their children's economic or political future or of the waste entailed in their ever-changing tastes and patterns of consumption. Our first glimpse of Netta merely novelizes this oft-central subject in Wylie's numerous political treatises: "Netta was pretty as a young woman; she was also durable and indomitable. Her personality was identical with her ambition which had been formed, delineated and defined to the utmost detail by American advertising. . . . She had found out, by the time she got her degree, that the style of man she wanted—rich, of course, important, social, urbane and worldly—would also have to be (if he were to marry her) weak and vain and somewhat gullible" (32–33). Significantly, Netta is a product of River City, the foolish virgin of the Sister Cities from Wylie's landscape, which neglects to prepare for civil defense and is thus left utterly disabled when nuclear attack actually comes. Although Netta has married over to the wiser, better defended Green Prairie side of the tracks, she still represents everything that is wrong with cold war society as Wylie sees it. Thus, the bomb dropped on her town, which disfigures her hideously and permanently, is the cleansing, cathartic antidote to the destructive, distinctly "un-American" momism she represents: had Netta not insisted on returning to the upper floor for her glamorous and voluminous wardrobe, she might have been spared the fate of "the blast [bringing] the window in on her. Her face, her breast, her abdomen were sliced to red meat. She was flung doll-like to the opposite wall" (278).

Of course the frenzy with which anticommunists sought to wipe out "sickness" in a weak national character only covered over their own debilitating infection—from a paranoia that had swept the nation so thoroughly that few thought to diagnose or treat it as such until years after it had subsided. Both Tim O'Brien and Maggie Gee have made studies of this fever of mistrust and hysteria, specifically its effects on average citizens who are much more inclined toward peace than the typical cold war militant ever was yet suffer just as severely the consequences of life lived in the shadow of a world-ending bomb. In response then to the large and influential probomb canon that burgeoned during the cold war, these recent novelists develop antibomb statements that nevertheless continue to depend on an equation between illness and the feminine. Importantly, however, instead of defining feminized illness as a *cause* of cold war madness, William (of O'Brien's novel *The Nuclear Age*) and Lorna (of Gee's *Burning Book*) are drawn as the symbol and *effect* of this madness, largely blameless and enormously instructive.

While perhaps not evident from my reading of this novel above, O'Brien's William *is* sympathetic to an antinuclear position insofar as his paranoia cum insanity is justified by the author's depiction of his traumatic early life. American baby boomers (though much more accurately here, "bomb babies"), like O'Brien and his protagonist William Cowling, had the misfortune to be extremely young, extremely impressionable, and extremely susceptible to nightmares and neuroses during an era that was terrifying to any thinking adult as well. As young adults they were further traumatized by the decision to accept, dodge, or protest the Vietnam draft, as well as the life-threatening trials attending each of these alternatives. In their early middle age, a Republican, bomb-happy administration refused to let the cold war go, drawing pictures of an "evil empire" to secure large funds for defense spending and subject their own children to more nightmares.

O'Brien's thesis, that all who have suffered through these times at these ages bear the unerasable scars with them yet, completes itself in the notion that to know oneself, to come to terms with the madness and violence inflicted on lives that were born and grew up with the bomb, is to succumb to the madness and violence that is the only "sane" response to it. Thus, William, while he might be eccentric and paranoid and, finally, even a danger to his family, is at least not in denial, not carrying out life in a self-delusory register that refuses to confront the nuclear threat (real or trumped up) in the enormity of its psychic debilitation. The early depiction is realistic and poignant, an effective antiwar statement:

> I was a child. There were few options.
>
> I scrambled out of bed, put on my slippers, and ran for the basement. No real decision. I just did it. . . .
>
> I went straight for the Ping-Pong table.
>
> Shivering, wide awake, I began piling scraps of lumber and bricks and old rugs onto the table, making a thick roof, shingling it with a layer of charcoal briquettes to soak up the deadly radiation. . . . I stocked the shelter with rations from the kitchen pantry, laid in a supply of bottled water, set up a dispensary of Band-Aids and iodine, designed my own little fallout mask. (12)

The seriousness and attentiveness to civil defense specification with which William labors to construct his shelter in the middle of the night is outweighed in pathos only by the ultimate futility of his efforts to be heard and understood. He is simultaneously a little crazy and (literally) the only one awake in a sleeping household, a sleeping society that would rather simply keep up with the Joneses and let the government handle the big questions. His family treats his construction project with belittling bemusement; finally William is sent to a psychiatrist, whom O'Brien quickly depicts as the crazy one.

William's increasingly nonconforming, antisocial life story is justified by its juxtaposition to a series of equally socially destructive historical events: the Korean War, the Vietnam War, nuclear proliferation, the conflict in Beirut. In the construction of an execution chamber/grave for his family (he digs an enormous, dynamite-rigged hole), William, with O'Brien's help, rewrites the "better dead than red" warmongering of the early cold war era: thanks to a largely delusional do-or-die mentality such as that characterized by the slogan, we have created a world in which we are only now, but undeniably so, better off dead.

Earlier in this chapter I discussed the homoerotics of O'Brien's novel, largely in terms of the male-male bonding that effectively erases the role of women in antinuclear politics, whether at the national level or in the grassroots sphere of one's own home front. We can align the "femininity" elicited in William by his queer counterpart (the seductive "talking hole") with his pacifism (albeit a peculiar brand) and liberal ideology; yet its potential association with William's paranoia and madness is intensely problematic for thoughtful readers: while we applaud William's eventual ability to overcome his murderous bent, we cannot receive William's simultaneous "restoration" to a heterosexual dynamic as any especially positive sign.

Still, while readable as madness and homosexual threat, the hole William digs is his true therapist, and his therapy as well. We note that he digs "in his own backyard," a cliché suggesting that the voice of destruction (and the silencing of it) that William perceives as coming from the hole actually comes from himself, echoing Dorothy's own prewar discovery in *The Wizard of Oz* that "there's no place like home" for the momentous journey of self-discovery she thought she would have to enter the stratosphere to undertake. Yet to stay at home, to choose life instead of death, is not a solution to the problem haunting William, but instead is a total reversal of its meaning for him. His conversion is complete and sudden, what Lee Schweninger in her reading of this novel calls a "radical epistemological shift," yet it leads into a meditation on the falseness of opposites (including those between life and death, knowledge and belief, insanity and madness) in a postmodern era that allows William to rebuild in the direction of secured physical well-being *and* mental health at once: "I will live my life in the conviction that when it finally happens—when we hear that midnight whine, when Kansas burns, when what is done is undone, when fail-safe fails, when deterrence no longer deters, when the jig is at last up—yes even then will I hold to a steadfast orthodoxy, confident to the end that E will somehow not equal mc^2, that it's a cunning metaphor, that the terminal equation will somehow not quite balance" (312). As inevitable as worldwide annihilation may be, we still live and love and daily save each other from smaller deaths, and the contradiction inherent in this postbomb condition calls even the opposite terms of an equal sign into question. The sameness of all opposites (and thus the imbalance of all balances) is a condition produced by the madness of the bomb and—since O'Brien tells us it is our only chance of survival—its simultaneous undoing.

If O'Brien breaks down the difference between present and future in an effort to preserve them both, Maggie Gee writes her antinuclear "case study" *The Burning Book* in wholehearted assault "against ending" by dissolving the boundary between present and past(s). Gee posits that wars (and particularly men of war) narrow the distance between entities meant to remain separate—the cultures of Japan and the United States, the "meat" of the *hibakusha* and its wrapper (the clothing that melted onto skin at Hiroshima), the present that holds the living and the future that brings only holocaust. While Gee describes as positive the empathy between the burnt and devastated *hibakusha* women and their British counterparts suffering from depression and paranoia in the postwar era, her novel speaks out against "unions" as overtakings, as storming through another's culture with superior weaponry and subjugating it.

In an effort to stave off this "ending" of the "beginning" begun at Hiroshima, Gee begins her chronicle of the Ship family over and over again, showing us the youth, adulthood, and old age of these related characters, yet rarely in that order and with repeated returns to earlier eras. It is as if the bomb has disrupted the normal progression of time, the linear movement of narrative itself, which has now developed an instinct toward planetary preservation by refusing to ever conclude. And yet the bomb (and again, specifically, war made by men) likewise incites narrative to produce a death drive as well: chapter after chapter the story of the family *does* advance, leaving off eventually with the stories of the elders, Rose and Frank, Prunella and Mervyn, and focusing more intently on the stories of the youth, particularly Guy, the middle brother of the youngest generation (the last generation to survive in Gee's nightmare), whose hatemongering ways are identified as the cause of World War III.

Like O'Brien's William, Guy's mother, Lorna, is almost exactly as old as the bomb—she was three in 1945—and, as in O'Brien's novel, the life of mental anguish this unfortunate timing bestows on her is a central feature of the story. As a child, some meat rotting in a case in her father's shop profoundly terrifies her, setting her off on a lifelong aversion to "raw meat," including everything from menu choices to dead bodies. Her decayed meat anxieties are brought horrifyingly to life through her father's death from cancer, and as a young adult Lorna realizes that war itself is the same such "rotten" endeavor: "She knew that people were meat, and other people were killers. She saw there was love, as well, but the two sides didn't balance out. . . . she didn't believe she was safe, and she knew that her babies weren't safe. Bodies weren't perfectly sealed: they could split and bleed like hers had. Or rot from inside like her Dad's. And so you were never protected" (75). Significantly, Lorna's family name is Lamb, allying her with the "meat" as opposed to the "killers" of the world, with sacrificial offerings being burnt alive in war-crazed nations everywhere.

Lorna passes on both vegetarianism and pacifism to her daughter, Angela, a politically aware product of several decades of women's liberation who comes of age during a time very close to our own, attempting to finish a dissertation on the postwar horrors her mother only sublimated through her paranoid fear of meat and meateaters. In Angela, who eventually overcomes this aversion with the help of her loving boyfriend, John, the paranoia emanates from a more abstract, unlocatable smell of *smoke*, of burnt cities and forests, the smell of sulfur and the sticky heat of August (in Acton or Hiroshima), during which it was "too hot to keep yourself separate. [Angela] felt swallowed up by things" (225). This fear of the blend, of the melting into, characterizes the condition of metaphor-as-illness as I have defined it, and here it coincides with Gee's overarching theme of the narrowing distance between worlds about to collide, between a present rushing forward to be engulfed by a future.

In fact, all of the women in Gee's novel suffer from depressions and manias brought on by loveless marriages and the inability to speak their minds about the various turns their society takes. Joanna is nymphomaniacal and in love with her brother; Rose is depressed and eventually loses her husband Frank. Prunella drinks too much and raises her daughters to be ladies when she in fact is hypocritically negligent of her marriage bond. Likewise, the peaceable, sensitive men of this family suffer emotionally as well—from alcoholism, depression, infidelity, and unnatural attractions to their daughters. That Angela is the first of her family to face her anxieties, through an investigation of the historical circumstances producing them and through an activist role enabling her to alleviate them, but is then cut off in her youth by the activity of warring men is the final tragic irony of Gee's story.

Lorna's other two children each joined an "army"—the bear-like but gentle George enlists in the regular Queen's army, and the hate-hardened, unlovable Guy joins a troop of black-shirted neo-Nazis creating havoc among the minority populations of the London suburb where they live. Guy is, of course, too young to have been instrumental in the atomic bombings that visit this world "during" (i.e., as an end to) this period—in fact he is the first to die violently in the novel, in an unrelated, neo-Nazi event. Yet the hatred stirred up in him by his despicable neighbor Big Ray (significantly, a butcher who "enjoys his job" entirely too much) is explicitly linked to the world-ending crises that follow through the meditations of Ray's abused yet self-possessed wife: "*Stupid old bugger,* she thought, as his voice droned on, *all acting.* A tide of pure resentment filled her: that they always had the power. They were just like babies, men. Inventing battles and fighting. It was pigs like him started wars. Then everything came to a halt" (172).

Guy's death signals an even larger ending, as shortly afterward news of escalating violence with Russia begins to reach the world occupied by Lorna and her husband Henry. They nevertheless plan a day at Kew Gardens and are amazed at the desertion of the urban surroundings, at the way the world has indeed, surprisingly, "come to a halt." Unaware of the exact magnitude of the danger at hand, Lorna and Henry have a picnic in the park and reaffirm their love for each other on this quiet yet seemingly charged afternoon. With the family scattered and in much disarray, no good-byes said, no offenses forgiven, the bomb strikes both Lorna's world and Gee's text itself. *The Burning Book* succumbs to smoke and silence as several of Gee's final pages of the novel proper are printed blank and blackened.[42]

To consider the differences between O'Brien's and Gee's postnuclear case studies of tormented bomb-children, whose neuroses only serve to make those of us less affected seem crazy, is to consider yet another issue of gender in this relationship between the bomb and (mental) illness. Martha A. Bartter, comparing women's and men's treatments of holocaust in science fiction and mainstream genres, notes that "women write more pessimistically than men about postnuclear reproduction" (261) and means by this not only reproductive rights but humanity's very chance for succeeding generations in a postholocaust world. She notes that men's optimistic treatment of apocalyptic themes is played out in various fantasies—genetic fantasies (humans remaining fertile) and technological fantasies (machines saving the day)—both variations of an underlying control fantasy in which women do not nearly as often indulge. In a similar vein, Paul Brians notes that "women generally depict nuclear war with more sensitivity and intelligence than male authors" ("Nuclear Family/Nuclear War" 135), citing concerns for family, children, and neighborhood that demonstrate the important fact that "in the atomic age science is everybody's business" (137). Interestingly, Brians notes that radiation sickness is an important issue in women's nuclear fiction, whereas with men "blast effects are far more often depicted" (135). This dichotomy reproduces not only the shift from violence to illness that characterize the move from modern to postmodern eras (see chapter 1) but also the traditional gender associations of men with explosion/orgasm (Bartter's "fantasies") and women with illness or weakness, an equation they have suffered within for centuries.

While certainly there are exceptions to these findings—Neville Shute's *On the Beach*, Whitley Strieber and James Kunetka's *Warday*, and the not surprisingly more realistic treatments of nuclear war by Japanese male authors, for instance—a sizable majority of postapocalyptic and science fiction texts authored by Western male authors during the cold war consists of these big-boom/regeneration fantasies. *No* women's nuclear texts that I have encountered (and this blanket assertion is easy to make since there are so few women's texts out there) have ignored the reality of nuclear catastrophe in this way. Cold war classics such as Helen Clarkson's *Last Day* and Judith Merril's *Shadow on the Hearth*, and more recent works such as Lynne Littman's *Testament* and of course Gee's novel, emphasize threats to the well-being of family and community and the challenge presented by material realities that women have always faced—providing food, shelter, medicine, and survival for children and neighbors, often with a husband missing or dead—as more difficult but more necessary than ever in the nuclear aftermath.

We can observe that of the two authors O'Brien has indeed produced the more optimistic, almost miraculously redemptive text, which relies, if not on genetic fantasies per se, at least on the powers of sexual and familial love to save not only William from madness but the world itself from the nuclear nightmare. Likewise his emphasis is on the explosion, the bomb that will go off in his backyard or over his entire nation, and the sexual connotations of this bomb and the hole he digs to avoid it have already been discussed. Meanwhile, Gee does not offer eleventh-hour reprieves but instead unleashes onto her characters the worst of all possible outcomes, sparing only her readers in a posttextual last warning. While she, too, depicts nuclear explosion in her final scene, the focus of the novel is on illness and deterioration processes—madness, rotting, family deception that worsens like a festering wound over the course of generations—that strongly resemble the radiation sickness that concerns other women novelists.

Additionally, O'Brien's male protagonist William is quite typically male in that he takes a much more *active* role in both the demonstration of the bomb's negative effects on him and of his response to this ever-present fear than does Gee's female central figure Lorna, who buries her anxieties amongst the distractions of marriage and motherhood, passing on both her fears and hopes to her children. While both authors argue that the joining of armies is explicitly counterproductive to securing peace for a nation, O'Brien suggests that the *male* bomb baby, be he veteran or draft dodger, is exposed to the trip wire paranoia suffusing his culture during the Vietnam era. Thus William's derangement is far greater and more violent than Lorna's, yet, says O'Brien, it is far more justified. The difference between their two statements lies in Gee's refusal to justify any such paranoid violence, despite its plausibility.

Thus, while O'Brien offers examples of both devastating, McCarthyite paranoia and the unexploded, less condemnable versions born in response to it within the psyche of a single male character, Gee divides these two pathologies into different characters, assigning, significantly, the violent fear turned into hatred to the ultraconservative male (Guy) and the inner-directed fears and anxieties to several of her women characters. While we might argue that Gee's essentialism is extreme, we must also argue that O'Brien's deconstructivism (William's craziness is "sane") is equally questionable; in any case, both authors have developed a profile of cold war illness that is chilling in its profoundly contagious effects: unlike the nuclear showdown that remains only an unrealized nightmare (or, horrifically, a dream for some), the cold war fallout of paranoia, accusation, and violence affected the most conscientious of cold war objectors and continues its weakening effects on the global condition through perpetuation of blind nationalisms, wasteful stockpiling, and the dangerous rhetoric of war.

TANTRUMS AND TIME BOMBS: GENDERED ILLNESS/ GENDERED BOMB IN AIDS TEXTS

Of course images of illness suffuse the intraepidemic text and run the gamut of physical, psychological, and psychosomatic manifestations; as in the nuclear texts, female and gay male characters embody these themes most often, although their positions of attachment to illness themes are, not surprisingly, reversed: sickness in AIDS texts is primarily a gay male issue and always only secondarily a narrative element used to define women. As was the case with several AIDS texts discussed above, women here are typically removed from the heart of this crisis by various devices that either "angelize" them into irrelevance or metonymize the illnesses they may have by removing them to the realm of inconsequence: women suffer here psychologically—from depression, paranoia, eccentricities, or even just overactive imaginations—and from an array of other "minor" (nonfatal) illnesses, so that the benignity of their situations, and their inappropriate overreactions to them, prevent these conditions from ever being construed as valid and instructive metaphors for AIDS itself.

As mentioned above, Tony Kushner's Harper Pitt from *Millennium Approaches,* the first part of *Angels in America,* conforms well to this profile. Her character, more than any other in the play, is controlled and defined by a symptom complex; finally she verges on being an allegory for illness itself, which has the effect of removing her from the realm of the human and minimizing our ability to care about her. Kushner's thesis is that, although hardly an unmediated decision, Harper's marriage to a gay man, the outrageous falseness of a love relationship she has exhausted herself trying to ignore, is the cause of her mental breakdown, that it is not Joe's lack of desire for her but her own (i.e., straight society's) pernicious homophobia that is to blame. Thus, her abandonment and deep depression at play's end are depicted as inevitable if not justified, the only possible outcome of a culture and a psyche so thoroughly entangled in self-deception.

In *The Weekend* Peter Cameron's Marian has suffered "skirmishes with depression" for many years and survived two suicide attempts in the middle-distant past. The wife of a rich man in upstate New York, Marian (with her husband, John) lives a life of cultured ease in a large, comfortable country house; yet John's half-brother, Tony, has died of AIDS, and this, coupled with the recent birth of a child, threatens to upset a precarious psychological balance Marian had only recently begun to regain for herself. Tony's lover, Lyle, who remains a close friend, comes one weekend to the estate but brings, much to Marian's dismay, his new lover, Robert:

> "This . . . this messes everything up. [. . .] I had invited Laura Ponti to dinner. [. . . Now] it will be five instead of four with this mystery friend of Lyle's."
>
> "And what's the problem with five? It's not as if you were trying to set up Lyle with the old lady."
>
> "That's not even funny," said Marian. "No, it's just that—well, there's a difference between four and five. Four is intimate, and five isn't. Everyone knows that." (47)

Marian's unfounded aversion to Robert's presence verges on paranoia and signals not only a resurgence of her underlying mental instability but also that its latest manifestation will indeed take the form of trying to "set Lyle up with the old lady"—herself. Unable to let go of Tony the way John and Lyle have quite appropriately begun to do, Marian would ensure that Lyle remains faithful to his memory (and his family) by preventing future relationships. Thus her protests here are not so much on Tony's behalf as her own, that is, her own version of grieving for her dead brother-in-law and her inability to let him go.

Marian as a stand-in for Tony fills out a "romantic" triangle initiated by Lyle and Robert's relationship, causing conflict in all directions. Awaiting Marian (and the past she represents) at the train station, Lyle suffers an attack of anxiety whose source he cannot name yet which is tied explicitly to Marian and her anticipated reaction to Robert. Marian and Robert's first exchange is testy and testing; she houses them in a room filled with old photos of Lyle and Tony and reacts overdefensively to Robert's remark about preferring museums to houses. Later, like a jealous wife, she resents Robert's intrusion into her conversation with Lyle, summing up her irrational attitude and accompanying disinclination to improve on it: "He's not a bad person. I just don't like him" (106).

Yet Marian's attachment to Tony is justified in light of the very good person he is revealed to have been and the magnitude of loss his passing represents. Marian recalls that "when she was in the hospital [for her suicide attempt] Tony was the only person she could really bear to see. She felt guilty with everyone else . . . as if she had to explain what had happened, explain her inability to live" (147). Tony in effect saves Marian by teaching her how to "believe that there was something present that could save you" (148); his inability to save himself in spite of this healing advice generates guilt within Marian now that he is gone. In many respects she owes her life to Tony and cannot give up the idea that he in some way exchanged his life for hers.

Thus, Marian's inability to complete her grieving for Tony and accept Lyle's new interest in another man is, though not fatal to herself, "AIDS-related" in a way that Harper's self-centered mental ailments were not.[43] Yet it is nevertheless contrasted to the admirably stoic acceptance of the men in the story, who emerge successfully from grieving for lost brother or lover or, in Robert's and especially Lyle's case, face the possibility of an early and tragic death from AIDS themselves. Marian's paralysis and hostility, in light of all the healing left to be done and of her own perfectly sunny physical prognosis, look absurd in comparison to the male reaction to the crisis: Robert leaves the estate feeling hurt and betrayed by Lyle in the middle of the night; their relationship seems all but destroyed, and Marian admits to the damage done by her unkindness only when it is well past the point of being able to do anything about it. Thus illness, even AIDS-related illness, in female characters like Harper Pitt and Marian appears as out of place, an irrelevant luxury, in male-authored texts. The hysterical symptoms these women exhibit reinscribe them as self-involved, spoiled, and immature, depicting their positions as paradoxically AIDS-"related" yet HIV-"negative."

Interestingly, the presence of bomb metaphors in these AIDS stories often signals a return from explorations of the metonymic (tangential/female) illness in general to a confrontation with HIV/AIDS itself: while these lesser illnesses play themselves out alongside of but removed from the larger crisis, acting not as metaphors for but as counterpoints to the tragedy of life and death with HIV/AIDS, the bomb emerges as an involving, productive metaphoric concept capable of speaking about the experience of HIV-positivity and the threat of AIDS in remarkable ways. In *Afterlife* Monette describes the various progressions of illness in those infected: "Some time bombs ticked louder than others, and some were hidden very deep in the caves of a man, but it was still only a matter of time" (149).[44] A chapter from Peter McGehee's *Sweetheart,* describing the growing anxieties of a group of HIV-positive men whose health is "fine, so far," is called "Time and Other Bombs." In works by both Paul Reed and Larry Duplechain, one character suspects another character of "dropping" this time bomb, damaging the relationship between them. In Reed's *Facing It* David fears an HIV-positive status and wonders whether "Andy [had] given it to him, and now, at this very moment, as his heart beat and his cheeks flushed, the virus was incubating, ticking away in his system like a time-bomb" (qtd. in Kruger 88). In Duplechain's *Tangled Up in Blue* HIV-positive Crockett accuses his healthy friend Harold of consigning him to death prematurely, as if Crockett "were some sort of bomb that could explode at any moment" (qtd. in Kruger 95). These many images of a time bomb running down its clock effectively convey a sense of the certainty of explosion that causes such traumatic uncertainty in the PWA characters themselves.

In an interesting cinematic variation, Gregg Araki's *Living End* reverses the assignments of bombed and bomber to turn the tables on traditional AIDS victimizers. In a pivotal scene, Luke, a handsome, HIV-positive drifter and petty thief, explains to his new lover Jon his guiltless amoralism: "There are thousands, maybe millions of us walking around with this ticking time bomb inside of us, making our futures finite. Suddenly I realize, we got nothing to lose. We can say fuck work, fuck the system, fuck everything. . . . We're totally free. We can do whatever the fuck we wanna do."[45] Trapped by the "neo-Nazi Republican final solution" that refuses to find treatments, to defuse the bomb ticking inside him, Luke turns his impending death into a weapon against the state and urges Jon to do the same. The lovers embark on a spending spree with a stolen credit card, play perpetrator and accessory to a violent assault, and later in the film flee from authorities after Luke shoots a cop. Significantly, the lovers are never caught or even chased by police during their "escape," which suggests that their inescapable medical condition has already judged and convicted them. As with the "walking time bombs" depicted in more traditional narratives, Araki's self-proclaimed "irresponsible film" places these HIV-positive heroes on a course of destruction that harms all others in their path yet engulfs themselves as well.

Andrew Holleran titles his collection of memories of and memorials to a changing, dying culture *Ground Zero* (a reference to New York City), casting the virus as a specifically nuclear bomb. The shift in metaphor—from the ubiquitous but provocative "time bomb" to the more intriguing nuclear explosive device—intensifies the crisis surrounding the disease: in this new light, the virus is revealed not as a random, isolated, inevitable surprise but as a politically motivated, demographically aimed, widely devastating weapon whose power finally threatens whole cultures and the planet itself: "World War I, we say, had causes, meanings, lessons. The Spanish influenza, which carried off hundreds of thousands after the war, did not. And yet because as long as it lasts, we must think of it as war and not some fatal flu, writing about AIDS will appear, and . . . inevitably be judged, I suspect, as writing published in wartime is: by its effect on the people fighting" (Holleran 17). Thus a "cold" war has transformed and escalated into a "flu" war with much more deadly effect. We must note that from this activist viewpoint it is impossible to dispense with the metaphors Susan Sontag and others have found so damaging to the cause of patients' rights. In Holleran's fully valid estimation, there is indeed a war out there—if not on AIDS then certainly on persons with AIDS, for patients are indeed "victims"—that is not of illness or uncontrollable circumstance but of an ignorant and indifferent social aggregate.

In several respects, Robert Ferro's illumination of the connection between the bomb and AIDS reverses and enlarges the efforts of the previously mentioned writers by moving from figural to literal representation of the bomb. His remarkable *Second Son,* ironically the last novel I came to in preparation for this study, is "finally" the foundation for it, a story that would have no doubt sent me in the exact direction I find myself to have taken had I come upon it first; nevertheless, it makes for a fitting conclusion to the literary portion of this project, an illuminating exploration of the relations between the nuclear threat and the AIDS crisis in our present age and of the solutions to these social ills that, while depicted as long shots so farfetched as to be "out of this world," have yet to be succeeded by completely effective alternatives.

Ferro's thesis, as mine has been throughout, is that both the potential violence of the nuclear crisis and the manifest violence of the AIDS epidemic are profoundly "environmental" issues that, Ferro argues, cannot be countered but only escaped by a radical change in environments. Like me, Ferro expands the concept of environment to include the natural *and* the social (i.e., political) spheres, both of which overlap and contend for the same space, with natural life (including humanity) losing most of the contests between them. Thus, AIDS is only the most recent in a series of environmental disruptions that began with the atom bomb but now includes the *Challenger* disaster, the toxic cloud from Chernobyl, and the failure of medical technology to contain the viral armies that are rushing in through the gaps caused by such disruptions and threatening the entire human race.

Recognizing this, Ferro's Mark and Bill, two lovers dying from AIDS, attempt to employ these disaster-producing technologies to their own ends, hoping to harness the potential emanating from them for lifesaving uses. In Rome the summer of the Chernobyl explosion, Mark and Bill take to the deserted streets, heartened by the possibility that "a mild dose of radiation might be good" in the effort to contain Mark's burgeoning Kaposi's sarcoma lesions (82). Indeed the two men are exposed to the toxic cloud, receiving "Iodine 131, Strontium 90, and Cesium 137, in unknown quantities" (87), yet they are too much in love with each other and Italy to be harmed by this. Indeed, Ferro suggests that their love for each other, and the inverted state brought about by their HIV-positivity (in a "normally" negative world), have in fact converted this toxic event from dangerous to curative: "Now, day by day . . . Mark watched [the lesions] fade. The bubble itself emptied and flattened, leaving a scarcely noticeable discoloration. . . . Headaches gone. This might mean nothing or everything" (103).

Likewise the *Challenger* disaster (a "bomb" that exploded going up instead of coming down) is a haunting and saddening presence throughout the story, underlining the shared early history of nuclear technology and space exploration, both advanced as weapons against the Soviet threat. As with the Chernobyl disaster, Mark and Bill would divert space technology to more benign and curative purposes, joining their friend Matthew in the financing of an expedition to the not-so-distant star, Sirius, inhabited by former earthlings, Matthew says, who welcome and await them. A group of "highly organized queens" in Austin, Texas, the Lambda Project, engineers and raises funding for the expedition, an all-gay tour of the galaxy that will allow its passengers not only safety from future uncontrolled meltdowns but a change in atmospheres profound enough to yield a cure for AIDS as well.

While waiting for the Lambda Project's ship to get off the ground, Mark and Bill enter into a new drug protocol that may prove effective in the containment or even amelioration of their enlarging spectrum of symptoms. A brother of each man must donate blood to be combined with a "new kind of interferon" and injected into their respective siblings as a kind of antiretroviral transplant. The novel ends with the lovers waiting, hopefully, for any one of these technological power sources to pay off. Yet Ferro, in aligning the Chernobyl effect and the medical protocol with the mostly ludicrous and financially ruinous trip to Sirius, forces us to question whether any of these solutions will work, whether the only thing keeping Mark and Bill alive after all is their love for each other: shortly after the physical improvement following the lovers' radiation exposure, new lesions appear on Bill, calling the reprieve into doubt. Likewise, a reading of this text several years after its publication reveals the interferon treatment Ferro describes to have been similarly inconsequential, if it ever existed at all.

Thus, the bomb-as-metaphor that Monette and Holleran feel is ticking within or blasting down on is not necessarily converted from illness to cure when depicted literally, as the "effects of radiation" we in the AIDS era must continue to deal with and suffer from in addition to more recent plagues. Indeed the Chernobyl cloud (as well as the weapons and space technology that continue to germinate from the same nuclear seed) is much more akin to illness than cure and, finally, makes a more successful metaphor for the AIDS virus itself than it does a metonymic "island" of security (recast in Ferro's novel as a distant planet) where we may, for the right price, find a perfect salvation. Not a spaceship but a house shaped like a ship, the beach house that Mark's family has owned for years and that is by far his favorite member of the family is his and Bill's final safe haven from the swirl of environmental disasters around them. Though his family wants to sell it to save his aging father's business, Mark recognizes that his own life, the quality of what life he has remaining, depends on this house, and he ultimately succeeds in securing it from their profit-seeking plans. Sheltered from, yet anchored securely within (both will start their new drug treatments shortly) the technological realities of life on earth, the men are enabled to pledge vows of unwavering love:

> "It's no good unless we both live." Mark sat up and looked at him. "I mean it."
>
> "I know. Don't you think I know that?"
>
> "Well, will you?" Mark asked again, now that the question was qualified.
>
> "I will never leave you," Bill whispered.
>
> "—Whatever happens," Mark went on. "No matter what."
>
> "No matter what," Bill repeated.

The question of their continued lives together must be "qualified" to include finally a spiritual union that allows for the possibility of their physical falling away, because neither their beautiful house nor a fantastic interplanetary voyage can protect them from their biological fates. Such safe havens or "spare planets" do not exist and thus cannot spare the lovers in Ferro's novel, nor would they spare any of us from a terminal disease or a ruined earthly ecosystem. Rather, they are more examples of the metonymic—the utopic, perfect island that is only a divisive delusion—as described in chapter 2.

• • •

Ferro and many others examined in this chapter point clearly to these islands' ultimate nonexistence, to the need during desperate days to turn inward to our spiritual resources and, perhaps finally, to technological advancements that will enable us to move beyond devastating plagues. To posit an "out there," a zone of order and control surrounding yet separated from the inner field of destabilized, triangulating chaos is to reestablish the false binaries (and false hopes) that have plagued not only the political progress toward peace and cure but relationships between sexes and genders throughout modernity. As demonstrated above, all the plague texts surveyed here depict heterosexual couplings and oppositions in sometimes subversive but often troubling ways; and interestingly, the introduction of a "third term" with respect to plague *imagery*—illness metaphors into the bomb image/nuclear text pairing, bomb metaphors into the illness image/AIDS text pairing—only helps to reinforce gender dichotomies along traditional lines: the "feminine" pathologized in nuclear texts, the bomb imagery defining male characters with "real" illness (AIDS itself) in AIDS texts.

Significantly, it is not third terms but "third wheels," triangulating characters themselves, who are the successful elements in challenging and disrupting these traditional pairings. These triangulating characters, featured in the AIDS-era novels discussed above, work effectively to redefine marriage, family, the committed relationship, the activist life, even psychic identity, and they often succeed in changing their fellow characters' smug assumptions about life, love, and sexuality. Always they have a destabilizing effect on the equally smug ideas of their readers, who must grapple with their definitions of the perfect couple, the happy ending, and new meanings of the heroic. Finally the gender instability found in these texts reflects the political and biological instability found there—and everywhere in the extraliterary world as well. It is a powerful symbol and reminder of the difficulty, if not impossibility, of stabilizing and containing the plague threat inside some expendable danger zone and of the vital need to eradicate through political and medical progress the indifference that propagates this threat.

4

Two Takes on a Scare: Cinematic Plague Texts and Their Remakes

THE RETURN AS THE REPRESSED: PLAGUE FILM REMAKES

In a climactic scene from Irving Yeaworth's cold war classic *The Blob,* the eponymous creature boils through the screen of a movie theater, where a monster movie is midway through its own project of horror and sensation. Their cinematic nightmare come to life, the audience of teenagers in Yeaworth's film runs from the theater on a screaming rampage, and the camera angle in this mad exit scene (faithfully reproduced in Chuck Russell's 1988 remake) is from above the heads of the fleeing teens, pitched to a moderately steep degree: the bird's-eye view "enworms" its objects below, reducing their size but emphasizing their frantic activity, causing the teens themselves to resemble significantly the slithering hordes of countless other horror classics in that era and suggesting an equation between their blind hysteria and the eerie, monstrous threat rolling out the doors behind them. The horror effect produced not by the blob itself but by its panic-stricken audience is due not only to the distancing and disorientation of the camera but to its sheer magnitude, to the terror as it is *repeated* body after body across the screen. In a macabre relay, the fright generated by the blob itself is handed off to the filmic audience and then to us, the viewers, moving finally as *contagion*—as a language that is so accessible to and accessing of our deepest fears and fantasies that it can leap off the screen and send us screaming—with fear or elation—into the night.

While it has been my aim throughout this project to examine the mark and meaning of contagion as registered in nuclear and AIDS-era novels, plays, and nonfiction, it is necessary at this point to turn to film as the most "communicable" of all genres—so widely attended, so enormously influential—

to complete our understanding of plague's effect on this postmodern era. Yet film is not only enormously infectious of its viewing audience but is also in deep and generative conversation with itself, the multiple cinematic texts that comprise its whole, especially through the original/remake relationship. Film's terrifically productive reiterability, its propensity to remake an "original" so often and so obliquely that this concept of originality is all but obliterated, lends itself well to my purposes here. In the cold war original/AIDS-era remake relationship we see more clearly than ever the complex cultural overlap between these two periods. The metaphoric or "blueprint" structure I have been describing throughout will become most evident in our comparison of these two periods, no longer through examination of their respective textual productions but through the lens of a single text, the "same" (original and remade) film(s).

Certainly film's massive influence has done even more to enlarge hysterical fears of reds, gays, HIV, and AIDS—the fears I have defined throughout as "plagues"—than many of the literary examples examined in preceding chapters. And as multiple film theorists have pointed out, the more mainstream, familiar, and familiarizing a film is—as many of those selected for inclusion here are—the more xenophobic and difference-eliding it is likely to be.[1] Meanwhile, films delivering positive challenges to the weakness and phobias at the heart of such hysteria create an effect worth delineating as well. While some of the remakes discussed here perpetuate the stereotypes and false assumptions plaguing their original versions, many of the AIDS-era remakes and even a few of the cold war originals approach audiences with the intent to clarify the mysteries dividing us from others, seeking to mitigate plague's negative fallout. I rely on psychoanalytic theories in many of the following discussions in an effort to connect postmodern hysteria to age-old *anxieties*—castration fears, trauma, and grief due to awareness of our removal from language, Oedipal "anxieties of influence" generated by the remake relationship (about which more will be said below). Perhaps more difficult to identify and acknowledge, the psychic anxieties underlying the very condition of human existence, and brought dangerously (or thrillingly) close to consciousness during the cinematic-viewing experience, may in part explain (though they certainly do not justify) the visible forms these fears have burgeoned into in the postmodern age.

The eight films chosen for discussion here are various in theme, style, and genre, though horror is, perhaps not surprisingly, the prevailing mode; and this prevalence reinforces our sense that what relates these two periods most complexly is primarily frightful and nightmarish. Original and remade versions of *The Blob,* hailing from this horror tradition, indeed constitute the purest remake relationship to be examined here, with the later film retracing the path of its predecessor carefully, respectfully, and completely. This discussion will come last for that reason. First, however, three film pairings selected from more mainstream genres—and these include, in various combinations, science fiction, comedy, satire, action, and drama—will be read so as to demonstrate the range and influence of plague films in both eras and to explore multiple ways in which AIDS-era films converse with cold war predecessors, remaking and redefining the terms of discussions initiated by these, even in the absence of a complete (or even rudimentary) remake relationship as it is traditionally conceived. As I therefore play rather fast and loose with the concept of a remake, I will also, again purposely, enlarge my definition of an "AIDS film" to include some of those appearing quite early in this period—the late 1970s and early 1980s, when the epidemic was forming in the bodies of its first victims, if not yet in the public consciousness: as I hope to have shown throughout, plague-related cultural representations not only *follow after* and *respond to* political and biological threats to the social body but in important ways *prepare* and *influence* our response to these very threats. Themselves products of the cold war that coincided with the sexual revolution and completed an outbreak of "bad sex" films produced throughout the 1970s,[2] these very earliest of AIDS films taught audiences to fear sexual identities and freedoms in new ways that would be tragically realized only a year or two hence. Ranging from silly to satiric to serious, all eight films partake of the dialogue that fueled or defused rational fears and uncontrollable hysteria in response to nuclear and epidemiologic threat.

INCREDIBLE SHRINKAGE: HAVING THE PHALLUS/BE(COM)ING A PENIS

In her study of midcentury "returning soldier" films, Kaja Silverman points out that the trauma produced by the war was strong enough to pierce the insulating "dominant fiction" of classical film narrative and erupt through a series of films dwelling on, instead of diligently disavowing, men's own castrated condition. She examines William Wyler's *Best Years of Our Lives* (1946), with its disillusioned, disengaged veterans as represented most vividly in the character of Homer, who has lost both hands in the war, played by Harold Russell, a real-life double amputee. Homer's obvious deficiency renders him helpless to provide for his family and initiate sexual activity with his girlfriend, turning him into a feminized "object of a probing social gaze" (121). Homer's and the other soldiers' stunted postwar condition invites a correspondingly "phallic" response from the women, who not only accept the men as they are but come to provide for them financially and rescue them from loveless marriages. While a postwar interpretation of this film, then, might have relied on a Freudian disavowal of men's castration, Silverman's more recent (AIDS-era) reading expands our recognition of "lack" and castration to implicate men as well as women.

In his reading of original and remade versions of *The Fly* (1958 and 1986), Adam Knee restates and concurs with this argument when he notes the difference between Helene's subordinated role in the original and Veronica's much more central function in the remake: "The [remake] is as preoccupied with male-female involvements as its predecessor, but we are here presented not with rigidly defined marriages but with the contemporary 'relationship' in which both genders have potentially commensurate social potency and in which sexual mores are not so rigidly codified" (24). Knee goes on to examine the explicitly antinuclear elements of the original version of the film, as well as the many AIDS-related implications of the latter, and the differences characterizing these two filmic contexts bear out his argument: where men shouldered most of the responsibility for (and thus enjoyed the power relationship to) the cold war nuclear threat, the gender blindness of AIDS has left each of us with our fingers on our own buttons, so to speak—that is, in roles of ever-increasing responsibility for our individual survival or demise. Indeed, we must recognize that women, in light of the escalating rates of maternal-child HIV transmission, may become even more centrally positioned than men with respect to diminishing or exacerbating this current epidemic. Thus Silverman's understanding of men—as "reduced" by their distance from the phallus as are women—seems even more valid in AIDS-era remakes than in the cold war films that are her focus: the enormous lack (of power, of immortality) that is all our lot is both democratizing and devastating, as our old source of salvation is, in this current crisis, unveiled and revealed impotent.

In discussing two films, Jack Arnold's *The Incredible Shrinking Man* (1957) and the 1981 remake starring Lily Tomlin, *The Incredible Shrinking Woman,* I will consider women's widening role from one plague era to the next as reflected in their complexifying relationship to castration anxiety, fetishism, being versus having the phallus, and, finally, representability within the Symbolic. Certainly, the notion of "shrinkage" is suggestive of multiple relevant issues—penile (and clitoral) disappearance or growth; fetishism; being the phallus (being reduced to a penis-sized creature); gender inequities and power struggles—and in the original film postwar conditions in general, not just those affecting returning soldiers, are blamed for reducing the potency of men's presence in the social order. Vacationing on a small boat in an isolated ocean setting, Scott Carey is contaminated by the radioactive dust coming from an underwater bomb test several miles away. Interestingly, Scott's wife Louise is spared from this danger, as she was throughout the war, by having been sent into the galley on a "woman's" errand, fetching her husband a beer. When she returns from below, we see the beginnings of an immediate role reversal, similar to that outlined by Silverman. "Look at your chest," Louise exclaims, shifting our gaze from its coerced fixation on the female star (and her chest) to the man's "breast," now covered with radioactive matter. Significant to my later argument, this fallout is sparkly and confetti-like, resembling much more Tinkerbell's fairy dust than anything ominous and organic associated with the bomb.

The incident is forgotten until Scott begins his shrinking process and the doctor questions him about radioactive exposure. I give the film much credit for acknowledging the multifactorial nature of so many postmodern syndromes; Scott has also been in the vicinity of pesticides (another 1950s cure-all/bio-nightmare), and this double exposure is determined to be the cause of his unfortunate condition. (I am also aware that the multifactorialism here has the effect of exonerating both global assaults in their singular forms. So long as you are not exposed to both within six months, the argument seems to go, you will be spared such horrific bodily crises and thus have no case against the use of either.) *The Incredible Shrinking Woman* also points out the multifactorial nature of our many mysterious and incurable late twentieth-century ills. In the early moments of the film Pat Kramer (Tomlin) is exposed to multiple noxious sprays and fumes that are indeed later determined to have caused her diminution. As opposed to the political and economic enormities that brought the radioactive clouds affecting Scott Carey, however, the story in the remake implies that the toxins that shrink Pat come from her dressing table and kitchen cabinet, that the banality of the "death rays" she atomizes onto herself daily is their most dangerous because most invisible aspect.

In both films our first glimpse of Scott and Pat as visibly smaller than the worlds around them (the first time camera trickery is employed to reveal the shrinking horror of it all) is almost identically produced. In living room scenes the camera is positioned behind a large, seemingly empty chair; family members and friends stare down sympathetically at the chair, addressing, it would appear, others around them but certainly not the nonpresence represented by the camera's point of view. When our gaze is swung around into the "empty" chair to reveal that, indeed, sixth-grader-sized Scott or Pat sits recessed therein, the films diverge again, this time along distinctly gendered lines. The moment in the original is rife with shock and horror: we cannot believe that Scott is so small. His voice and manner are preserved but his reduced physical state in the apple-pie suburban setting makes him seem doll-like and subhuman; the scene is, even today, disorienting and surreal. In the remake this moment is radically downplayed; Pat sips from a brandy snifter, now huge in her diminutive hands, and looks with mixed resignation and irony at her husband and his boss, who has come to visit. There is no emphatic chord of background music as accompanies the original, no sudden swings of camera positioning to reveal her size as especially shocking. As the film will imply throughout its remainder, women's smallness is, in fact, nothing much out of the ordinary.

Thus Tomlin here is not only riffing on the oversized chair and props of her well-known character Edith Ann but also on the classically understood position of women in their relationship to the castration complex, to its concomitant psychic baggage of loss and lack. We must read this film as arguing that women are always already in a position of smallness (if not nonexistence) with respect to ownership of a penis and the castration anxiety that threatened loss could produce. The earlier film says just as emphatically that men retain the penis as the tiniest promise for fulfillment in the Symbolic and therefore suffer enormous anxiety when castration is threatened. Its dreaded enactment, as begins to occur in this scene, is only shocking and unspeakable. We might note, then, that the difference between men's and women's relationship to the phallus is the difference, in this case, between dark horror and broad comedy.

From here the films continue on their diverging paths—Scott running off to join the circus and tarrying with a pretty carnival worker his own size, and Pat finding her fifteen minutes of fame on "The Mike Douglas Show," where even in her amazing smallness the "typical" insignificance of her role as housewife cannot be surmounted: Mike almost immediately ignores Pat's low-key narrative, answering his own questions with trivial remarks meant to keep the laughs coming. Despite his continued diminishment, Scott remains the controlling husband figure, growing more "tyrannical" and "monstrous in [his] domination of Louise" with each inch he loses. While the narrative moment describing this tyranny is clouded with sorrow and regret, Scott hardly amends his bullying ways but instead, by film's end, resolves to "dominate my world" as "man had dominated the world of the seen." His elemental struggles with house cat and hairy spider, his return to "instinct" and "clear thinking" at once suggest that he has regressed to a purer, even pre-Symbolic, caveman-type self. In the final scene his clothes are torn and bloodied, he is armed with spear and hook, he is small enough to at last escape through the screen of the basement, where he has been imprisoned for days—into the wilds of his suburban lawn. The music swells and the perennial reference to the Almighty and His universe salvages a happy ending from this most dismal and diminished situation: the last frontier is not the infinite but the (nuclear) infinitesimal. "To God there is no zero," Scott proclaims. "I still exist."

On initial analysis, then, the films support a traditional, gender-divided reading that would counter Silverman's equalizing efforts, suggesting that the very generic distinctions between the two, the irony and even comedy that enable Tomlin's film as both indebted remake and irreverent spoof, are integral to the differing relationships of men and women to the phallic order: Scott's loss of power is a tragedy, while Pat's is yesterday's news. And yet Silverman's argument prevails upon a second look at the original and remake, upon investigation of Scott and Pat not as entrenched in their normative heterosexual roles but as dependent on radical cross-gender episodes for the resolution of their respective stories. In the original film, for instance, the position of the ultranatural ur-male, destroyed by but also reborn of uncontrolled nuclear activity, is questioned and undercut by the explicit feminization he undergoes throughout the film as well. From the first scene, Scott's role as husband and provider is threatened when it is learned that the couple vacations on his brother's boat, not one Scott has purchased for himself. His position in his brother's advertising firm seems additive and extraneous even when he is of normal size; his shrinkage severs his business ties and his ability to provide, and his brother moves more and more clearly into the role of householder and husband figure. Likewise Scott is threatened by "Baby," the male cat that Louise holds in her lap and that later usurps Scott's position as master of the house by threatening his life and banishing him to the basement. Trapped in this underworld Scott pulls a nail almost as long as he is from some debris and points it, in a mystifying self-castration gesture, toward his own crotch, demonstrating minutes later that he is using it to cut off the legs of his trousers, turning his pants into a sort of toga. His weapons are in actuality pins and thread from his wife's sewing kit, and the climactic death scene with the spider leaves his skirt bloodied and torn, a use of mise-en-scène that would complete the most traditional of deflowered-virgin narratives. Finally Scott is most feminized by being shifted from the register of having to that of being; he is for most of the film no bigger than a penis, and equally as powerless.

Conversely, Tomlin's character in the remake, running off neither to the circus nor the backyard, prefers to stay at home in her domestic situation but is dragged by her profit-minded husband into the world of showbiz and best-sellers, leaving her exposed to the plots of evildoers. While Scott becomes isolated and elemental, Pat is hypersocialized and enmeshed; she becomes the prisoner of would-be world leaders who want to *inject her blood* into unsuspecting populations, shrinking them and capturing this new "small world" for their own control. Thus, Pat's shrunkenness is not prized as the purifying fallout of nuclear proliferation but is redrawn as a blood-borne, communicable condition that can produce a "global village" through radical population "reduction."[3] As Silverman would point out, then, that the feminization of men (returning soldiers) provides a prevailing theme in postwar films, I would argue concurrently that the masculinization of women—not only their increased proximity to plague-related threats but also their intensifying relationships to power, violence, and the ability to affect social change—marks the AIDS-related subtext of 1980s remakes, as demonstrated by Adam Knee and in the readings I present here.

For all these films' differences, we must note that protagonists of both, in their return to embryonic states, enact a retreat from normal (heterosexual) development—as it is depicted, at any rate, in classic Freudian, homophobic terms—revisiting the position of the other sex that was passed successfully through on the way to "normalized" gender roles. Scott is "returned" to the realm of the feminine, the life of the weak male child who is bested and controlled by his father (although this aspect of his journey is downplayed), while Pat retreats down the "circuitous path"[4] that brought her to femininity, reassuming a position of paternal identification to access and eventually overturn masculine provinces—international intrigue and world politics. While gender-switching by characters may be read in other films as provocative, even subversive, the overriding theme of shrinkage here recasts such steps sideways as steps backward, as regression—pathologic, presexual, out of control, and animalistic (at their smallest Scott is closely associated with a cat and spider and Pat with a laboratory ape)—and is thus intensely problematic.

While Scott remains, by film's end, in his shrunken, feminized state, Pat is restored to her normal size when she is doused in a pool of the multiple feminine sprays, creams, and gels that shrunk her in the first place. Yet the film's last laugh, born at the expense of its status as remake, is a shot of Pat's foot, bursting through her frumpy shoe, taking the film, literally, in an entirely new direction. This choice of the highly fetishized woman's foot as the viewed site of Pat's impending colossalization finalizes the equation between the feminine and phallic power: as far as heterosexualized roles are contrived and coerced, a woman's access to phallic representation is never fully severed. Savvy of smallness when it is forced on her, human (gender equal) and even superhuman (phallic) roles are part of her psychic past and cannot, therefore, be fully eliminated from her present experience.

PARASITES WITH SUBMARINES: SOME SMALL, SICK, SCIENTIFIC SPIES

Shrinkage as a theme continues into more mainstream plague films, although we note in this mainstreaming a recasting of shrinkage-as-pathology into a military-controlled "miniaturization"-as-science. In the same way that many beginning writing students insist that "utilize" has a smarter, more sophisticated ring to it than "use," one can put "miniaturization" to militaristic use, as in "Put them in the miniaturizer!"—when the command to "Put them in the shrinker!" would never be obeyed. This active, directed use of miniaturization continues in the vein opened by Tomlin's treatment of phenomenal smallness not as casualty of war but as political weapon; yet since shrinking suggests inner worlds, underworlds, buried secrets, and disappearance, we find ourselves in the register of espionage and information warfare, not in the semiotic of exploded bombs but the feverish underside to explosion—cold war spy games.

Richard Fleischer's *Fantastic Voyage* (1966) provides as useful an example as there is of the immunological dynamic that controlled cold war strategic thought. An Eastern Bloc spy's body becomes both friendly and hostile territory, as the gains to be derived from his defection to the West are canceled almost immediately when snipers from the "other side" wound him with a near-fatal gunshot to the head. A collection of cold war regulars—scientists, generals, and government bureaucrats—gather for an excursion in a markedly miniaturized state through the veins and arteries of the dying spy. Tension builds throughout the film through a remarkable realization—that the "good guys" are in fact themselves the enemy, that they will, should their inevitable regrowth take place while they are still within, be recognized as foreign invaders (in Soviet territory) and destroyed by the spy's immune system.

As with the cold war original of *The Incredible Shrinking Man,* the impending smallness of the scientific crew is associated here with a feminization, with castration and a loss of identity. The manly Stephen Boyd plays Grant, a communications expert who is hesitant about his call to service. "How much can a man give to his country?" he asks snidely upon entering the miniaturizing chamber, suggesting that the shrinkage, reversible though it may be, is also a sacrifice, that upon his restoration to normal size something will have been taken from him and not returned. That this sacrifice is linked to the castration threat is borne out by the female technical assistant's easy but eager attitude toward the mission. Grousing about "being shrunk" early in their journey, Grant is met with a quip from the assistant, Cora Peterson (Raquel Welch): "you may learn to like it." Again, as was implied in *The Incredible Shrinking Woman,* women's ties to a diminutive state place them in a position of relative power when miniaturization is not only a condition both genders must undergo but, here, the test of their patriotism.

Ironically, smallness is not an attribute that has ever attached itself to descriptions or images of Raquel Welch. In typical Hollywood fashion, her "bigness" is emphasized in this film by a tight jumpsuit, an even tighter diving suit for the underwater scenes, and camera shots that follow her movements so closely they are only the most subtle of her many second skins. Interestingly, coinciding with Cora's feminine large-breastedness is her masculine largeness of mind, as she is knowledgeable, unafraid, and, as the film eventually confirms, innocent of the sabotage plot afoot on board the sub. Instead the feminine gap on board is filled by the character of Doctor Michaels (Donald Pleasance, the perennial cinematic creep throughout the 1960s and 1970s), who is at first thought to be the most patriotic and motivated of the crew members but ultimately is revealed as a sissy and the true saboteur. Tellingly, his position of operation (he navigates the ship through the patient's arteries and organs) is at the feet of, literally between the legs of, the skipper of the ship, who sits above yet facing Michaels. When the two men speak Michaels looks directly into the skipper's crotch; his hands can be seen tracing routes on maps in a teleprompter in the skipper's perch—again, just at groin-level.

Doctor Michaels's early panicky outbursts in the enclosed, claustrophobic ship are forgiven when they are revealed to be the product of an old war injury. A two-day air raid in London during the last war has left him shell-shocked and weakened; his previous show of bravery now excuses and obscures his inability to handle the current crisis. Interestingly, the film overflows with weak, dependent men. The military types hanging around the control room, watching the ship's progress on radar, smoke like fiends and tank up on oversugared coffee. By film's end they are so overwrought by the fantastic voyage that the general cannot even kill an ant that frolics in the nervously spilled sugar. His colonel says warmly that the general will "wind up a Hindu," orientalizing, feminizing, and declassifying his superior in one move.[5]

While smallness was a nearly insurmountable problem in the earlier film pair, the inevitable return to normal size that marks these characters' situations signals an equally assured return to heterosexualized norms: when several of the crew have been swimming about in the spy's ear canal, Cora is singled out by the invading antibodies and covered with their sticky, weblike organisms. In a rape-like frenzy, the men drag her back to the ship and drop to the floor around her, clawing away at the suffocating antibodies (with their odd propensity to adhere to her chest). The feminized Doctor Michaels is treated to a similar ravaging: attempting to abandon the rest of the crew, he commandeers the ship and lodges in a gland, where he is immediately overcome with mounds of oozing lymph. When the four surviving crew members are fully restored, they return to their normalized roles as well: Cora is hanging limply on the arm of Grant; the secondary males Doctor Duval and the skipper slump or sit at a slight remove, granting the heterosexual couple its position of primacy. Any previously suggested equation between patriotism and gender role-reversal is jettisoned at this point, Cora's scientific abilities forgotten, Michaels's limp-wristed machinations soundly punished, and the miniaturization undergone by the masculine heroes plainly inscribed as a temporary, already surmounted state.

It would have been difficult to introduce *The Fantastic Voyage*'s AIDS-era counterpart into this discussion any sooner, largely because the Steven Spielberg–produced *Innerspace* (1987) is not so much a studied remake as a loose and widely digressing rip-off. I caution, however, that I do not (for the most part) use this term pejoratively; to insist that a remake be only overt or obeisant in its copying of an original is to forget that all films to some degree borrow and recycle themes, plots, and concepts with as much disregard and self-interest as *Innerspace* has here. While in fact Spielberg has only borrowed the doctor-within-the-patient concept to fuel an entirely different plot, these films are indeed in dialogue on plague themes, on the nature of infection and cures emanating from within. Most importantly here, the body invaded by the tiny scientist Tuck Pendleton (played by the rambunctious, eternal fraternity guy Dennis Quaid) is not passive and comatose on a surgical bed but walking and ranting about the San Francisco area in the skittish and hypochondriacal person of Jack Putter (Martin Short). Enormously suggestive for our reading here, the rebellious and aggressive Tuck (also the name of a well-known hemorrhoid treatment) enters the unsuspecting Jack's body, during a chaotic escape from evildoers bent on stealing Tuck's miniaturizing capabilities, through a syringe to his behind. Tuck spends the lion's share of the film "inside" Jack in this manner, both "riding" and "driving" the feminized Short to new heights of unabashed self-expression and manhood.[6]

Yet Tuck also "rides" Jack in the sense of Jack's being his only vehicle to rescue. Tuck is dependent on Jack not only for movement but for sight and sound, and his experience is as consummately controlled by Jack's actions as Jack's transformation is the product of Tuck's proddings from within. As one might expect from Spielberg, homosociality fostered by the men's bodily attachment is tempered (at least that is the attempt) by a popular, attractive female presence, Lydia (played by Meg Ryan, who later married Quaid in real life). In classic conformity to the triangle investigated by Eve Kosofsky Sedgwick in *Between Men,* the intensity of the relationship shared by the men is refracted through their mutual attraction for Lydia. Ironically, Jack's attraction for Lydia (Tuck's former girlfriend) is both the inspiration and barometer of his increasing masculine capabilities—that is, his ability to bring himself and Tuck to the proper authorities and effect a separation. Thus, Tuck must encourage Short's "growth" at the same time he is ever watchful of and threatened by it. The conundrum is emblematized in the kiss shared by Jack and Lydia; in true AIDS-era fashion Tuck is transmitted between them during their saliva exchange, acting as the "germ" that aborts their sexual relationship and, once inside Lydia, "spying" the previously undisclosed fetus that seals Tuck and Lydia's romantic reunion. Through a convoluted plot device, Tuck must be transferred back to Jack through another kiss and is thus rescued through one of Jack's tears (one of the few *Fantastic Voyage* elements resurrected here), thus being reborn Athena-like from the head of his unlikely father. To emphasize the rebirth motif, Jack hands Tuck a cigar as he is reunited with Lydia; not only are Jack and Tuck proud fathers of each other, but Tuck looks forward to the birth of his still-unannounced child and reclaims the phallic symbol, as taker of the feminine prize, that Jack cheerfully remands.

Comparing the positions of Cora/Welsh and Lydia/Ryan, especially as they are worsened or relieved by the "other women" (feminized men) in their respective romantic triangles, is telling. In chapter 3 I noted that the strength of a female character corresponded inversely to the strength of the interloping male other: the more dangerous or threatening the presence of the male buddy or adversary, the more intact the woman's position in relation to the leading man at the story's end. With the cinematic examples here, the positions of these corresponding figures are directly, not inversely, related; and we might identify this shift from inverse to direct relationships as a smoothing of the complexity that is simply more often found in novels than popular films. These latter can be (and in fact here are) so reinforcing of the fears and tastes of their audiences, that *The Fantastic Voyage*'s scapegoating of all things feminine only reflects the paranoia of weakness that defined cold war culture, while *Innerspace*'s comparative valorization of both women and effeminate men is the result of the women's and gay rights movements that have forced audiences to at least a moderate degree of acceptance of both.

Thus both Cora and Doctor Michaels suffer a death blow from Grant: Michaels literally in the lymph-engulfed ship, and Cora figuratively in that she is reduced from knowledgeable scientist to clinging damsel by film's end. Of course, Cora the character was trapped from the start when the decision was made to cast Raquel Welch, the actor who more or less made a career out of playing a body, in the role. Conversely, casting the boyish, light-comic Meg Ryan in the AIDS-era remake considerably freed up the character of Lydia. While Lydia, like Cora, ends up hanging on the leading man's arm, she is throughout the film stuck inside neither Tuck nor his enmeshed relationship with Jack. It is she, in fact, who issues the command to "put [the bad guys] in the miniaturizer!" that is duly carried out by the submissive Jack. In direct relationship, Lydia's visibility is tied to Jack's corresponding centrality: he is not a threat (either to Tuck or his sexual bond with Lydia) but a victim and a savior. He is allowed to survive the adventure, largely because he happily resumes his role as "third wheel" in the triangle but also because his effeminacy no longer represents the intolerable "menace" it once did. While the original concerned itself with hidden, buried secrets, the remake acknowledges and explores several open secrets—the miniaturization process sought after by several enemies, Lydia's unborn child, and most especially the homosocial attachments of the two men.[7] This opening up of the film's focus mirrors the shift from local to global identified in the *Shrinking* films above: the blood-borne phenomena of both the Tomlin and Spielberg remakes eventually threaten the world population, while both originals contained and cured their respective medical crises in enclosed and secret places—in *The Incredible Shrinking Man,* the home; in *The Fantastic Voyage,* the submarine. The liberation of Ryan's Lydia, as was the case with Tomlin's Pat, is also a product of this outward filmic thrust.

While *The Fantastic Voyage*'s engineering of bodily organs, physiologic processes, and small-scale illusions was striking enough to snag it an Academy Award for best special effects, Spielberg (elsewhere a master of such filmic tricks) spends almost no time on the fantastic quality of Tuck's voyage through Jack. The driving faith in science so characteristic of cold war fantasy films is replaced in Spielberg's New Age remake by a sentimental interest in psychology and romance—not Jack's ear canal and coronary arteries so much as his head and his heart. Nevertheless, Jack is still a patient in the film, a hypochondriac who keeps his doctor in business, and Tuck the scientist (he is a former astronaut) is sent in to cure him—not of his version of "HIV" (his hypochondriasis) but his version of queerness (his effeminacy) that, once effectively treated, will, it is assumed, cure his physical symptoms as well. Thus in spite of the relative sympathy and autonomy granted to both Jack and Lydia in this more recent film, it proves as problematic as its original in terms of treating serious social issues (nuclear espionage/blood-borne illnesses) with the most bogus of Band-Aids (restoration of the heterosexual couple): the potentially subversive triangulated dynamic in both these films, as constituted by a heterosexual coupling and an intervening feminized male, is recouped by traditional forces through the obvious subordination of this third figure, the psychosexual challenge and the societal disruption that he represents.

PANIC IN THE STREETS OF SAN FRANCISCO: CROSS-METAPHORIC TREATMENTS OF PLAGUE THEMES

As I hope I have demonstrated throughout this study, the conditions defining one plague period are by no means irrelevant to the crises in other periods that have generated or will follow from it. The metaphors developed during the cold war still enable powerful statements during the AIDS era, while our understanding of and reaction to the AIDS crisis come in part from the disease-related imagery and discourse that sprang from the cold war. Elia Kazan's *Panic in the Streets* (1950), for instance, examines apathy, bureaucracy, and hysteria in the postwar era as manifested during a hypothetical epidemiologic nightmare. Kazan, whose message here may have been complicated by his own shifting political attitudes,[8] found the metaphor of the epidemic accessible and instructive. In more recent decades, a nuclear nightmare like *The China Syndrome* (1979) anticipated not only the accident at Three Mile Island but the devastation of HIV and AIDS about to be realized by the general population. Granted, *The China Syndrome* "remakes" *Panic in the Streets* only in terms of some important shared themes—especially citywide panic, resulting from and exacerbated by government apathy and corruption—with the latter owing nothing to the former in terms of plot, character, or subject matter. The films, however, function almost identically during their respective plague eras, depicting a barely avoided biological disaster while identifying the misinformation and disinformation surrounding the near miss as a bigger threat than the "explosion" itself. The films invest to varying degrees in issues largely unrelated to their historic contexts, with the issues becoming metaphors for these historic contexts, enabling the films to comment indirectly and provocatively on the forces controlling and threatening their respective periods. In both films the movement, suppression, and exchange value of *information* forms a second level of metaphoric discourse that facilitates the translation between epidemic and nuclear crises and back again.

Thus, in Kazan's *Panic in the Streets*, information, the story of the impending epidemic and the danger it presents, is a bomb that must not be dropped on the unsuspecting citizens of New Orleans at any cost. Public health official Clinton Reed (Richard Widmark) fights to make his medical findings important to an indifferent city council and then to keep them from a hungry and hysterical press. The identity of a small-time gangster ravaged by plague, and his circle of contacts during his last contagious days, is a mystery to city officials because he is established from the first as a "foreigner" without a history. In keeping with (yet also critical of) the red-baiting stereotype of the outsider as disease carrier, the dying man speaks with a heavy accent and alienates his new gangster pals by becoming sick just after winning several poker hands. When his bullet-ridden body is discovered at the river, the cop identifies him as a "foreigner" even though his accent is obviously no longer giving him away, suggesting a certain tangibility to his outsider status that identifies him clearly—as a total enigma. Doctor Reed knows he must find the information he needs—the identities of the man and his contacts, including the killers who merely beat the virus to the punch—quietly and directly, by offering cash rewards for information to the circles of men who may have known him.

Thus Reed finds himself in one world of men after another—gangsters and police, military enclaves, dockworkers, ship crews, and flophouse denizens—on the trail of solving his mystery. As this is the story of a growing contagion, scenes of unwitting transmission through close and intense physical contact between the men are interesting and suggestive tension-builders. The hiring house at the dock and the flophouse on the wharf are packed with men pressed against each other, waiting for job calls or settling down for the night. As Poldi, one of the gangsters who killed Kochak (patient zero), lies dying from plague, Finch cradles his sweating chest and head, caressing him and leaning over him as protector. Threatening for a second time to beat the disease process to the finish, Blackie climbs onto Poldi's bed, grilling him about hidden money, literally breathing down his neck to scare the sick man into talking. Reed (who may or may not have become contaminated during his search) also shares many close moments with Captain Tom Warren, who looks warmly at Reed during their first time alone yet hangs back hesitantly when Reed insists on taking him for coffee. While at first on opposite sides of the issue, the two men become close associates. After the climactic "new community" speech (see below), Reed is offered the traditional "postcoital" cigarette by his new sidekick, Tom, and accepts. Significantly, Reed is rough (in typical Widmark fashion) and distant with his wife, calling her a "mushy dame" with looks that are barely passable and insisting that she stay away from him during what could be an incubation period for him, even when she informs him that she is incubating her own surprise, their second child. Thus, the mysterious and contagious disease not only circulates almost solely among communities of men but has the effect of bringing these men into ever-tighter, even fatal bonds, distancing them from the women in their lives.

As metaphor for information (i.e., power), the epidemic is not surprisingly an all-male issue.

Throughout the film, Reed's city hall adversaries lean on the easy distinctions that controlled modern (as opposed to postmodern) civic rule and civil defense: city council members brush off the death of the foreign gangster, whose body on autopsy is found to be ravaged by the effects of pneumonic plague, because of the violence that outpaced and thus occluded his fatal illness. "He died of two bullet wounds," insists one councilman. "He died of plague," Reed returns, yet the administrators refuse at first to take action because the bullet wounds are crime-related and uninfectious, the marks of business as usual in what was a new and unusual age. As crime-effect, the body is in demand by the police for evidence, possibly providing information about the killers, yet Doctor Reed, knowing full well who (or what) the man's real killer is, has had the body cremated. In the just-passing era, then, the body is information and cure (solution) to a murder mystery, while in the midst of a postmodern plague the information available reveals the body, information itself, as part of (the root of) the problem.

Late in the story a recalcitrant mayor insists on bringing in the press to protect the community by informing them. Reed cuts off his outdated argument: "Community, what community? You think you're living in the Middle Ages?" After a bit of business about advanced technology and being able to be in Africa within ten hours, Reed concludes to the mayor, "we're all in a community—the same one." Aside from the film's remarkably progressive outlook, as demonstrated by this exchange, we can see again that in the film's lexicon, information would not flow but would, moving too fast and too frantically, explode.[9] Peter Biskind calls Reed's "Big Picturism," his abstracted, international perspective, the true focus of this film, whose pro-U.N. tendencies were in absolute keeping with the interests of its time (29, 31). Thus the press, with a brief nod to the First Amendment, is portrayed largely as a parasite, an exacerbating influence too in league with defamation and rumor-mongering to enjoy its usual freedoms in panic-stricken times.

In *The China Syndrome*, information is even more centrally considered and is closely associated with not only sex and disease but the best available treatment of the sickness as well. Significantly in the earlier film, plague serum could be used to counter the effects of illness, making the language (information) surrounding and compounding it extraneous and dangerous. In the field of nuclear energy big profits and limited alternative resources prevent a "cure" (plant shutdowns) from possibility, and accurate information is the only means of controlling what could one day be a devastating mishandling of power. Thus, where the press in the previous film was peripheral and parasitic, in *The China Syndrome,* it is essential to the packaging and movement of vital information and assumes a positive role. Jane Fonda plays Kimberly Wells, an attractive reporter stuck on the fluff beat of a Los Angeles news affiliate. She happens onto a phenomenally close call at the Ventana Nuclear Power Plant and must use her sex appeal to obtain information from Jack Godell (Jack Lemmon), the right-thinking shift supervisor who is immediately attracted to her, and to obtain permission to follow the story from her womanizing boss. For reasons I will consider below, Kimberly's sexual charms fail her on both counts: Jack is so reluctant to "put out" for her and her camera crew that it is too late when he finally does, and her bosses at the news station want nothing to do with her story; they are eventually revealed to be in bed with Ventana big wheels.

The information Jack needs to pass on to Kimberly is both a story about sickness (a breakdown in plant operations that could mean biological and environmental disaster) and a disease itself (ruin for the plant, its wealthy owners, and the prospects of nuclear energy as a safe source of energy). Interestingly in both this film and the similarly themed *Silkwood* (1983), X rays, as for a sick patient, are taken of the plant's workings, "doctored" (not cured but tampered with) by wrongdoers with access to them, and ultimately used as evidence against the greed-driven technicians who endanger a city's health by endangering that of the facility. Jack has found these X rays and realizes that cracks in the sealings have gone unrepaired, threaten the entire southern California area, and have caused the near-meltdown witnessed by Kimberly and her crew. The burden of the undisseminated information drives Jack to a distracted state: finally he has a mental breakdown while holed up in the control room of the plant; the cameras are running, Jack is killed in a hail of bullets, and his story is discredited by the plant's owners as the ravings of a madman.

This disease-as-information is sexually transmissible (though never transmitted), as Kimberly uses her feminine wiles to wins Jack's confidence, and Jack's attraction to Kimberly is what inspires and enables him to make the limited stand he does. He demands to have her delivered to him in the control room, where they will "interview" together before the watching world; their first experience in that room was even more explicitly sexual: in the near-meltdown, Jack, his technicians, Kimberly, and her cameraman, Richard (Michael Douglas) all feel a powerful, unnameable "vibration" that, once survived, is less terrifying than exhilarating. In the clinch, however, Jack is unable to deliver the goods, due not so much to his own failings as to the inability of the medium (and its slow-witted consumers) to receive complex information for more than thirty seconds at a time. No talking hairdo, Jack stutters and shakes and finally is only babbling and digging his own grave. While the information is present, its avenue of transmission is about as fail-safe as the Ventana plant itself; the breakdown in this pipeline cuts off solutions (cures), and Jack is assassinated by a SWAT team minutes later. I would add that the cameraman Richard is a sexual interest for Kimberly as well, but neither man consummates his desire for her. Despite the waning days of sexual freedom that are this film's context, something (the story of sickness itself) keeps all three players focused on their work and celibate.[10]

Thus Kazan's *Panic in the Streets* is a cold war film about a contagious disease that as information is both bomb and dud (false alarm, or "panic") and that as biological actuality is "sexually" transmitted—in that it confines itself to circulation in the male sex, due to the men's homosocial contact and their propensity for the corruptions attached to power in that era. Conversely, *The China Syndrome* is an AIDS-era film about a nuclear explosion that as biological event can only be defused (because never disarmed) through press-generated information, while this information, due to its dependence on successfully executed sexual interaction in an age when sex was already potentially fatal, weakens and dies before it can do any good. That the relationship of this "remake" to its "original" is deeply imbricated yet entirely unintentional reveals the intense similarity and interdependence of their respective plague periods themselves: perhaps many (if not all) films produced during these periods that address themes of social illness and upheaval, the information circulation that contains or exacerbates them, may be seen as participants in this overarching conversation.

KIDS THESE DAYS: THE OEDIPAL AND EXTRA-OEDIPAL IN REMAKE RELATIONS

Thomas M. Leitch has pointed out that the homage to an original film or to the oeuvre of a preceding auteur is partially intended to revive interest in the work or works of the earlier filmmaker, to generate audience demand for the rescreening of original work(s) at the expense of the remake itself, the inevitable sense of something missing that defines it. A remake's reverential backward glance can push a near-forgotten or previously dismissed original into classic-film status, sacrificing itself to its artistic father's knife even as it must be credited with raising this father from the dead. Yet Leitch describes the "aporiac" position of the remake with respect to its cinematic forebear, a position that can be stated as "I am just as good as the original—only better" (142). The tension arising from this contradiction produces a love/hate relationship that is duplicitous, parasitic, and classically Oedipal: "The exemplary case is that of a Thorold Dickinson's *Gaslight* (1939) which MGM remade in 1944 under George Cukor's direction after purchasing and destroying the negative of the British film. The true remake admires its original so much it wants to annihilate it" (145).

This love/hate Oedipality governing the remake relationship explains in part the widely varied relationships between these several cold war films and their respective "rebellious children." For it should be fairly obvious that this chapter about cold war plague films and their AIDS-era remakes has yet to focus on a film pair joined by anything like a typical remake relationship. A spoof/satire, a thematic rip-off, and a cross-metaphorical connection neither require nor demonstrate the care, reverence, and explicit restatement of an original that constitutes the studied remake of literary greats or cinematic classics; yet the remake's "patricidal" impulse to replace its cinematic parent with its usurping self is missing as well, due no doubt to the thematic and formal distances separating each of these near-remakes from the originals that in some way or another spawned them. These cinematic stepparents, then, are denied the emulation of children who strive to be worthy of their name yet also are spared the threat of being challenged, equaled, and ultimately replaced by them. Meanwhile, their stepchildren are bound to them through if not specifically Oedipal conflicts then pre-Oedipal or extra-Oedipal ("perverted"), equally complex ones. Thus all the remakes in this chapter may be positioned along the same spectrum, bound on one end by desire, on the other by identification—by the polar conditions of a remake wanting to *have* its cinematic original (either for partner or for dinner) and wanting to *become* its cinematic original.

Near-remakes gravitate toward the pole of desire (wanting to have) as opposed to that of identification with (wanting to be) their originals, where we will shortly find the true remake.[11] In the remake relationship between *The Fantastic Voyage* and *Innerspace,* for instance, the child does not so much *want* (desire) its parent as *want from* it—to ingest parts of it for nourishment and reject or regurgitate what is not pleasing to its taste—in a way resembling less an Oedipal desire than an oral or anal fixation. Indeed, Spielberg eviscerates the body of its cinematic forebear yet is able to build a nearly unrecognizable exterior around these scavenged innards by feeding off the fuel they provide. The rip-off resembles the self-centered and inner-directed pre-Oedipal child, in that he looks to his parent not with love or desire but only for what needs of his she can gratify. In a similar way the remake of *The Incredible Shrinking Man* ransacks the cold war original for its theme, special effects, and campy potential, challenging the view of the original to secure its own validity.

Yet *The Incredible Shrinking Woman* has its Oedipal as well as pre-Oedipal shadings. Significantly, this "girl-child" stands ambivalently in relationship to its cinematic father, revealing a desire to couple with it by regendering title, characters, and situations so as to be the mate for, to stand in heterosexual complementarity with, the cold war original. Ultimately, however, the remake thumbs its nose at the father-original through its satire, irreverence, and feminist social commentary, as discussed above. The role of androgyne that Tomlin has developed for herself elsewhere coincides perfectly with the Freudian daughter's dilemma—the choice between masochism (identification as feminine/desiring the father) and "pathology" (identification with the father) that the film settles uneasily around throughout.

If the first remake relationship I describe here figures the remake as a needy and self-centered son, aggressively ravaging a correspondingly feminized parent (breast/site of oral gratification), and the second relationship depicts a daughter-remake locked in Oedipal struggle with her father-original, one could go on to argue that the third relationship discussed above reverts to a mother-son configuration, but one that has now graduated to the Oedipal stage. What characterizes the bond between *Panic in the Streets* and *The China Syndrome* is simply the negation of a bond, a nonrecognition or disavowal that describes castration anxiety or, when developed in the extreme, fetishism. In similar fashion those who "remade" *Panic in the Streets* as *The China Syndrome* would disavow a relationship to the "original" ("That's not what I look like; I have something my (m)other doesn't"), which only seals the identity between them ("I *am* like my (m)other; we are both without the phallus") that much more firmly. The remake takes itself as its own fetishistic object (and therefore we see here not so much fetishism as an especially active case of castration anxiety), perceiving a gap in the previous plague era that it tries to fill in or surround safely with its AIDS-era alternative. Of course there is no such gap, such unspoken statement, in the previous era (and neither is mother really "missing" anything), while the remake fruitlessly fills its space (insisting on difference between it and its predecessor): "he" is (as are all of us trapped in the Symbolic) already castrated.

A fourth, as-yet-to-be-disclosed remake relationship is one of a cold war original and its "true" AIDS-era remake, appropriately figured by the most traditional of Oedipal children—a "son" that not only takes the exact name of its father but grooms itself in the fashion of its forebear and seeks a strong identification with it. Not unexpectedly, Chuck Russell's *Blob* (1988) admires, emulates, and ultimately overtakes Tony Lyn's 1958 original of the same title; multiple critics have hailed the technically generated horror effects of the later film, to which those of the first can only pale in comparison.[12] I myself did not find the remake to be in any way more memorable or artistically superior to its cinematic "father" but thought only that the second, when viewed in relationship to the first, had the effect of canceling out the original, of confusing the viewer as to which scene went with which film and making such distinctions seem useless shortly thereafter. This cancellation effect allows the viewer to shift her attention from the films themselves to the context that bore each one respectively—in short, the plague eras under consideration here and the nature of the blob produced by each. In fact, both the original and remade versions of *The Blob* are hokey, campy, intriguingly bad films, with the original (the already evident star quality of newcomer Steve McQueen somewhat aiding this) coming out a slight favorite in all contests. Thus it is possible, and productive, to ignore the lion's share of plot, character, and setting that define and differentiate these films, to focus not on *The Blob*s but the blobs—two fine, scary, and telling monsters terrorizing different but significantly related plague periods. Recalling a Barthesian style of analysis that often discovered and interpreted a single thread running throughout an otherwise complex and multidimensional film, fashion, or cultural event (especially in *Mythologies*), I would like here to extract these blobs from their positions as supporting actors in a large and expansive horror genre to dissect their appeal to contemporary audiences, their underlying semiotic of cultural pronouncement, and the significance they hold for audiences years or decades later.

NOT *THE BLOB*S BUT THE BLOBS

"Myth," says Barthes, tracing the path of ideology in culture, "is a semiological system which has the pretension of transcending itself into a factual system" (134), and he uses semiology, whose systems could also be deployed antimythically, as in poetry or in the active language of political revolution, to ferret out the mythemes that enable ideology to do its work. In film Barthes opened up his targeted mytheme—"The Romans in Films," the landscape of *The Lost Continent*—to reveal the multiple levels at which ideology works in a single cinematic component. The blobs running rampant through the two films named for them are similarly multilayered, ideological, but also to some degree antimythic or "politicized," speaking a language that, if not pure action ("I speak the tree," says the woodcutter, and only the woodcutter [Barthes 145]), at least advances a strong critique against and in spite of the mythological forces that gave them life.

An initial comparison of the two blobs reveals the dramatic change in technological effects that have supported films from one era to the next. Note that

I use the word "change" when "improvement" might have been chosen by other film observers; the blurb on the remake's video packaging promises that "the oozing gooey killer is back with a whole new high-tech '80s look." Yet the technology that enabled the original's effect was in many ways perfect—not only thoroughly suited to its B movie quality and the B-quality context of 1950s horror consumption but also to our ultimate understanding of the "real" monster the cinematic blob (and countless creatures from other films of that era) only symbolized on screen—Russian/communist ideology. As the original blob/Russian threat was terrifying then, it is revealed now as a false and phony monster, an easily seen through, heavily contrived "bogey man" dancing in front of an uncertain audience so as to entertain but also control it. Indeed, improved technologies—filmic and strategic—have enabled us to realize that this monster is, in retrospect, about as disquieting as a truckload of liver pudding, that (cinematic and political) audiences scared pretty easily back then and in fact led lives in beds of roses compared to what faces American society today. In contrast the 1980s version of the blob, more "lifelike" (and thus deathlike), does not metaphorize into a false bogey but an actual, as-yet-unsolved problem, the AIDS crisis. Again, the advanced technology performs the double function of illuminating a problem in all its horrific detail and simultaneously suggesting the enormity (beyond the best of technology thus far) of its solution.[13]

The cold war blob of the original is indeed a glowering, undecipherable, dull-red menace that falls from the sky in meteorite form in a patch of woods one evening, threatening the sleepy town that adjoins it. In contrast, the blob of the 1988 remake is not dull or red but glistening and a pearly gray, like a mucous membrane. While the original rolled and lumbered like a clumsy Russian bear, the remake slides and strikes aggressively; it lashes out with phallic tentacles that attack both men and women. The original blob is a domino theorist's worst nightmare; discovered as a creature no bigger than a fist, it devours one man and then another and in so doing increases its size, strength, and velocity. Finally it is large enough to cover a diner. While the remake blob also enlarges throughout the film, it is not a unified organism depending solely on a single trail of food for expansion. Instead it is an atomized, *balkanized* blob that attacks minutely at different sites—an old man in a hospital in town, a couple necking in the woods. Eventually the bulk of the blob comes together to be frozen and trucked away to the "icehouse," but the remake's final scene—of the now religion-crazed preacher hoarding a few unclaimed and thawed out shards of blob horror—promises a *Blob 3* at the very least, the unchecked progress of the current crisis at the very worst.

The original blob attacked in random, unreadable patterns whose very randomness was part of the terror it (and the Russian menace behind it) represented, while the remade blob seems bent on an implausibly specific mission—attacking only single men and boys and sexually engaged heterosexual couples—whose specificity is part of its terror. In both films, an old hermit living in the woods is the first victim. In the hospital where the "can man" in the remake dies we realize that this monster, in a significant shift from the cold war original, invades its victims' bodies and attacks its next victim *by springing out from the recesses of its previous host.* Also, in contrast to the zealous medical professionals who attend the old man in the original (they are that blob's next victims), the old man's worsening condition and eventual death in the remake are blamed in part on the indifferent healthcare system that admits him to a hospital for indigents and then allows him to waste away indefinitely in an exam room. In the long intervening period, the invading monster explodes the old man like a bomb, and Paul, the town kid who found him and goes in to check on him, is the next to be attacked. The monster moves on to get the projection man in the moviehouse, who is a friend of Meg's little brother's and a sheriff's deputy. Significantly, the effeminate and freakish reverend is injured by fire but left unharmed by the blob; his obsessive relationship to it at the end of the film positions him as its brainwashed victim but also as the origin of its next wave of terror.[14] In scenes equating this blood-associated danger with sexuality, the blob infiltrates Vicky, then deflates her like a balloon and engulfs Scott just as he is reaching to touch her breast. It simultaneously surrounds and suffocates Herb and Frannie, whose budding romance is consummated only by their final gaze into each other's eyes. In both films, the primary heterosexual couples—Jane and Steve in the original, Meg and Brian in the remake—are spared, as are, importantly, their immediate families. Both films then suggest a relationship between solid family ties and the avoidance of blob-wielded disaster, while both would condemn the solitary life of, say, the doctor in the original, whose lack of ties prolongs the mystery of his death and thus a solution to blob-related problems, or the crazy preacher of the remake.

Yet for all their fearmongering and exaggeration of the threat posed by Russians, gays, and HIV-positive individuals, both films comment almost as effectively, however obliquely, on opposing ideologies—the dangers of red-baiting and McCarthyism in the original, of the environmental abuses responsible for HIV and other global threats to humanity in the remake. Significantly, it is the stake in the heart, the blob's intolerance of cold, that opens up these countercommentaries in both. The blob retreats from his attack on Jane and Steve and on Meg and Brian when each couple is trapped in a cooler, and it is driven back and contained, however temporarily, when the town is able to amass enough dry ice and carbon dioxide on the front line.

In the original, the suggestion is that the cold—that is, the cold war and icy relations between superpowers—is even more deadly than the blob (Russians/communist ideology) itself. This anti-red-baiting theme is reinforced by the subplot concerning Steve and the rest of the town—their inability to believe his story—and Jane's initial betrayal but ultimate support of him. Throughout, Steve has struggled to get his community to believe the "truth," the reality of a threat (in political context, the relative lack of one), and is labeled as a radical and a troublemaker. Solving the problem, both Steve and the film attest, lies not so much in doing something about it but understanding the true nature of it. At one point he outlines his plan of action to Jane: "We're gonna find this thing, and we're gonna make people believe us." Thus communal acknowledgment of a problem and the acceptance of outsiders are presented as substitutes for, the most effective way to minimize, violent action.

The couple moves from the disbelieved fringe of the community to the center of it as the terror they forecasted becomes a reality. By the end, they are surrounded not only by the monster (who is wrapped around the diner they are trapped in) but by the concerted effort of the town itself, which battles the monster to save them, *under* the direction of Steve, who is issuing instructions from within the diner. The film centralizes the couple even more by cobbling together a trapped, surrogate family (the diner owners as parent figures, Jane's little brother as Steve and Jane's son) in which they are both chronologically and ideologically centered as "our greatest hope."

The cold air that blasts the blob of the remake into submission is also laden with a surprisingly liberal social comment, specifically regarding environmental abuse leading to global warming and the biological, even economic, damage this can cause. Arborville is a ski resort town whose tourist season is threatened by an unnaturally warm fall. Frequent references are made to the "boiling" temperatures, even at night in October, and Herb worries to Frannie that the town (i.e., the ideal of small-town life) will not survive if the warming continues. In supplemental fashion, the film suggests both that the warmth is caused by the red-hot blob-containing meteor that crashes to earth *and* that global warming itself is responsible for producing such freaks of interplanetary nature. The destruction of the blob with blasts of cold air from a snowmaker results in an atmospherically balancing, economically revitalizing snowfall that settles like a benediction on the sadder but wiser townsfolk, who would resolve to go forth and emit fossil fuels no more. Thus the equation between global warming and the unleashing of an overpowering, fatal organism (blob/HIV) onto an unprepared population suggests that both stem from the same origin—the disruption of delicate biospheres to exploit the land and inhabitants—and condemns both equally.

• • •

The multiple remakes of cold war originals that proliferated throughout the 1980s and continue to the present, including the four more or less obscure examples I investigate here,[15] demonstrate, I hope, the complex dialogue between the film pairs and their respective plague periods, the significance of cold war cultural expressions as curative commentary on the crises we face today, and the propensity for AIDS-era filmmakers to resurrect these cold war themes to comment, helpfully or detrimentally, on the fears plaguing their own eras. Significantly, while all four plague originals I examine here treat the themes of cold war and the nuclear threat as overt and central, none of their AIDS-era remakes treat HIV-infection, or even issues of sickness itself, directly in any fashion. *As* disease (and not merely "social ill," as the cold war and nuclear proliferation may be seen to be), HIV/AIDS in discourse must be recognized as largely internalized and extremely infectious: not only does the sexual ennui that wound down the "swinging" frenzy of the 1970s enable the production of "AIDS films" as early as 1979, but even those films produced several years later, at the obvious (first) peak of the AIDS era, talk undeniably about this illness—through themes of male-male relations, blood-borne disease, the infectiousness of (mis)information—while never mentioning it. Not only their production during this period but also, and most especially, their remake relationship to cold war predecessors marks them as discussants in this continuing conversation about postmodern plagues, directs the viewer's gaze toward identifying the AIDS-related discourse that in fact lies readily discernible below their respective surfaces.

While both original and remade films may have only incited or reinforced hysterical fears of seemingly unknowable others for their respective original audiences, the remake relationship itself disrupts this status quo by the *pattern,* the spatial marking this remake propped against its original automatically creates, by the insight that observation of this pattern may eventually produce. At the conclusion to the first chapter of *Postmodernism,* Fredric Jameson proposes an "aesthetic of cognitive mapping" to counter the "negative and baleful effects" of multinational or late capitalism on postmodern space (50). Appreciated for its "pedagogical dimension" and potential for "radical internationalism," cognitive mapping grounds and orients postmodern "travelers," establishing for each a relation to the totality that mirrors the unrepresentable Real for Althusser. As pedagogy (illuminating to observers) and as spatial structure, the remake relationship resembles this cognitive map, which Jameson correlates with the Lacanian Symbolic, a "representational dialectic of codes" (54) that is well suited to a reading here of the heavily coded cinematic.

Jameson argues that we are yet to realize "the new political art" that would have to include and surpass its opposite—"the world space of multinational capitalism" (54)—in classic dialectic fashion. Yet his very articulation, not only of the problems before us but of the several solutions to them that his cognitive mapping affords, suggests that in fact this sort of activity is not only in the future but is already part of our present moment. Hopefully, the spatializing carried out here between these plague film pairs begins the kind of grounding and orienting necessary to "getting around" (affecting positively) one's town or planet. In this case, the AIDS-era remake casts a backward and insightful glance not only on its cold war original and the relationship between their respective eras but on problems and solutions from an earlier period that may bear significantly, curatively, on those of our own.

Conclusion: One Fine Day—Toward a Realization of the "Eutemporal"

Throughout this study I have found suspect and ultimately untenable the notion of the "utopic"—a metonymic island or other secured place where the "innocent" find unbreachable safety from the trials of the fallen world. I have criticized this idea, whether found in literature, national legislation, or the columns of conservative pundits, for the boundaries around a "healthy" society that it promises but in fact can never deliver, for the impulse to ignore and reject those among us already afflicted that these false promises encourage. Yet an equally politically conscientious thinker such as Fredric Jameson retains the "utopic" (largely in its denotative meaning as "no-place"[1] but also to a certain degree its connotative shading as a "beautiful" or "better" place, the "*e*utopic") in his vision for political and economic justice, as traditional marxist teaching insists that Utopia is the realm of the collective that one day will triumph over the reign of individualism.[2] In the conclusion to *The Political Unconscious,* Jameson places the "negative hermeneutic" of ideology in dialectic relationship with the Utopia of collectivity, imbricating them while opposing them, identifying himself as a proponent of the Utopic—that is, as a believer in its eventual realization.[3]

In an explicitly queer-theoretical context, Ephen Glenn Colter and his coeditors of *Policing Public Sex* oppose utopianism to conservatism, while in separate pieces contributors Wayne Hoffman and José Esteban Muñoz oppose utopianism to escapism by insisting that it describes "the vision of how things *could* be, not just how they *were*" (Hoffman 338; see also Muñoz 357). Throughout his essay Hoffman interchanges "utopia" with "fantasy," and this latter term (with its subversive associations with sexual fantasy and the "fairy" tale) for me better describes the politically powerful goal setting and daydreaming that gay- and AIDS-rights activists should be engaged in. Meanwhile, Muñoz's theory-inflected reading of utopianism includes quotes from a relevant dialogue between Bloch and Adorno; again, the marxist influence leads Muñoz to his pro-utopian position.

All politically concerned theorizers of the postmodern face the dilemma of action (a positive, unilateral movement) in an age they understand to be ruled by negativity, elusive or nonexistent meaning, and the "death" of agency. In an effort to resolve this dilemma for myself, I find it important (and have tried to demonstrate this importance through many of the preceding pages) to resist the comforts of utopic fantasy, marxist or otherwise, not because I believe progress and societal improvement are impossible dreams but because they are not to be found in a beautiful (i.e., radically other) *place.* The utopic and its emphasis on different spaces conjure images of not only philosophically "alternative universes" ("our world," just without sick people) but also technologically abandoned planets—images not of planetary responsibility but of artificial living environments that allow and forgive planetary destruction, not of disarmament but of bomb shelters, not of cures but of quarantines. The spatial aspect of the utopic lies at the heart of its problematic nature; its falseness is not in the concept of beauty it promises but in the idea of alternative space that it imagines and promotes.

I suggest in its place the alternative fantasy—as such dreams are vital to action and activism—of the *eutemporal,* neither a no-place nor a beautiful place but a beautiful and better *time* that maintains and rejuvenates the place we are in right now, that includes not only all of us in this space but the space itself in a vision of a safer, a more just and equal future. We see in Derrida's writings on the nuclear that time is of the essence in slowing and reversing the arms race, while even Jameson, observing a postmodernity all but taken over by the spatial and the surface-deep, looks for the restoration of history, of the depth of temporality itself, to alleviate the amnesia and schizophrenia debilitating us. While I have often throughout this study considered the supplemental, interdependent relationship between space and time, I have in fact only embraced the spatial as it enabled the (temporal) relationship between these two plague periods—that is, I have mapped or palimpsested two or more entities in an illuminating and instructive *pattern.* Whenever the spatial has served not to join diverse elements but instead to separate and divide (the "island," the pure "metonym"), I have suspected and challenged this phenomenon, working to undercut or deconstruct it. Here, I will do what I can to problematize the notion of another place, of an edenic island waiting for us, and to valorize the temporal as a constant reminder that we have only one space, one planet to inhabit yet time enough to improve and preserve it.

In terms particular to this study, we must note that time—uncontrollable and inevitably upon us—bears an important *infectiousness,* a condition that is shared by and thoroughly democratizing of all who live on earth, that counters the comparatively divisive concept of space, with its immediate shadings of nationalist "territory" and capitalist "property." Space forces the kind of dichotomizing activity—through its "hereness," which automatically refers to and subordinates "thereness"—that poststructural theory has effectively challenged if not yet completely terminated.[4] While space has been at the heart of almost any war, coup, or gangland battle you could name, time (except for the antitemporal concept of a fundamentalist "eternity") is rarely the cause of spilled blood, forced takeovers, or lost fortunes. Indeed, whenever we attempt to "buy time" we throw our money out the window—always a delightfully subversive act of philanthropy. Our awareness of a markedly limited span of time (as opposed to a sense of an ultimately limited space that is yet to fully hit home) causes us to consider and conserve the spaces of our present that will only enrich the times of our descendants.

Time is in fact the very seed of activism, the realization that there is time enough in our brimming lives to visit HIV patients in a clinic or ward, take calls on a hotline, chain ourselves to the fence of a reactor site, e-mail our congressional representatives, or march on Washington. In this case time must often be controlled (i.e., "created") when the understanding becomes strong enough that, time enough or not, something must be done. This kind of time—literally, the *realization* of it—is the kind that breaks through and dissolves spatial boundaries between the "enemy" (fear, of course) and the "within" (all of us) that define it. It is also the kind that can "buy" time—not extensions of our individual natural lifespans but the preservation of a global time, spared from abrupt truncation as threatened by worldwide epidemics and nuclear holocaust. This stretching of "five minutes" into "all the time in the world" is not only possible but vitally necessary; as the eutemporal must be our future, it will (as all futures inevitably will) be upon us one fine day, a thought, I hope, that can inspire and move us safely through our present.

Notes

Introduction

1. In her preface Henriksen cites 1980s studies by Boyer, Brians (*Nuclear Holocausts*), Lifton and Falk, and Jonathan Schell (*The Abolition*). Elsewhere, H. Bruce Franklin has determined that "neither the achievements at the negotiating tables nor the awesome new arsenals appear to have had a dramatic impact on American consciousness during the years from around 1965 to 1979. . . . After the post-Sputnik burst of fiction and film that climaxed in *Dr. Strangelove* and other works released in 1964 . . . cultural activity overtly dealing with the nuclear threat receded into its original home of science fiction" (qtd. in Stone 68).

2. This year was not the authoritarian nightmare that Orwell predicted it would be; in fact it witnessed the publication of multiple works that seemed designed to ensure his prediction would be never realized. Interestingly, while Orwell never mentioned a specific nuclear threat, all of these texts contain an explicitly antinuclear message: novels and plays published during this year include Susan B. Weston's *Children of the Light,* Ryder Stacy's *Doomsday Warrior* and *Doomsday Warrior No. 2: Red America,* Kim Stanley Robinson's *Wild Shore,* Whitley Strieber and James Kunetka's *Warday: And the Journey Onward,* and Arthur Kopit's *End of the World.* An anthology of poetry, short fiction, and creative essays, *Writings in a Nuclear Age* (edited by Jim Schley) was also published. Nonfiction and scholarly inquiries include Freeman Dyson's *Weapons and Hope,* Alwyn McKay's *Making of the Atomic Age,* and the influential "Nuclear Criticism" issue of *Diacritics.*

3. Peter Ruppert notes that utopia is defined by its "landscape that can be traced to the ever-present barriers that enclose it" (27) and thus escapes the ravages of history in this way. By contrast, dystopia includes "the necessity of history" (98).

Chapter 1: Counting Down—To Catastrophe or Cure?

1. In a similar vein Eve Kosofsky Sedgwick has read paranoia in literature to trace the path of homophobia and heterosexism in society. Significantly, in "Paranoid Reading and Reparative Reading" she finds that "paranoia tends to be contagious" (6), that it can spread from writers to readers and among readers in the act of reading itself.

2. I am aware that multiple feminist and queer theories challenge the pathologizing of pornography, especially as found in feminist-based treatments by Andrea Dworkin and Catharine A. MacKinnon. I use Jonathan Schell's reference only for completeness' sake, not to argue for a correlation between pornography and social problems.

3. William L. Leap argues that English-language users do not want to touch even the word "AIDS" for fear of being contaminated by it. Using linguistic prophylaxis like indirect reference, ellipsis, and euphemism, people "find ways to minimize the occurrence of such encounters [with AIDS], refocusing in the process the meaning of the discussion into other 'safer' domains" (141).

4. Along similar lines, Douglas Crimp has argued that "AIDS does not exist apart from the practices that conceptualize it, represent it, and respond to it. . . . This assertion does not contest the existence of viruses, antibodies, infections, or transmission routes. Least of all does it contest the reality of illness, suffering, and death. What it *does* contest is the notion that there is an underlying reality of AIDS upon which are constructed the representations, or the culture, or the politics of AIDS" (3). See also Treichler's "AIDS, Gender, and Biomedical Discourse."

5. This theory will be discussed later (see chapter 1, note 14).

6. Edelman argues interestingly in a similar vein in "The Plague of Discourse" (302).

7. Hinds and Windt point out that while the term "Iron Curtain" was not coined by Churchill, it had no cultural currency before he adopted it, and it is speech acts such as this, they argue, that brought the cold war into existence: "the cold war was a rhetorical state of mind rather than a description of Soviet-American relations, a rhetorically constructed ideological reality that was first accepted within the ruling circles of government, then publicly conveyed through major speeches and writings to Americans who generally accepted it as the reality of both foreign and domestic politics" (5).

8. See also Arthur Kroker and Marilouise Kroker's introduction to *Body Invaders: Panic Sex in America,* where they define late-millennium "urinal politics" as that which tests for and punishes crimes against "pure bodily fluids" in its citizenry. They argue that "the politics of urination under observation are a *recyclage* of the McCarthyism of the 1950s which . . . insists on the (unattainable) ideal of absolute purity of the body's exchanges as the new gold standard of an immunological politics" (11). Although the authors make a case here primarily against enforced drug testing, McCarthyistic urinal politics certainly include the policing of gay sexual activity to control it and the disease it is blamed for spreading. Later they describe "panic science" as the "deep relationship between AIDS and Star Wars research" (15) and note that "the rhetoric surrounding both AIDS and Star Wars focusses on the total breakdown of immunity systems: AIDS can be perceived in such frightening terms because its appearance indicates the destruction of the internal immunological system of the body (the *crisis within*); while the rhetoric of Star Wars creates, and then responds to, generalized panic fear about the breakdown of the technological immunity systems of society as a whole (the Bomb as the *crisis without*)" (12). Of course I hope to demonstrate my reasons for defining here both these postmodern plagues as crises—or "enemies within"—yet I appreciate these authors' formulation nonetheless.

9. The unnerving unidentifiability of gay men during the cold war is incisively treated by Edelman in his discussion in "Tea Rooms and Sympathy" of the case of Walter Jenkins, who served in the 1960s in the Johnson administration.

10. The Foucauldian distinction between doing and being that has been guiding this discussion mirrors exactly the difference that Michael W. Messmer makes between modern (pre–World War II) and postmodern warfare in "Nuclear Culture, Nuclear War." Discussing Michael Walzer's distinction between the "aimed" attacks on offending populations that defined modern warfare and the "unaimed" kind that characterize postmodern conflicts, Messmer notes: "The moral difference Walzer sees is one between 'aiming

at particular people because of things they *have done or are doing,* and aiming at whole groups of people, indiscriminately, because of who they *are*'" (167; emphasis added). Rephrasing this distinction in terms of the militarily defined "conventional war" versus the now-prevalent "total war," Messmer concludes: "The history of the twentieth century provides overwhelming evidence that total war is now the mode which the conduct of war inescapably assumes, and this is especially the case in our times as the distinction between conventional and nuclear arms is increasingly eroded in terms of both technical sophistication and destructiveness" (163–64). The "surgical strike"—clean, ethical, and devastating—is the ultimate military goal but also, as Messmer implies here, the ultimate military-generated myth. The more powerful or "pseudonuclear" weapons become, the less likely it is that those unleashing that power will be able to control the size and scope of their targets or apprehend the fading modernist distinction between soldier and conscientious objector. As with the collapse of distinctions that may have once protected the innocent from charges of traitorous or "indecent" behavior, the slippage between being and doing under postmodern war conditions now turns every war into "total" war, every civilian into a soldier, and every local skirmish into a planetary threat. See also Derrida's "Rhetoric of Drugs" (esp. 20–22).

11. A new, more accurate reference to HIV has become widely used in the popular press, that is, "the virus that causes AIDS." Now and then the appositive construction "HIV, the virus that causes AIDS" can be found, but overall the media correctly assume that reference to HIV plain and simple will still be largely misunderstood by the public.

12. I am in vigorous disagreement with Leap's argument that the substitution of this narrower, more particular language for the umbrella term "AIDS" represents some sort of "distortion" or denial on the part of users of this language (142). Leap's references to this more accurate terminology, even in healthcare contexts—doctors' offices, training manuals for hospital personnel (142, 145)—as "synonyms," "code words," and "jargon" suggest that he is unaware of the realities of the HIV-related clinical setting. At one point Leap favors the "straightforwardness" of the thoroughly incorrect formulation "I caught AIDS"—of course one does not catch the syndrome or symptom complex but rather a virus, HIV—over the more accurate "I have AIDS," since in his opinion the "have" is too neutral and obscures the transmission event that caused the disease's appearance.

13. Much from the subsequent discussion is from Radetsky.

14. Political and scientific breakthroughs coincided remarkably at this time. It was the Russian scientist Albert Sabin (significantly, a Russian emigré to the United States) who quickly challenged Salk with an oral form of the vaccine, then tested it with great success on populations in Eastern Bloc countries and some parts of equatorial Africa, where the injectable vaccination—which had to be stored at near-freezing temperatures—was unfeasible. In June 1961, the American Medical Association (AMA) approved Sabin's version for use in the United States before it was even licensed, which did not occur until winter 1962.

Just as Sabin was countering Salk's achievement with his own more distributable vaccine, the Soviets launched Sputnik into orbit, astonishing American aerospace experts, who were sure they would send the first craft into space. The resulting "missile gap" was only worsened by the "polio gap" created by Sabin's success. The AMA's official recognition of Sabin's vaccine came within a year of the breakdown in relations between Cuba and the United States; and by November 1962, when the Cuban Missile Crisis reached a peak and then began to ease, the licensing of Sabin's drug in America seems in retrospect to have been a much-needed peace offering. Yet while the United States stood up to the Soviet threat in Cuba, Sabin's successful crusade against an internationally dreaded disease undercut Salk's position as an American hero as well as America's faith in its own invincibility. Thus development of the field of immunology was not only coincident with the heart of the cold war era; it was in many ways directly responding to it, being simply another theater of conflict, with its own generals, strategies, and casualties.

15. Perhaps Mary Douglas's widely influential *Purity and Danger* (1966), also published during this period, aided the dissemination of these ideas. Observing hygiene and religious ritual among "primitive" groups, Douglas notes the widespread perception that a "polluting person is always in the wrong. He has . . . crossed some line which should not have been crossed" (qtd. in Quam 38). She observed elsewhere in her study that "the body is a model which can stand for any bounded system. Its boundaries can represent any boundaries which are threatened or precarious. . . . Why should body margins be thought to be specially invested with power and danger? . . . all margins are dangerous. If they are pulled this way or that the shape of fundamental experience is altered. Any structure of idea is vulnerable at its margins. We should expect the orifices of the body to symbolize its specially vulnerable points" (qtd. in Quam 39).

16. While space does not permit a full survey of the several similarly structured biohysterical scares intervening between only the first and most recent of these postmodern plague periods, we can include in this list the polio epidemic of the 1950s, Agent Orange during the Vietnam war, environmental assaults such as pesticide use and global warming, and a host of recent viral and bacterial threats to vulnerable populations worldwide, including hantavirus, necrotizing fasciitis, "mad cow" disease, E. coli, and the dreaded Ebola viral strains. With the exception of the first crisis mentioned here, which we might read as a disease vestige of the modern era, high technology is/was no alleviator of these problems but rather a direct and exacerbating influence on their careers of global contamination. With the exception of the second crisis, all struck/are striking middle-class populations of "first-world" nations in addition to the more traditionally affected disempowered worldwide. All are silent and insidious killers; many on this list would be denied by government and even medical officials as presenting a significant threat or even actually existing, reinforcing their illness-effect as invisible invaders, as enemies within. For a general overview, see Garrett's *Coming Plague* and, from a different perspective, Showalter's *Hystories.*

17. MacCannell's theory is corroborated in part by Elaine Tyler May's research on this same issue. In *Homeward Bound,* May cites a *New York Times* 1950 finding that "a boom in rural real estate was directly linked to civil defense concerns" and that brokers of that period had advertised "'country properties for this Atomic Age'" (107). Early editions of Philip Wylie's novel/manifesto of civil defense entitled *Tomorrow!* included an illustration in the center of the book—a map of the story's soon-to-be-bombed twin cities, River City and Green Prairie, stamped with widening rings of destruction. Ground zero is the "negro district" situated at the center of the complex and abutting a "slum area" that would also sustain heavy damage.

18. Peter Dickinson points to Sontag's own writing as well as that of gay activists like Larry Kramer and Tony Kushner when arguing that "abstract theorizing about AIDS . . . frequently lacks a body, a corpus, a corpse" and "threatens whole groups of marginalized peoples . . . with erasure, if not complete annihilation" (219–20). Likewise, Lee Edelman, after an intensely theoretical spin through the figurality of the literal, acknowl-

edges in "The Plague of Discourse" that "as much as I would insist on the value and urgency of examining the figural inscriptions of AIDS, I am sufficiently susceptible to the gravity of the literal to feel uneasy, as a gay man, about producing a discourse in which the horrors experienced by my own community . . . become material for intellectual arabesques" (316).

19. Judith Wilson Ross has made a similar argument. And in *Inventing AIDS* Cindy Patton considers the damage done by the notion of "winning" against AIDS, when the category of victory may never apply here. She even reads "vaccine" and "cure" as language too heavily slanted towards a "good" (moral) outcome, which automatically designates those who have the illness as "bad," "failed," and "deviant." More recently, Heather Schell has surveyed emerging virus narratives and challenges the metaphoric language proliferating therein, specifically the associations between virus-discoverers and big-game hunters (116–19). See also chapter 1 of Kruger's *AIDS Narratives* and Martin's *Flexible Bodies.*

20. In his survey of postwar American novels, Tony Tanner determines such themes to be definitive of the period: "Clay, jelly, jelly-fish—what this image cluster suggests is the dread of utter formlessness, of being a soft, vulnerable, endlessly manipulable blob, of not being a distinct self. The nightmare of non-identity, of no-form, is a recurrent one. On the other hand, any one adopted armature which will contain and give shape and definition to the jelly or clay is at the same time felt to be an imprisoning deathly constriction . . . ; and in the name of liberty these . . . constructions other people build around us are to be cast off or broken through. . . . But then follows the risk of a return to formlessness" (*City of Words* 19).

21. Brian Patton has made a similar argument, citing the military metaphors in Emmanuel Dreuilhe's *Mortal Embrace* as "conscious . . . attempts to turn his illness into metaphor for *therapeutic* ends": "Here, perhaps, in the use of metaphors (including the military ones condemned by Sontag as destructive) for self-reconstructions and self-empowerment by persons with AIDS and their caregivers, lies a solution to the dilemma that arises from our recognition of the inevitability of metaphoric thinking in response to new phenomena" (282; see also Morris 269–70). Along similar lines, D. A. Miller critiques Sontag's antiviolent bent and points out that certain aggressive terms such as "polemic" and "militancy" are empowering even to "patients" like herself (Sontag has had cancer in the past): "'Fight back, fight AIDS' is a chant of this activism, one of whose many organizations calls itself Mobilization Against AIDS" (101). Meanwhile, I do not agree with Miller that "it is almost unspeakably insulting to suggest that 'fighting AIDS' sooner or later means people with AIDS in a context where the notion has authorized the pursuit, *by* the people with AIDS, first among others, of such very different goals" than those held by mainstream, homophobic society (101). In fairness to Sontag, we must first acknowledge that this gay-affirmative context is not at all the one Sontag imagined as she denounced the notion of a "War on AIDS." Instead she aimed her comments directly against mainstream society, which has remained largely indifferent (and openly hostile) to the "carriers" as well as the disease. Additionally, Edelman has shown in "The Plague of Discourse" that even AIDS terminology as seemingly proper and secure as "Silence=Death" produces "discourses that reify and absolutize identities" (309) such that no group is immune from the damage language can do. For a survey of recent gay fiction largely supportive of Sontag's antimetaphor arguments, see Jones's *Plague and Its Texts.*

22. This defense of violence presents itself often, almost in every case, in conjunction

with some genderized reading of the terms in play, borrowed perhaps from the vocabularies of those he explicates, but transcribed by Derrida without so much as a raised eyebrow. In a chapter from *Of Grammatology* entitled "The Violence of the Letter," Derrida reads Lévi-Strauss's "invasion" of a native tribe, specifically his "violation" of the play rituals of a group of little girls. Elsewhere, language is portrayed as the "mother tongue," who should be allowed to submit herself to the aggression of a now masculinized writing, to be invaded "by any outside": "Why should the mother tongue not have a history . . . in a perfectly natural autistic, and domestic way, without every being affected by any outside? Why wish to punish writing for a monstrous crime . . . ?" (41–42). Derrida also discusses Rousseau's understanding of the passions as "the mother" of language as well as language's inevitable tendency away from the passions, the figurative. This movement toward the literal not only ends in the death (of language) but begins with death (the mother's murder): the "obliteration of . . . the 'maternal characteristics'" (*Of Grammatology* 271).

23. The destruction/transformation binary, used here to describe the shift in warfare from the modern to postmodern age, is reflected in key conceptual moments of postmodern theorists: Althusser delineates the destructive and transformative nature of Repressive and Ideological State Apparati, respectively; and Foucault uses this distinction to explain the repressive hypothesis and the movement of power in his *History of Sexuality.*

24. For instance, Derrida argues that two historical opposites, *doxa* and *episteme,* have now become utterly interrelated, as there can be no more "knowledge" of nuclear "experience" that is not also the end of knowledge, of truth. Yet this blend itself forces a break—in the activity of stockpiling (repetition) of weapons and language ("No Apocalypse" 24).

25. Elsewhere in this important "Nuclear Criticism" issue, Ferguson determines that the nuclear, whenever it is cast in its role as "the unthinkable," takes on the dimensions of a twentieth-century version of the sublime. This experience, like that of the surreal, is metaphorical in its double move of joining and dividing at once. The sublime is traditionally characterized as the feeling of being subsumed into nature or, in the anthropocentric version Ferguson favors, of our own borders expanding to include the awesome example of nature before us. Simultaneously, however, Ferguson points out that while this dissolution of boundaries profoundly threatens our existence, it is the most self-affirming of all experiences, as the sublime "quickly comes to be defined as no object at all, because it gets defined . . . as that which cannot stand alone without a supplementary human consciousness" (6). Quoting Kant, Ferguson notes that "'we must seek a ground external to ourselves for the beautiful in nature, but seek it for the sublime merely in ourselves'" (6). For another reading of the nuclear sublime, preferring Edmund Burke's "passive" sublime to Kant's "active" one, see Messmer's "'Thinking It Through Completely'" (408–12).

26. At the end of chapter 4 I will return to this theme, specifically as it is advanced in Fredric Jameson's theory of "cognitive mapping."

Chapter 2: Four Corners of a Crisis

1. I am therefore in disagreement with Emmanuel S. Nelson, who hears only "silence" on the issue of AIDS in several of the texts (e.g., White's and Whitmore's) that I am defining here as "AIDS-related." Accounting for this silence, Nelson posits: "Perhaps to some writers the burden of creating art out of horror seems too heavy to bear, the proportions of the calamity too large to be contained within the boundaries of fiction" (48). But where

Nelson bluntly distinguishes between ignoring and confronting AIDS, I think the more complicated, supplemental relationship that I develop here, between the "pre-epidemic" text and the epidemic that spawned it, as opposed to Nelson's antiepidemic and some clear-cut opposite, is necessary to a full understanding of these literary works.

2. In *Monopolies of Loss* Adam Mars-Jones concurs with this assessment with his provocative suggestion: "Surely the truly responsible thing to do now would be to write sexy nostalgic fiction set in the period before the epidemic, safe-guarding if only in fantasy the endangered gains of gay liberation?" (2).

3. Minute strains of this novel are recognizable in *Mad Max beyond Thunderdome,* but the adaptation is so loose that the two versions serve markedly different cultural functions.

4. In an interesting counterpoint to this argument, David Román has warned against "nostalgic retreats into a formulated and artificial collective memory" as enabled by the camp performances of Lypsinka (315).

5. In a similar vein, Derrida notes in "The Rhetoric of Drugs" that "the virus . . . may *always already* have broken into any 'intersubjective' space" (20).

6. This reunion of spatiality—the superficiality of postmodern existence—with temporality—an all-but-lost historical consciousness—is Fredric Jameson's main project in *Postmodernism.* Elsewhere Linda Singer includes spatial and temporal metaphors to define the postmodern problem she seeks to describe: "the sexual epidemic [i.e., the viewing of sexuality *as* epidemic, as illness out of control among 'our youth,' gays and lesbians, etc.] temporalizes the erotic and eroticizes the temporal in the direction of profit intensification, similar in strategy and effect to the profit intensification of spatiality in the 1970s under the name of the 'condominium'" (41). No doubt enjoying the play on this revived notion of "going condo(m)," Singer here reads the spatial earlier and the (eroticized) temporal now as subjected to the same demands of the capitalist machine: both must turn a profit due to demand created through the "myth of scarcity"—that city space was disappearing in the 1970s and that now life itself, threatened by deadly epidemic from every bodily contact, is being unnaturally foreshortened and can only be enjoyed erotically through costly, surface-deep, throwaway sex. Interestingly, and in part echoing Jameson, Singer notes that "the depth of the body and history" are feared as "explosions ready to happen" (41).

7. I depict "repetition" and "return" in opposition here, mainly to emphasize the differences these several readers ignore. Finally, the two concepts are corollaries of metaphor and metonymy, and I mean to argue ultimately that the motion of repetition *includes* the motion of return—as I argued earlier that metaphor *includes* metonymy, and as Lee Edelman shows here that heterosexuality *includes* homosexuality as its primal gesture.

8. In chapter 3 I will explore the opposition between a masculinized "mastery" and a feminine principle in Schwenger's (and Derrida's) arguments, but suffice it to say here that as far as these masculine principles *are* opposed to feminine ones, they partake of a heterosexist paradigm that is distinctly opposed to any construction of queer sexuality as well. While impressed with the feminist ethic and methodology employed in Schwenger's earlier *Phallic Critiques,* I am only surprised that the same author has produced such a "masculinist" reading of nuclear criticism and literature.

9. I appreciate Clum's further distinction between two "pasts" in recent AIDS literature: the "ancient" past of gay life before AIDS and the recent past, which includes the potentially terrifying narrative of infectious sexual history.

10. Will notices of an old crony of Charles's, Ronald Staines, that "his wrists were very thin, and I saw that he was smaller than his authoritative suiting" (50), suggesting the image of an AIDS patient with wasting syndrome whose clothes no longer fit. Another aging friend, Firbank, is described in Charles's 1920s diary as suffering from tuberculosis, a description that resonates with modern HIV-related TB infections (178–79).

11. Richard Dellamora points out that the novel's selective use of the past mirrors its avoidance of confrontation with the more immediate present as well. For instance, nothing is said in the novel about "the prosecution of upper-middle-class and aristocratic homosexuals in London during the early 1950s" (173). Noting a similar phenomenon in his reading of this novel as AIDS text, Joseph Bristow states, "*The Swimming-Pool Library* finds itself unable to face the unutterable trauma that brought its story into being" (172).

12. Ross Chambers, defining the history of "loiterature" that has taken over in the gay canon from the classical picaresque, describes Will as a flâneur and a loafer, a parasite on the system he both disdains and depends on (207–8). Here again, however, the parasite-host relationship is supplemental through and through: Will both leeches off a repressive and homophobic grandfather and the system he represents and, as leech, provides finally the purgative measure—the opening up of ancient but unhealed wounds, acknowledging (and thus resuming) the progress of history.

13. Dewey has, interestingly, read and responded to an entirely different novel than the one I found upon my encounter with Whitmore's same text. His emphasis is almost entirely on Craig's relationship to his uncle Wayne and Wayne's thwarted romance with his navy buddy Vernon. Dewey only explicates the scenes involving Craig and Wayne, leaving off with the story when Uncle Wayne has disappeared after his trial and picking it up again with Craig's journey to and settling in California. His father is mentioned in little more than a phrase, and no mention is made of his female family members or the conflicts they create for him. Having constructed a gay coming-of-age story out of what is in fact a much larger novel, Dewey is able to assert that "without regret, without apology, without anger, without pity, Whitmore launches Craig, his sexual identity now powerfully asserted, into the breaking dawn of a day that would within a scant decade unleash a most absolute night" (38). This depiction of such a vibrant dawn, the very dawning of it, is, says Dewey, an important contribution to "that countermovement of eros" that is so important to "AIDS fiction" (38). I do not set my reading against this one but wish only to add mine to it. Whitmore's novel has both "nothing" and "everything" to do with the AIDS crisis.

14. Kruger points out similarly empowering narrative devices employed by Paul Reed, whose dying character Andy has the last word in *Facing It: A Novel of A.I.D.S.*, even as it is the last word in his own life (Kruger 87), and by John Weir, whose "declining" Eddie Socket, in *The Irreversible Decline of Eddie Socket*, "kept talking" even until his last moments (Kruger 182).

15. Bartlett reads from a 1960 study entitled *Oscar Wilde: Was He a Genius or Just a Pervert?* which argues that "Oscar's moral decay was evident in his conspicuously terrible skin, that he was as wide-hipped as the mother who made him homosexual by dominating him" (27).

16. In "No Apocalypse," Derrida writes that "'reality,' let's say the encompassing institution of the nuclear age, is constructed by the fable [of nuclear war, as yet only imagined]" (23) and therefore not only resembles literature (itself "fabulously textual," without external referent) but *is* literature—part of the vast archive of rhetoric and opinion ("doxa") that constitutes textuality from ancient literary forms to modern-day nuclear

diplomacy. In a reversal that would be total and itself irreversible, this archive of all language forms would be destroyed at the moment of realization of the nuclear "fable." "That is why deconstruction [post-referentiality]," adds Derrida, "at least what is being advanced today in its name, belongs to the nuclear age. And to the age of literature" (27).

17. I have, of course, violated several Derridean parameters in formulating the preceding sentence as I have. Not only have I posited a prize resembling "truth" beyond the law (and the lie) that is language, I have equated this trap with heinous political dictatorship (instead of the much more acceptable, even comforting trap of, say, human consciousness), thus suggesting that a move past language is both as possible and as desirable as is freedom. As ultimately unreachable (even nonexistent) as this outer zone may be—in these novelistic worlds or in our own—the alternative vision I locate in the texts provides nevertheless a provocative challenge to the prevailing standard—to the linguistic game-playing ever insisted upon by Derrida (though perhaps more damagingly by text-analyzing Derrideans in an ever-lengthening line behind him), even when the stakes are enormously high. While he speaks out frequently and effectively against social injustice, the harm done by capitalism, and even nuclear weapons, Derrida's unrelenting assault on the "metaphysics" of meaning makes it impossible to valorize, to even understand, the challenge to totalitarianism undertaken by the novelists investigated here: even the overthrow of the "apocalyptic tone" in philosophy must come, says Derrida, from the "apocalyptic tone" itself (Carpenter 129).

Thus, for example, in typical deconstructive fashion, Joseph Andriano congratulates Atwood's Offred (in *The Handmaid's Tale*) for "frequently pun[ning words] to assure their multiplicity of meaning. An anarchy of words, as on a Scrabble board, is infinitely preferable to a rigidly inscribed monolithic text" (91–92). Elsewhere, he notes that "the system" has "a crack in the tablet that assures the ultimate crumbling of Gilead," while Magali Cornier Michael celebrates the "gaps" in Offred's world that assure her escape. But should we really promote such playfulness in readings of political oppression and resistance? Why even worry about the fate of Offred or societies like hers under authoritarian rule when the tenets of deconstruction assure us that no evil is sustainable, that slavery *is* freedom after all?

In a countering argument, Albert E. Stone has applauded the grim outlook of authors like Poul Anderson, Edgar Pangborn, and J. G. Ballard. For Stone, these writers "achieved more jolting effects—and possibly more effective education—by not letting readers off the hook with jokes, parodies, or absurd fantasies" (38). Similarly, Patrick D. Murphy has identified "the didactic signals of [dystopia authors'] chosen genre" and distinguished the sublimated response—produced by "dream literature" (Joanna Russ's term), which "lead[s] simply to a cathartic reduction of anxiety" and "enables escapism or reinforces smug assumptions"—from the cognitive response—produced by fiction, which "encourages discomforting reading and social action through implicitly or explicitly commenting on the reader's contemporary predicament" (26). Quoting Darko Suvin, Murphy notes that this "'significant utopia'" is formally closed but "'thematically open: its pointings reflect back on the reader's "topia"'" (26). Closure—narrative, philosophic, but also here the closed-off world of total totalitarianism—is anathema to the savvy postmodernist within us, yet shall we delight in the havoc-wreaking properties of "doublethink" (deconstruction in its earliest incarnation) when it has been much more accurately defined as "the Party's ultimate goal of thought control" (Macklin 176)?

18. See also David Seed's "Flight from the Good Life," which links similar theories of

Baudrillard's to Bradbury's *Fahrenheit 451* in a remarkable reading of Montag's wife Mildred's "disappearing mouth" (231–32).

19. For Auster, see Howard (92–93), McCaffery and Gregory (18), Washburn (63), and Woods; for Bradbury, see Seed ("The Flight from the Good Life" 225, 240), Wayne L. Johnson (84, 86), and Touponce (79–80); for Atwood, see Michael (138); for Orwell, see Howe (321), Rose ("Eric Blair's School Days" 89), and Rothbard.

20. Discussing *1984* (though his remarks are widely applicable here), Murray N. Rothbard describes a "perpetual but peripheral cold war" which "as pursued by the three superpowers of *Nineteen Eighty-Four* was key to their successful imposition of a totalitarian regime upon their subjects" (5).

21. The novels under consideration here were selected for the fullness of the example they provide. Often the alterapocalyptic is a subgeneric strain in postwar texts, so we may recognize not only alterapocalyptic narratives but also the alterapocalyptic *in* narratives. Examples include Arthur Koestler's *Darkness at Noon,* Anthony Burgess's *Clockwork Orange* (discussed elsewhere in chapter 2), and even Samuel Beckett's mostly postapocalyptic *Endgame* and *Happy Days.* Likewise, film and literature about the Vietnam War, whose historical raison d'etre was itself a conscripted, miserably failed alternative to nuclear war, demonstrate elements of the alterapocalyptic.

22. Comparing the potential for resistance in *1984* and *The Handmaid's Tale,* Ruud Teeuwen points out that "remembrance is a much vaguer presence in *Nineteen Eighty-Four:* Oceania has been in place for decades at the time we join Winston's life in it, and memories or a prerevolutionary life have, for the most part, lost the intensity of the personal. Gilead exists for just three years. . . . In *The Handmaid's Tale* memories are still suffused with detail. Where despair is a dull presence in Winston's life, it is an acute pain in Offred's" (117). Adding the idea that memory is tied to resistance, that totalitarian authority cannot be acquired "without a transitional phase of rigorous repression of the memories, desires, and idiosyncrasies of old, original contexts" (118), Teeuwen widens this discussion to apply nicely to the situation of Auster's novel as well.

23. More than one reader of this novel has indeed described this segment of Orwell's vision as a surprisingly wide hole in the net, which a true big-brotherian regime would never allow. See Rahv (315) and Deutscher (338). In defense of my positioning of *1984* at the end of this study—on account of its being the most dystopian, and thus the most alterapocalyptic of the four texts examined here, I would point out that while Orwell, who felt revolution would come from the most gifted among the proletarian class, includes proles in his vision, they offer no escape for Winston and Julia (recall that the room over Mr. Charrington's shop is a trap) and no permanent alleviation of the difficulties shaping their lives.

24. A number of readers recognize thinly veiled representations of modern-day New York in this novel's landscape, and while this reading is plausible, Tim Woods's discovery of "beauty" in the setting itself (109) and graceful movement ("cursives and strokes") in its inhabitants certainly surprises me. See also Howard (93).

25. Dennis Barone has argued that even this sphere is successfully reentered, if not by Anna herself then at least by the letter she writes: "We know that [Anna's message does get through] because the novel is actually told in a third-person narration. Someone has received Anna's story-as-letter, had read it, and, in turn, is now telling Anna's story to us. This is a story of triumph, not of disintegration" (8). Other readers of this novel, meanwhile, are less optimistic. Katharine Washburn calls Anna's letter (the entire narrative)

"a document cast into the void, mailed to some sort of dead letter zone at the end of the world" (62), and Sven Birkets insists that "if I'm right about the gated city and what it represents, these words are the last Anna will ever write" (68).

26. Again, Baudrillard's terminology is relevant here, as "obesity"—of communication systems, of signification, even of American bodies—is not so much the symptom but rather the cause of our enslavement to these systems and is for him synonymous with "obscenity."

27. While depicted in the narrative as a most willing consumer of the diet of inanity and inertia fed to her by her society, Montag's wife, Mildred, has been described by Donald Watt as a victim suffering physical symptoms due to socially induced repression, just as is Montag himself. Following her suicide attempt with sleeping pills, and the authorities' cold and mechanical stomach-pumping treatment, Watt notes that "the poisonous darkness within [Mildred] has become endemic to their way of life. The darkness suggests all the unimagined psychic bile that builds up in people, to embitter them, alienate them from one another, snuff out any inner light on their mode of existing" (201).

28. This phrase is Patrick D. Murphy's, employed in his description of Offred's universe as suffering "the aftermath of nuclear war and women's oppression" (27). In the novel itself, Offred puns the biblical "balm in Gilead" as "bomb in Gilead" (218), again reinforcing the implied nuclear prehistory and cohistory of the narrative.

29. In spite of what I will argue to be the novel's ultimately bleak ending, enormous gaps like these in Gilead's supposedly watertight system of control foster optimistic readings such as Lucy M. Freibert's, in which the writer declares that "Offred promises to come off a winner" and that the novel "offer[s] women a measure of hope," even though she curiously posits only moments later that "the system brooks no resistance or dissent" (281). Thus Freibert insists on an impossibly difficult challenge to overcome which our superheroine Offred successfully overcomes anyway. In note 17 (chapter 2) I discuss Andriano's and Michael's equally overenthusiastic assessments of Offred's many powers (see also chapter 2, note 12).

30. As with Orwell's Oceania, Gilead is a place of severe deprivation, frequent and unwitting encounters with spies, and technological excellence in home observation/invasion methods. Atwood's all-seeing "eye" over her bed corresponds to Orwell's telescreen. The armoire in which Offred reads the revolutionary note equates with the desk in which Winston hides his journal and the alcove where he makes his entries. Riffing on Huxley's *Brave New World* as well, Atwood's citizens of Gilead are stratified according to social role and identifying uniform, as were Huxley's alphas, betas, and gammas; and the reproductive function of women is taken over in both texts (though in different respects) by an intervening government authority.

31. Remarks from Laurence M. Porter underline this point: "In most such [apocalyptic] works, an element of hope subsists, because the hero differentiates himself from the surrounding chaos through (physical or mental) escape (Vonnegut), resistance (Camus), or both (Grass). . . . Thomas Mann's composer is engulfed, but leaves a legacy of genius. Orwell's mediocre hero, in contrast, is engulfed and leaves nothing" (62). In the midst of his study of Ray Bradbury, Wayne L. Johnson makes a similar point, with relevance to the genre-based discussion underway here as well: "Pessimists about the future of mankind have not always envisioned atomic extermination. An uncomfortable survival under a worldwide totalitarian state has also been suggested as a grim possibility. George Orwell's *1984* represents the hub of such writing" (83).

32. Readers of Atwood scholarship are familiar with the debate, entered into by almost everyone who publishes commentary on this text, as to the meaning of the historical notes appended to *The Handmaid's Tale.* Similarly, discussion as to the meaning of Orwell's appendix has centered around whether it represents some sort of liberation—if not for Winston himself, then at least for the seemingly doomed world of Oceania. Larry W. Caldwell has argued that the novel's grim ending is of only "apparent finality," since in the appendix "a voice from 'outside' the narrative, evoking a world altogether distinct from Winston's" (339) reassures the reader that Big Brother did not in fact have the last word. Richard K. Sanderson points out, however, that the moving final scene of the novel proper and not the dry technicality of the appendix is what readers remember as the "ending" of *1984* and that, even when considering the appendix as the novel's official last word, the fluent doublespeak understood and demonstrated by its author makes him or her seem anything but a reliable harbinger of a post–Big Brother age. Using the same terminology as does Caldwell, although reaching an opposite conclusion, Sanderson argues that, "by trying to reconcile the novel and the Appendix, we *experience* for ourselves—'outside' the novel as it were—what it might be like to inhabit a world in which the authenticity . . . of all documents is in doubt" (594). Thus while the "Historical Notes" of Atwood's text have the effect of closing off the Gileadean empire (in addition to Offred's role as storyteller), the appendix to Orwell's has the opposite effect—of opening out the Orwellian nightmare described previous to it to include and engulf the reader.

33. Meanwhile, M. Keith Booker has interestingly positioned at least Pynchon's *Vineland* as a direct descendant of the dystopian tradition that includes Orwell's *1984*, Zamyatin's *We*, and Huxley's *Brave New World.* Booker notes that *Vineland* is set in the year 1984 and that surveillance and detainment camps conducted by government spies are a way of life in Vineland, a place largely reminiscent of these earlier dystopias.

34. For example, see Friedman and Puetz, Ozier, Weisenburger ("The End of History?" and "Pynchon's Hereros"), and Seed ("Further Notes").

35. This phrase is borrowed from Joseph Slade, who puts it to much different purpose in "Communication, Group Theory, and Perception in *Vineland.*"

36. Several critics have made the case for Pynchon's novels as referring directly to events of the cold war period. For instance, Richard Pearce insists that *Gravity's Rainbow* "is [the experience] of more than the terror that pervaded England toward the end of World War II" ("Where They're At" 224) and includes within this larger experience the atomic bomb, the cold war, and the Korean and Vietnam Wars—yet offers no support for this claim. Frederick Ashe argues that multiple anachronistic elements in *Gravity's Rainbow* reflect Pynchon's connection to the 1960s "youth movement" but describes his role as a civil rights and antigovernment protester, not as a specifically antinuclear activist. Paul W. Celmer Jr. notes that "communist plots" were much in the news as Pynchon composed *V.* and contends, plausibly, that a notorious female spy, Vera Micheles Dean, may be yet another namesake for the multiply identified "V." Celmer, however, can push his comparison only so far, noting Pynchon's use of "apocalypse" and "an omnipresent, insidious conspiracy," which are for Pynchon, as I argue in chapter 2, concepts more philosophical and metaphysical than historically specific. McHoul and Wills's overly clever study of Pynchon's work concludes with a chapter titled "Fall Out." After several pages of Derridean wordplay, the authors happily fail to make the connection between Derrida's nuclear writings and a specifically nuclear theme in Pynchon: "We have not through all this

forgotten our nuclear umbrella question. What marks the nuclear question and all the apocalypse asks in coming, is an answer still falling after the end" (221).

37. For readings of the character of "V." along these lines, see Henkle and also chapter 4 in Berressem.

38. Some critics have stepped into this same contradiction. While opposing the science and philosophies of Pointsman and Mexico, Pearce describes the "limits of probability" that divide the two men, yet notes that Roger can "predict the striking pattern of the V-2 rockets with extreme accuracy" ("Introduction" 5). Friedman and Puetz contrast statisticians' views of a "truly random state of nature" with determinists' strict rules of cause and effect, yet they introduce the issue by describing "randomness *governed by the laws* of probability" (349; emphasis added).

39. For a fine overview of conspiracy versus anarchy in Pynchon's work, see Sanders.

40. For example, see Safer (159) and Sanders (188).

41. Lawrence Wolfley describes "Pynchon's hostility to the Calvinist tradition . . . that . . . divides society, on specious and hypocritical moral grounds, into two unequal classes" (108). Thus it is surprising that Pynchon conforms to this Puritan/Poinstmanian dichotomy of "here" and "not here" by disappearing Slothrop into preterition as soon as The Firm loses interest. One could argue that Pynchon is simply acknowledging, not embracing, such a system, yet the oddness of Slothrop's abrupt and anticlimactic disappearance sixty pages from the novel's end seems specially designed to reinforce the either/or of existence/salvation as set down in Puritan tracts.

42. Terrence Holt has considered *all* nuclear-related novels and short stories as preapocalyptic, arguing that these fictions reveal our subconscious death wish to detonate and unleash radioactive destruction upon the world (207).

43. Weber describes an exchange between David and his mother, who asks about his sexual relationships: "'You're careful, aren't you?' David responds, 'Of course'" (71). Weber notes that this is the closest we come to any mention of AIDS in Cameron's novel and then acknowledges, "That 'of course' may sound glib to some in the gay community who have seen numerous friends die . . . several years after male homosexuals started to follow safer sex guidelines" (71). Weber tries to head off an objection like this by noting that "neither Cameron nor any of his characters seems unnerved by the threat of AIDS—at least no more so than other educated Americans their age, male and female, straight and gay, *the majority of whom* do not share needles or *engage in unprotected sex*" (71; emphasis added). Sensing the numbers of Americans who *always* use condoms might be a little less than "the majority," after all, Weber continues: "At the very worst, I suppose the characters in Cameron's fiction could be said to conform too closely to standards of 'proper' gay behavior," and "that stain of propriety might be enough to draw charges from some gays" (70–71). In short, since Weber is unable to put down this charge of "glibness" coming from other quarters, we must assume he himself cannot dismiss it entirely either.

44. Based on statistics of the Gay and Lesbian Service Center in Los Angeles, Todd Simmons reported 200 new infection cases for people under age twenty-five in center records: "Those infections reflect a national rise in the rate of infection for gay teens and young adults—a group that lacks the personal experience of AIDS common to older gay men" (30).

45. While Michael Dorris and Louise Erdrich have argued that "a majority of postnuclear war novels of the last 25 years are irrationally optimistic, if only in their lack of true realism" (54), these reviewers' criterion is too simply met. "Irrational optimism," by their

definition, must include the depicted survival of *any* characters, even those "degraded, mutated, and dazed—or some facsimile of them— . . . to tell the tale" (54).

46. The notion of permanence and the safety this brings is undermined again and again in Cameron's novel through multiple references to issues topical in the year it was published but now largely irrelevant: Manuel Noriega, Burt Reynolds and Lonnie Anderson, "L.A. Law," fat jokes about Oprah Winfrey (reincarnated here as "Orca"). These many already archaisms produce the postpublication subthesis that nothing is permanent (or even older than "5") in postmodern society, that everything that goes around almost simultaneously comes around.

47. I am using this term in its typically pejorative sense here, as opposed to the "vacations" from full confrontation with plague crises offered by the pre-AIDS and alterapocalyptic genres. Both of these genres use their sidestepping gestures to speak to and alleviate these crises nevertheless and not simply ignore or forget them.

48. Whitmore warns early in *Someone Was Here,* his account of three AIDS-related medical settings that the real story of AIDS is about "blood and shit." The stories he tells are of the urban poor and the recently impoverished due to the high cost of living and dying with HIV, and the neglect endemic to the big-city technocracies supporting them turns their respective hospital beds into chambers of horrors.

49. Jones locates this original reference to a "gay space" in *The Gay Academic,* in which Jacob Stockinger describes a "homotextual space." In contrast to the closet, a space that gays by 1978 were well on their way to demolishing, the site of gay writing resembles, says Stockinger, Woolf's "room of one's own" (142).

50. Kruger describes a similar gap between speakers of different "languages" and the heightened anxiety this gap creates in his reading of early AIDS fiction whose characters'—patients' and doctors'—acquaintance with medical terminology, and the increased medical knowledge of AIDS accompanying this, does not match that of the more seasoned, educated reader: "As the novel [Reed's *Facing It*] progresses—with Dr. Branch gaining medical knowledge, Andy gaining knowledge of experience, and David, a journalist, beginning to research the illness and its manifestations—the characters' expectations become bleaker and bleaker, approaching congruence with the informed reader's" (84).

51. Hoban made this remark during an interview with Natalie Maynor and Richard F. Patteson, who circle around that comment for most of the paper, suggesting several ways in which language in *Riddley* is "particular" and "linguistic" without ever really delineating why it is heroic or good (protagonistic). At least Jeffrey Porter embodies (if not valorizes) Hoban's language, noting that in *Riddley Walker* "language knows things people do not. . . . [It is] essentially intelligent" (451–52). Porter demonstrates this with his focus on new "fissions" or explosions of words that in their splitting have added a sublayer of meaning to our search for the old one. Thus "soar vivers" are not only "survivors" but "sore live-ers"; the "Ardship" is the privileged "archbishop" but also the bearer of much "hardship"; "breaving" is not only "breathing" (inspiration) but "grieving" and "bereavement" (expiration) as well (457).

52. Holt observes that bombs were not only envisioned as babies, the one dropped on Hiroshima having been named "Little Boy," but also that babies were perceived in postwar America as bombs, or at least as weapons—the "fodder" of a population explosion that would outnumber enemy ranks (206). Also, however, Holt notes that babies were positioned as a central "potential victim of nuclear weapons" (207).

53. Martin Baker notes that "in the comic form, there is an interaction between the

pictureness and verbalness of the speech-balloon, to produce the meaning of sound. We 'hear with our eyes'" (11).

Chapter 3: Three Points of Sight

1. On the (homo)erotic nature of Donne's sonnet, see Rambuss, Klawitter, and Mueller.

2. On the use of "man" and "he" in criticism of Pynchon, see LeClair, Friedman and Puetz, Golden, Sanders, and Simmon.

3. Tony Tanner's assessment that in *V.* there are "figures" since "one can hardly speak of characters" (*City of Words* 164) holds true for *Gravity's Rainbow* as well; yet even the masculine figurations are more engaging and dimensionalized than the female ones.

4. I appreciate John W. Hunt's more specific formulation: "It is the narrator, not Stencil, who for the reader is making Stencil's quest into a quest for a metaphysical absolute, and he does this by forcing V. to mean everything and thus nothing" (36). For another of the many meanings behind V.'s "V," see Henkle.

5. Schwenger's hipster reference resonates with his later comment on the work of Mailer, whose "'language of men'" (Schwenger's term)—"conversational, even colloquial; slangy; occasionally even foul-mouthed; and above all anti-literary" (*Letter Bomb* 107)—reminds him of William's own voice in *The Nuclear Age.* His description of a "style [that] must then be evolved that will fend off the threat of emasculation, that will turn pen into penis" (107) applies to the hole's speech and even to Sarah's, which is also macho, off-putting, and stereotypically masculine.

6. Not surprisingly, Sarah's most interesting quality is the way in which she dies, the literal and permanent absenting that only completes the vacancy marking her character throughout the novel. A bombshell in earlier days, Sarah appears in the novel's present as sick and weak, a potential carrier in need of quarantine who "coughed and rubbed her eyes. She'd lost some weight . . . and . . . seemed skinny and poor-looking. Unhealthy, too. The blister at her lip was hard to ignore" (289). The blister is, finally, the sole indicator of fatal encephalitis; significantly Sarah has been toting an armed nuclear warhead around the country before reuniting with William, the implication being that if she did not "catch" encephalitis from nuclear contamination, the mortifying stress of existence literally in the bomb's shadow played a crucial role in her undoing.

7. Virginia Carmichael has pointed out anal fixation themes in several, specifically male-authored, cold war novels, including Doctorow's *Book of Daniel,* Coover's *Public Burning,* and Pynchon's *Gravity's Rainbow.* Carmichael notes that "misogyny, gynophobic homosocial bonding, and narcissistic anal aggression are predominant . . . as figures for U.S. cold war states of mind . . . [and] as evidence of the costs to the individual, the family, and the society of state abuse" (187).

8. On male-to-male trafficking in women, see Rubin.

9. In "Nuclear Culture, Nuclear War," Michael W. Messmer notes the effects of "nuclear culture" on children of Melinda's era: "Not as an apocalyptic horror to haunt their daydreams or rouse them screaming from nightmares [as was the case with William's own cold war childhood] but rather, like radiation, silently, and initially painlessly, penetrating the very marrow of their developing awareness of the wider world around them" (176–77). This shift from violence to illness that Messmer observes reproduces the trend that I argue is definitive of the entire postmodern plague period.

10. In what is probably the strongest defense possible for Wylie's depiction of women

in this manner, Clifford P. Bendau blames society (not Wylie's own narrative, as I am doing here) for "forcing men and women into separate psychological and material domains" (45). Yet what Bendau defines as Wylie's corrective response to this separation is marked with the problematic and dichotomous logic by which society removed and oppressed women in the first place: "there is [according to the thesis of *The Disappearance*] only one sex, with men and women being halves" (45).

11. Carol Cohn has documented the multiple language-based efforts of nuclear strategists and intellectuals to position themselves as birth-givers and creators of life since the inception of nuclear weaponry at midcentury. The bomb dropped on Hiroshima was named "Little Boy," and congratulatory telegrams between scientists and politicians were exchanged like cigars between proud fathers. The atom bomb at Los Alamos was named "Oppenheimer's baby," and the hydrogen bomb at Lawrence Livermore "Teller's baby." Interestingly, the feminine principle is dismissed as utterly irrelevant to the creative process: Teller was denounced after all as only the "mother" of the hydrogen bomb who merely "carried" the ideas of Stanislaw Ulam to fruition; early tests determined bombs as "boys" if they exploded and "girls" if they were duds (700–701).

Elsewhere in that article Cohn questions the heavy percentage of domestic terms also emerging in nuclear-planning discourse, and Gillian Brown offers a smart analysis of domestic imagery as entirely in keeping with a capitalist society's emphasis on individual survival and women's "burden" to repopulate the world after an enormous crisis such as nuclear holocaust. Brown notes that "what gets affirmed in the effort to cope with nuclear disaster is not gender equality but the domestic sentiments still attached to women. The association of femininity with futurity registers and allays anxiety about the displacement of human functions by human inventions" (183).

12. Like many of the utopias I discuss in chapter 2, Piercy's free town of Tikva ranges from the unbelievable to the unbelievably boring in nearly all of its manifestations. For largely unexplained reasons fresh flowers and vegetables and live animals flourish in this otherwise ruined ecosystem, the air is breathable with only minimal filtering, and disease and nuclear radiation effects remain at survivable lows. In contrast the remainder of "Norika" (formerly the United States and Canada) rages with plague, deprivation, and violence in the large, unpoliced expanses of "Glops" (megalopolises) where the non-techie population is forced to carry out its mean existence. Yet marauding bands from these burnt-out zones never threaten the free towns, and the encroaching multis are kept successfully at bay by the thinnest of economic leverage. Likewise everyone in Tikva is perfectly on top of his or her (especially her) game: Avram is successful, productive, and healthy in his old age; Malkah is a font of spiritual wisdom, gentle humor, vibrant sexuality, and hard-to-find gourmet delicacies any hour of the night or day; the town council is for the most part cool-headed and prudent. Interestingly, Yod himself, an all-providing, all-problem-solving "utopia" of security for Shira and her family, is an island of technology in a sea of humanity, controlled, as were many of the islands of chapter 2, by the metonymic. Yod's early language facility is thoroughly concrete; he cannot imagine how love is like a red, red rose, and all "metaphorical thinking seemed to stymie it" (92).

13. As the title itself already promises us, Piercy's novel fairly writhes with the kind of love couplings and triangulations that make up any good daytime drama. "He, she and it" refers to the years-old "affair" between Shira and Gadi as it is interrupted by the cyborg Yod, with its own attractive characteristics. There is a secondary triangle between Shira, Yod, and Malkah—who is considered by Shira to be "too old" for an affair, yet whom

Yod considers as attractive as a younger woman, since he was programmed (by Malkah herself) to not notice the differences of age in women. There are oedipal triangles formed among Avram, Gadi, and Shira (both father and son having measures of desire for Shira); among Avram, Shira, and Malkah (who has desires for Avram and is tired of battling Shira for the eligible men); and among Malkah, daughter Riva, and granddaughter Shira (who worries that "Malkah preferred Riva to her" [200]).

14. This list includes Aldous Huxley (*Brave New World*); Philip Wylie (*Tomorrow!*); Pat Frank (*Alas, Babylon*); Bradbury and Vonnegut, whose relevant novels will be discussed shortly; and Martin Amis ("Thinkability") as read by Adam Mars-Jones in *Venus Envy.*

15. Victoria A. Brownworth's findings on this issue are close to my own: "gay male writing differs very little in its portrayal of women from its straight male counterpart. Gay male writing runs the gamut from ignoring women altogether to presenting a hatred not dissimilar from that of its hetero twin" (7).

16. HIV infection rates among lesbians are remarkable for their statistical absence from most data samples. In 1995, the Centers for Disease Control (CDC) attributed infections for women overwhelmingly to heterosexual contact and intravenous drug use. Frustratingly, the CDC groups its percentage for women's "other rates of infection" (possibly lesbian contact) with multiple other factors—patients pending medical review, patients who died, who were lost to follow-up or declined interviews—so that this slice of the pie is quite large but impossible to subcategorize. A 1995 survey by Lemp et al. groups lesbians and bisexual women in its findings, although certainly the documented increased risk of bisexual activity should not be allowed to indicate a heightened risk of lesbian activity as well.

More recently Laurie Fitzpatrick, in an article for *Arts and Understanding,* strenuously rejects the "persuasive myth of lesbian immunity" (23) but can only go on to cite infection rates for populations similar to those I describe above: lesbians *and* bisexual women and, even more broadly, the population of "women" who are dealing now with skyrocketing infection rates. Try as she might, and for whatever mystifying reasons she may have, to enlarge the perception that lesbians are at high risk for HIV, Fitzpatrick can only resort to circular reasoning: "The truth is that lesbians are probably more at risk for AIDS. Why? Because we perpetuate the myth of 'Lesbian Immunity'" (25). Later she lists the ways in which lesbians (and in fact all of us) are at risk for HIV, none of these, significantly, involving sexual contact with other women: "We have unsafe sex with men, trade sex for money, food, drugs, and shelter. We inject IV drugs and share dirty needles. We receive artificial insemination and blood transfusions, and we risk occupational exposure" (25).

17. A flyer circulated some years ago by a campus student health service demonstrated this new challenge to binary systematizing by featuring a background split diagonally between a field of tiny pluses and a field of blank space. Thus the opposite to positivity was not negativity but nothingness, nonpatient status. For an interesting related discussion, see Savoy (67).

18. An important, however solitary, exception to this argument is John Weir's *Irreversible Decline of Eddie Socket,* which remarkably represents both men's and women's roles in the AIDS crisis, bettering some of the work done by even the most open-minded of the lesbian authors I will investigate momentarily. As with these women-authored texts, Weir's novel depicts a leading female character, Polly, as compassionate, strong, and fully human. No "angel" by a longshot, she midway through the novel emotionally abandons Eddie, who is HIV-positive, while she tries to secure a relationship with a self-centered

boyfriend, and while Eddie suffers unrequited feelings for an older man. The pain of impending death brings out the selfish side of Polly, who admits that "suddenly she wanted a refund on all the time they spent together. She wanted their moments returned. She wanted Eddie carefully extricated from her life, . . . air-brushed out like a Soviet diplomat excised from history" (214). But at novel's end she returns to him in his hospital room, visiting and thinking of him constantly in the final weeks. On their last day together, she bathes him and changes his soiled sheets, holding him in her arms as he dies. Despite his critique of the "consistent erasure of women from the public discourse on AIDS" (57), Steven F. Kruger, in his lengthy and otherwise helpful reading of this novel, does little to emphasize the important role played by the female character here.

19. Referring to the theories of Eve Kosofsky Sedgwick, Ross Chambers insists that *The Swimming-Pool Library* is a homosocial novel "in which relations between men are mediated by women—who as a consequence of that mediating role—are excluded" (312). After describing several romantic triangles in Hollinghurst in which the compulsory heterosexual (the woman) is replaced with another, less-favored man, Chambers concludes that "mediating men can be stand-ins for the women who are absent from the novel" (313). Joseph Bristow later quotes this last statement from Chambers in his own work and declares it an "astute observation" (179) with central importance for Hollinghurst's novels.

20. Richard Fung has pointed out that the hyposexualization of Asians in Western culture is no less endemic to the gay population. In gay porn iconography, a mere handful of Asians have reached the status of "porn star," and even in this situation they remain passive or resisting figures in sex scenes in which white men do the penetrating and whose pleasure is the cinematic focus. In the queer paradigm, says Fung, the Asian is the classic anonymous trick, faceless and "inscrutable," whose very unknowability fosters erotic attraction toward them and is emblematized in the stage name of a leading Asian porn star, Sum Yung Mahn.

21. In part 2 of Kushner's play, the angel describes herself as being "hermaphroditically equipped" with eight vaginas and a "Bouquet of Phalli" (44), but this reference to the angel being biologically male is singular throughout the play's seven hours and contradicted by the fact that, according to David Savran in "Ambivalence, Utopia, and a Queer Sort of Materialism," the angel has always been cast as a female. As I will note below, a female figuration of the angel is vital to the play's meaning on multiple levels: not only is she, like Lady Columbia, an allegory for America itself; she is also part of the radical gender upheaval going on throughout the play—in the form of gay Prior's erection and wet-dreaming and motherly Hannah Pitt's enormous orgasm—so clearly a part of Kushner's core project. She "concludes" the two-part production by making an entrance late in part 1, appearing on the cover of the Sarabande Press edition of part 2, and solidifying into the Bethesda Fountain angel—"*She's* my favorite angel. . . . Louis will tell you *her* story" (145; emphasis added)—at the end of this second half.

22. In "Ambivalence, Utopia, and a Queer Sort of Materialism," Savran points out that "amidst all the political disputation [in *Angels*], there is no talk of social class. Oppression is understood not in relation to economics but to difference of race, gender, and sexual orientation. . . . There is no clear sense that the political and social problems with which the characters wrestle might be connected to a particular social class" (224). Meanwhile, Savran describes Kushner's "avowed commitment to socialism, an alternative to capitalism" (224), and in the afterword to *Perestroika* Kushner blames "Individualism and the

political economy it serves, Capitalism" (150) for America's many social crises. Finally, however, even Kushner admits that "we're at a point in American political history where it's much easier to say 'I'm a homosexual' than it is to say 'I'm a socialist'" (interview with Lowenthal 12). Perhaps in fear of antisocialist retribution (though perhaps in fear of nothing of the kind), Kushner broke contracts and promises so as to maneuver his production into the most lucrative Broadway venue possible (See Brustein [30–31] and Lyons [57]). Here class consciousness seems to have won out over the playwright's disdain for class distinctions, as it does in his rendering of the play itself.

23. The angel, reprising her moment of descent from part 1 in the opening act from part 2, even hails Prior as "long-descended, well-prepared" (36), implying that his impressive pedigree has specially qualified him to receive angels with all the decorum they deserve and thus receive the gift of longer life that angels are singularly authorized to bestow. Likewise, these terms are double entendres (long-descended/"well-hung," well-prepared/sexually ready) that refer indeed to the sexually vibrant state Prior is about to work himself into, thus signaling his return, however temporarily, to healthy and active life (see chapter 3, note 25).

24. In both productions documented in a 1996 anthology of Vogel's work, male, not cross-dressing female, actors were cast as the "third man" who is constantly bedding Anna.

25. Even though Prior is not cured of his illness in the way Frazier miraculously is, he assumes a vibrancy and strength that is distinctly counter to his role in part 1. Interestingly, Vogel describes Anna's increased sexual activity as an "urge to fight the sickness of the body with the health of the body" (29), and our first picture of Prior in *Perestroika* is as potently sexual: he is wet-dreaming during the night and having a waking orgasm at the words of the angel shortly after that. Later he successfully wrestles the angel for her blessing and an extended stay on earth and concludes the play not only very much alive but also centralized by the dramatic narrative.

26. I appreciate Eve Kosofsky Sedgwick's formulation of the phenomenon many critics have observed: "What goes on at football games . . . and at climactic moments in war novels can look, with only a slight shift of optic, quite startlingly 'homosexual'": "For a man to be a man's man is separated only by an invisible, carefully blurred, always-already-crossed line from being 'interested in men'" (*Between Men* 89).

27. W. Russel Gray has pointed out that in *1984* O'Brien's "Christian name is missing, unknown, or irrelevant" (125). In what is probably no small coincidence, all of the male characters in the three novels under consideration here—save one (Winston himself)—are referred to by their last names, while all of the major female characters are addressed only by their first names. Of course the assumption that Mildred and Anita had taken their husbands' last names at marriage may have released Bradbury and Vonnegut from having to state the obvious, but Julia is unmarried throughout Orwell's narrative and on a first-name basis (only) with Winston and with the reader. Sue Lonoff points out that in earlier drafts of *1984* Julia had the last name of Vernon (by which she would have been tagged with the diminutive form of the name of Orwell's predecessor dystopist, Jules Verne) but that, for reasons Orwell never felt compelled to defend, this was cut in the final version.

28. While Jonathan Rose has speculated in "The Invisible Sources of *Nineteen Eighty-four*" that O'Brien may have persecuted Winston out of sexual jealousy over Julia (139), Lonoff's reading that "O'Brien unmans Winston—in the text's words, gets inside him" (33) positions O'Brien's desire more accurately, especially in light of several readings delineating a "homoerotics of Room 101": Laurence M. Porter notes that "the dreaded Room

101 symbolizes the original personality ('1') annihilated ('0') and then replaced with another ('1') totally subordinated to the Party" (70). Since Porter is in the middle of a psychoanalytic reading of *1984*, we are easily reminded of the orgasmic *jouissance* responsible for this dissolution of the subject and may further read "101" as shorthand for the one-"on"-one torture games played by O'Brien and Winston in their sadomasochistic closet. W. Russel Gray, citing a helpful passage, draws an important conclusion: "Also, toward *his* violator Winston develops not only dependence but strange affection: 'a blissful, healing warmth spread all through his body. The pain was already half forgotten. He opened his eyes and looked up gratefully at O'Brien. . . . He had never loved him so deeply as at this moment'" (119).

29. Donald Watt has discerned even more triangulation among Bradbury's characters: "Beatty and Faber . . . are the poles between which Montag must find his identity, with Mildred and Clarisse [the young neighbor who inspires Montag early in the story, then disappears] reflecting the same polar opposition on another level" (197). Not surprisingly, Watt finds that "the men are the intellectual and didactic forces at work on Montag, while the women are the intuitive and experiential forces. Beatty articulates the system's point of view, but Mildred lives it. Faber articulates the opposition's point of view, but Clarisse lives it" (197).

30. On the triangulation of male-male couplings in Mailer, see Ellmann, Hardwick, Millett, and Radford.

31. I appreciate Richard Poirier's formulation that there exists "a curious connection in his mind between sexual careers and the career of the novelist, between sexual creativity and the creative effort to shape history" (86).

32. Jean Radford marks a similar shift in attitudes toward homosexuality between Mailer's first two novels and his third: Teddy Pope "is shown, as in the scene in which Teppis tries to force him to marry Lulu, capable of honesty and affection in contrast to the hypocritical morality of the 'straight' world represented by Teppis. The homosexual in Mailer's third novel is no longer the agent, the striking force, of totalitarianism, but is another victim" (132).

33. Andrew Gordon points out that Mailer's descriptions of the aurora borealis as electromagnetic force field resemble Reich's own theories of electrical charges, specifically a "form of tangible, measurable libido" called "orgone energy" (49).

34. Indeed Michael K. Glenday has read "Alaska" in this novel as "a rehearsal for the killing fields soon to be visited by two of the huntsmen, D.J. and Tex" (106), and Philip H. Bufithis develops the analogy even more plainly: "The hunting party is the American military in miniature, replete with commanders and their GI subordinates. The crazed animals being annihilated by aerial machines are the people of Vietnam napalmed by the Air Force" (76).

35. For other negative responses to Pynchon's work see Morgan, Henkle, Sanders, and Friedman and Puetz.

36. I much appreciate Francine Prose's recent consideration of the "inferiority" of women's writing, especially her survey of the negative response to Leslie Marmon Silko's *Almanac of the Dead*, a "wildly ambitious, epic, gritty, and violent novel" (68). Covering a Pynchonian range of events and elements from American history and culture, Silko's book contends for canonical status but is so far having horrible luck. I quote Prose's interesting, and here relevant, findings at length: "From the horror that greeted Silko's book, published in 1991, one might have concluded that she herself was plotting insurrection

or confessing to all the bloody crimes committed in her novel. How upset reviewers were by this 'very angry author' seething with 'half-digested revulsion,' by her inability to create 'a single likable, or even bearable, character,' her bad judgement and 'inadequate craft,' the 'nonexistent plot,' and worst of all, her 'emphatic view of sex as dirty, together with a ceaseless focus on the male sex organ, suggest[ing] that more than the novel itself needs remedial help'" (68). Of course these same terms have been applied, these same "ceaseless foci" (though on *female* sex organs) expected, whenever critical attention is turned to Pynchon's work, although in his case these observations always manage to spell out acclaim instead of disgust.

37. On the connection between an exploding and an explosive female sexuality, see also Whitfield, D'Emilio, and Weart.

38. I realize I am condensing the two images offered in this scene from Pynchon's novel, in which the "clairvoyant" (though more accurately "clairectile") Slothrop comes upon a shred of announcement regarding the bomb dropped on Hiroshima. The scrap is part of an army-generated newsletter whose logo is of a large-breasted woman straddling a long, pointed cannon, while the image in the newsphoto, of a mushroom cloud, is depicted by Pynchon as hermaphroditic—phallic and vaginal at once. In his reading of this scene, Peter Schwenger makes the same condensation—"a woman with a penis powerful as a steel cannon, explosive as a bomb" (*Letter Bomb* 62)—and both our conflations result no doubt from the proximity of Pynchon's destructive, phallic cannon to his destructive, phallic bomb.

39. One exception is Margot A. Henriksen's review of multiple films, novels, and even paintings that described life as a "snake pit" in this period.

40. Bérubé cites a 1948 U.S. Navy campaign to tie homosexuals to a series of grisly murders (262) and a 1953 U.S. Navy memorandum that exonerates homophobic witch hunts and dishonorable discharges in the postwar period by defining homosexuals as "dangerous security risks" (269). Bérubé notes that this and other such military policies incited similar paranoia and hostility throughout Washington, resulting in the persecutions and firings of hundreds of government personnel. Ultimately society as a whole contracted the hysteria: "The media and government propaganda associated homosexuals and other 'sex psychopaths' with communists as the most dangerous nonconformists—invisible enemies who could live next door and who threatened the security and safety of children, women, the family, the nation" (258).

41. Both May and Whitfield single out the vitriolic anticommunism of novelist Mickey Spillane, who evidently despised women and Soviet operatives with equal vigor yet reserved the brunt of his narrative violence for the worst of both these worlds—women who were also communist sympathizers or spies. Whitfield notes that Charlotte Manning in Spillane's early *I, the Jury* "is easily overwhelmed by the force of [Mike Hammer's] machismo, yet continues to run a heroin ring, thus must ineluctably die at his hands" (35). A tougher customer, Ethel Brighton, continues in her procommunist ways after spending a night in Mike's apartment, "so he strips and whips her" (36). Whitfield documents the enormous popularity of Spillane in this era, noting that even McCarthy was stealing lines from his titles ("my gun is quick") to swagger among his political opponents. Thus Spillane's multiple and complex hatreds were widely disseminated, and his violent, vigilantist response to a threat he perceived to be "everywhere" became accepted as the only means of combating this pervasive threat to the health of society.

42. Peter Schwenger provides an illuminating reading of Gee's postscript, "Against

Ending," in *Letter Bomb* (16), yet I am disappointed by her pulling back the curtain from this final scene of total destruction to inform us that things are really not so bad. I find such saving grace too easy and inappropriate in a text such as hers, exactly the kind of forgiveness sought after by readers looking to ignore or forget her message.

43. Marian is only one of the more complex and thus attractive among a large representation of women in AIDS novels suffering from this kind of AIDS-related phenomenon. In Peter McGehee's *Sweetheart* and Edmund White's "Running on Empty" (in *The Darker Proof*) both HIV-positive male protagonists come from large families of women who were always a bit strange but whose inability to deal with the homosexuality and HIV-positive status of a loved one has only worsened their eccentric or neurotic ways. McGehee's cartoonish, dysfunctional family drinks too much, speaks in brain-deadening clichés, and all but refuses to acknowledge the presence of homosexuality or AIDS in their universe. In White's story, the aging, lonely women of Luke's family do attempt to come to terms with his sexual orientation and illness, their evangelizing spirits bent on loving him, yet loving him *in spite of* the "sins" he has committed. Finally Luke's visit wears on him and actually advances, however slightly, the process of his deterioration, and he realizes that he has come to assuage their guilt—yet also break through their denial—at the expense of his own health.

44. In "Manifesto" (*Love Alone*), Monette writes literally and figurally about the bomb at once, referring to actual bombings AIDS activists might carry out against government offices but couching this suggestion metaphorically, and negatively, as lament: "every tent revival mantra / is one less bomb tossed in the red-taped labs / of the FDA" (40–41). Interestingly, this question of whether to bomb or not to bomb (to instead succumb to the enervating influence of new-age pop philosophers like Louise Hay), recast by the poem's end as the decision between "the mirror" and "the tank," has come to form the grounds of debate within the gay community about which path of activism is more effective. See Edelman's *Homographesis* and Crain.

45. In this paragraph I quote from my own viewing of a videotape of *The Living End.*

Chapter 4: Two Takes on a Scare

1. For example, see the seminal essays by Baudry and Metz and the more recent psychoanalytic-feminist work by Friedberg, Doane, and Copjec.

2. By this time, several influences had coalesced to produce the sexual ennui depicted in popular films: a winding down of the sex boom of the 1960s, the growth of Reaganism and the religious right, and a string of medical "scares" (Legionnaires' disease, toxic shock syndrome, and contaminated bottles of Tylenol) combined to create the realization that we had moved into a new and noxious age. Multiple films portrayed "swinging" and other forms of loose or "perverted" sexuality in graphic terms, only to demonstrate the mortal dangers surrounding these. They include *Midnight Cowboy* (1969), *Taxi Driver* (1976), *Looking for Mr. Goodbar* (1977), *American Gigolo* (1980), and *Cruising* (1980).

3. Interestingly, multiple critics disliked the film's final twenty to thirty minutes, during which this AIDS-suggestive plot develops, regarding it as a falling away from or slowing down of the film's earlier comic-satiric momentum. Indeed, the film does get quite silly and strange at this point—we might even say that it is "infected" or at least weakened by its entanglement with this issue (see the reviews by Ansen, Corliss, O'Toole, Denby, and Kael). Elsewhere in her review, Kael uses sexually suggestive terminology already

reflective of AIDS and queer cultures, describing Pat's "promiscuous use of chemicals" and Pat herself as "a masochist who just goes from one cage to another" (110).

4. The phrase comes from Freud, who notes that little girls, whose leap from mother to father as object choice is complex and precarious, are therefore much more susceptible to failing in this leap, thus falling back into a stunted, permanent preoedipal state (230).

5. In her *New Republic* review of *The Fantastic Voyage,* Kael smirks at "the medical and military men outside [the patient's body] with their homey little ironies. 'What a time to run out of sugar,' says government-man Edmund O'Brien, like a 'housewife' in a commercial" (34).

6. I am rather obviously in disagreement with David Ansen's request in his review of *Innerspace* that we "say good-bye to the sex comedy (this is post-AIDS Hollywood); action comedies are the name of the game" (60). Meanwhile, I appreciate his suggestive description of this film as a "biological buddy movie" (60).

7. In *Epistemology of the Closet,* Sedgwick describes not just homosocial activity but queer subjectivity itself as structured (within the confines of a homophobic society) as an open secret—the closet that, to be opened fully, must be reopened to every stranger passed on the sidewalk and that, when not (yet) opened at all, almost inevitably reveals the closeted nevertheless (1–22).

8. In a seemingly anti-McCarthyist gesture, Kazan's film speaks against panic and hysteria but advises the use of lies (the withholding of information) instead of truth (the dissemination of information) to preserve public order. For the record of Kazan's own confused history as a member of and informer on the Communist Party in America, see Maltby.

9. Reminiscent of my observation in this study's early pages about the ways in which the cold war was made largely out of language, one reviewer complained about this cold war classic that it "needs more medical curiosity and less vigorous gab" (Farber 214). Another reviewer diagnosed the same trouble in the original *Blob* (discussed later in chapter 4): "Unfortunately, [producer Jack H. Harris's] picture talks itself to death, even with the blob nibbling away at everybody in sight" (Thompson 23).

10. In his review of *The China Syndrome* Ansen makes this remarkably coincident observation: "This is a movie about how jobs compromise and define people, in which all the characters are always at work, even at parties, and [director James] Bridges' style—cool and un-sensual—is right for the subject. It is a movie notably devoid of romance" (103). Commenting on the new seriousness he had sensed in several recent films rebounding from a fluff decade, Richard Corliss says that *The China Syndrome* may signal that "movies may once again *mean* something to people" ("Chain Reactions" 27).

11. In describing a similarly desirous relationship within cinema, that of the spectator to the actors on screen, Christian Metz notes that a certain *distance* is required and offered by cinema, a temporal distance separating actors' moment of presence (during the profilmic episodes) and spectators' (during the viewing episode). This distance enables viewers to watch in a clandestine, "unauthorized" manner, heightening their voyeuristic pleasure as it recalls for them their similarly hidden and unauthorized position as witnesses to the primal scene (62–64).

12. See the review by Magid and "Chuck Russell's *Blob* May Be the Most Sinister Slime of All Time."

13. Making her own semiotic comparison, Janet Maslin observes that the remade *Blob* is "very much a film of the moment. It is more violent than the original, more spectacular, more cynical, more patently commercial" (6).

14. As analog for the disease-carrying queer in this unsuspecting society, the reverend corresponds to the feminized disease carrier as more perpetrator than victim in a disease's progress. Sander Gilman, in his reading of syphilis-related images in previous centuries, notes that "by the eighteenth century, the image of the patient . . . becomes the corrupt female. . . . It takes over two hundred years for the image of the syphilitic to shift from male 'victim' of the disease to its female 'source'" (254–55).

15. While the *Incredible Shrinkings* and the *Blobs* often make it into discussions of the cold war–1980s film connection, even more obvious examples include *The Fly* (discussed earlier in chapter 4), *Little Shop of Horrors, The Invasion of the Body Snatchers, It,* and Romero's *Living Dead* series (*Night of the Living Dead, Dawn of the Dead,* and *Day of the Dead*), which has spanned both periods.

Conclusion

1. In "Progress versus Utopia," Jameson emphasizes the "impossible" nature of Utopia's realization and argues that the writing of Utopia is its "miraculous" realization nevertheless, a literary feat that should inspire readers of this genre to strive for the utopic in their own lives.

2. Elsewhere Jameson has described Utopia as "a transparent synonym for socialism itself" ("Of Islands and Trenches" 3) and a "radical strangeness and freshness of human existence and of its object world in a non-commodity atmosphere" ("Progress versus Utopia" 155).

3. Not only is Jameson a vigorous and prolific defender of the utopian as a literary genre, but he is likewise overtly hostile to the genre of dystopia, specifically the kind produced by Orwell and other midcentury alterapocalyptic authors. Writing for *Diacritics,* Jameson declares that "anti-utopianism constitutes a far more easily decodable and unambiguous political position: from religious arguments about the sinful hybris of an anthropocentric social order all the way to vivid 'totalitarian' dystopias of the contemporary counterrevolutionary (Dostoyevsky, Orwell, etc.), . . . the enemies of Utopia sooner or later turn out to be the enemies of socialism" ("Of Islands and Trenches" 3).

Of course, my entire project is in disagreement with Jameson on this point. I contend that Jameson's critique of Orwell is brief and based largely on a "technicality": the "technology" present in Orwell's universe signifies the presence of "science," negating the thesis that what is indeed described is total totalitarianism. As Jameson writes, "if science and technological mastery are now hampered by the lack of freedom, the absolute technological power of the dystopian bureaucracy vanishes along with it and 'totalitarianism' ceases to be a dystopia in Orwell's sense" ("Progress versus Utopia" 155–56). Setting aside this problematic, traditional marxist faith in the saving powers of science, I still wonder what Jameson is referring to by the presence of "technology" in the novel. Beyond the presence of the telescreens in the lower Party members' rooms, the entirety of Oceania society is run (into the ground) by hand: Winston and his fellows manually remove and rewrite the pages of offending history, their most sophisticated equipment being antiquarian vacuum tubes to transport messages; and "hate" sessions featuring newsreels of Emmanuel Goldstein are conducted using simple projection equipment. Granted, the technologically complex bomb is a constant if peripheral presence, but in fact the bomb and all the lesser elements of technology are not improving or even moving in the story but have come instead to a grinding halt. Instead of being deployed and developed, the few technological advancements made before the onset of Big Brother's regime are used for what they are worth, then discarded or forgotten.

Likewise I am unhappy with Jameson's defense of Utopia as a superior literary genre (for the inspiration of political activism) and sociological theory, as Jameson admits that "sophisticated American readers" are "bored" with the reading of Utopia ("Progress versus Utopia" 154) and therefore, we must conclude, unlikely to be moved to action by this. Jameson himself admits to "nod[ding] over the more garrulous passages of the classical Utopias" ("Of Islands and Trenches" 16) and acknowledges that the flat, static description that defines the genre often outweighs and overwhelms the narrative that might salvage it for a wider audience. Most disturbing to me is his argument that the founding gesture of Utopia, the digging of a trench that effectively transforms a "promontory" into an "island," results only in the expulsion of "wealth" and "violence" from the now-separate society ("Of Islands and Trenches" 20). As I have tried to prove throughout this study, much more and many more are expelled or excluded during such retrenchments; in Jameson's own words, this utopic faith in the Solomon-like powers of division by "King Utopus" are of "a simplicity indistinguishable from naïve sentimentalism" ("Progress versus Utopia" 155).

4. We could conceivably argue that time gets slanted and hierarchized in similar fashion, with "nowness" always obscuring and thus lessening the import of ever-approaching "thenness" (U.S. consumers' continent of credit card debt being a recent relevant example). Meanwhile, appeals to "our grandchildren" are among the most effective when teaching environmental awareness to an indifferent society; even conservative politicians will occasionally pay lip service to planetary causes in the name of this family-values subcategory that resonates so strongly with many constituents. For a related discussion, see Lenzen (68).

Works Cited

Aaron, Daniel. "How to Read Don DeLillo." In *Introducing Don DeLillo.* Ed. Frank Lentricchia. Durham, N.C.: Duke University Press, 1991. 67–81.

Althusser, Louis. "Ideology and the Ideological State Apparatus." 1970. In *Essays on Ideology.* London: Verso Press, 1984. 1–60.

American Gigolo. Dir. Paul Schrader. Paramount/Pierre Associates, 1980.

Andriano, Joseph. "*The Handmaid's Tale* as Scrabble Game." *Essays on Canadian Writing* 48 (1992–93): 89–96.

Ansen, David. Review of *The China Syndrome,* dir. James Bridges. *Newsweek,* 19 March 1979, 103.

———. Review of *The Incredible Shrinking Woman,* dir. Joel Schumacher. *Newsweek,* 9 February 1981, 97.

———. Review of *Innerspace,* dir. Joe Dante. *Newsweek,* 13 July 1987, 60.

Ashe, Frederick. "Anachronism Intended: *Gravity's Rainbow* and the Sociopolitical Sixties." *Pynchon Notes* 28–29 (1991): 59–76.

Atwood, Margaret. *The Handmaid's Tale.* New York: Ballantine/Fawcett Crest, 1987.

Auster, Paul. "Interview," by Larry McCaffery and Sinda Gregory. *Contemporary Literature* 33.1 (1992): 1–23.

———. *In the Country of Last Things.* New York: Penguin Books, 1988.

Baker, Nicholson. *Vox.* New York: Vintage/Random, 1993.

Barker, Martin. *Comics: Ideology, Power, and the Critics.* Manchester: Manchester University Press, 1989.

Barone, Dennis. "Introduction: Paul Auster and the Postmodern Novel." In *Beyond the Red Notebook: Essays on Paul Auster.* Ed. Dennis Barone. Philadelphia: University of Pennsylvania Press, 1995. 1–26.

Barthes, Roland. *Mythologies.* New York: Noonday Press, 1972.

Bartlett, Neil. *Who Was That Man?: A Present for Mr. Oscar Wilde.* London: Serpent's Tail, 1989.

Bartter, Martha A. "The Hand That Rocks the Cradle." *Extrapolation* 30.3 (1989): 254–66.

Baudrillard, Jean. *Fatal Strategies.* Trans. Philip Beitchman and W. G. J. Niesluchowski. New York: Semiotext(e), 1983.

Baudry, Jean-Louis. "Ideological Effects of the Basic Cinematographic Apparatus." *Film Quarterly* 28.2 (1974–75): 39–47.

Beckett, Samuel. *Endgame.* New York: Grove Press, 1958.

———. *Happy Days.* New York: Grove Press, 1961.

Bendau, Clifford P. *Still Worlds Collide: Philip Wylie and the End of the American Dream.* San Bernardino, Calif.: Borgo Press, 1980.

Berressem, Hanjo. *Pynchon's Poetics: Interfacing Theory and Text.* Urbana: University of Illinois Press, 1993.

Bérubé, Allan. *Coming Out under Fire: The History of Gay Men and Women in World War Two.* New York: Plume/New American Library, 1991.

The Best Years of Our Lives. Dir. William Wyler. Samuel Goldwyn, 1946.

Birkets, Sven. "Fiction, Reality, and *In the Country of Last Things.*" *Review of Contemporary Fiction* 14.1 (1994): 66–69.

Biskind, Peter. *Seeing Is Believing: How Hollywood Taught Us to Stop Worrying and Love the Fifties.* New York: Pantheon, 1983.

The Blob. Dir. Irving S. Yeaworth Jr. Paramount, 1958.

The Blob. Dir. Chuck Russell. TriStar, 1988.

Booker, M. Keith. "*Vineland* and Dystopian Fiction." *Pynchon Notes* 30–31 (1992): 5–38.

Boyer, Paul. *By the Bomb's Early Light: American Thought and Culture at the Dawn of the Atomic Age.* New York: Pantheon, 1985.

Bradbury, Ray. *Fahrenheit 451.* 1953. Rpt., New York: Ballantine Books, 1973.

Bray, Rosemary L. "Please Mr. E-Mail Man." Review of *Virtual Love,* by Avodah Offit. *New York Times Book Review,* 7 August 1994, 9.

Brians, Paul. "Nuclear Family/Nuclear War." *Papers on Language and Literature* 26.1 (1990): 134–42.

———. *Nuclear Holocausts: Atomic War in Fiction, 1895–1984.* Kent, Ohio: Kent State University Press, 1987.

Briggs, Raymond. *The Tin-Pot Foreign General and the Old Iron Woman.* London: H. Hamilton, 1984.

———. *When the Wind Blows.* New York: Schocken Books, 1982.

———. *When the Wind Blows.* (Dramatic version, adapted by the author). New York: Samuel French, 1983.

Bristow, Joseph. *Effeminate England: Homoerotic Writings after 1885.* New York: Columbia University Press, 1995.

Brown, Gillian. "Nuclear Domesticity: Sequence and Survival." *Yale Journal of Criticism* 2.1 (1988): 179–91.

Brown, Rita Mae. *Venus Envy.* New York: Bantam Books, 1993.

Brownworth, Victoria A. "Someone Has to Say No!: Women in Gay Male Writing." *Lambda Book Report* 2.7 (1990): 6–9+.

Brustein, Robert. "Angels in America." *New Republic,* 24 May 1993, 29–31.

Bufithis, Philip H. *Norman Mailer.* New York: Ungar Publishing, 1978.

Burdick, Eugene, and Harvey Wheeler. *Failsafe.* New York: McGraw-Hill, 1962.

Burgess, Anthony. *A Clockwork Orange.* 1962. Rpt., New York: W. W. Norton, 1987.

Caldwell, Larry W. "Wells, Orwell, and Atwood: (EPI)Logic and Eu/Utopia." *Extrapolation* 33.4 (1992): 333–45.

Cameron, Peter. *Leap Year.* New York: Harper and Row, 1990.

———. *One Way or Another.* New York: Harper and Row, 1986.

———. *The Weekend.* New York: HarperCollins, 1994.

Carmichael, Virginia. *Framing History: The Rosenberg Story and the Cold War.* Minneapolis: University of Minnesota Press, 1993.

Carpenter, Mary Wilson. "Representing Apocalypse: Sexual Politics and the Violence of Revelation." In *Postmodern Apocalypse: Theory and Cultural Practice at the End.* Ed. Richard Dellamora. Philadelphia: University of Pennsylvania Press, 1995. 107–35.

Caws, Mary Ann. "Singing in Another Key: Surrealism through a Feminist Eye." *Diacritics* 14.2 (1984): 60–70.

Celmer, Paul W., Jr. "Pynchon's *V.* and the Rhetoric of the Cold War." *Pynchon Notes* 32–33 (1993): 5–32.

Chaloupka, William. *Knowing Nukes: The Politics and Culture of the Atom.* Minneapolis: University of Minnesota Press, 1992.

Chambers, Ross. "Messing Around: Gayness and Loiterature in Alan Hollinghurst's *The Swimming-Pool Library.*" In *Sexuality and Textuality: Reading Theories and Practices.* Ed. Judith Still and Michael Worton. Manchester: Manchester University Press, 1993. 207–17.

Chelsey, Robert. *Jerker; or, The Helping Hand.* In *Out Front: Contemporary Gay and Lesbian Plays.* Ed. Don Shewey. New York: Grove Press, 1988. 449–91.

The China Syndrome. Dir. James Bridges. Columbia/IPC, 1979.

"Chuck Russell's *Blob* May Be the Most Sinister Slime of All Time." *People,* 28 August 1988, 114–15.

Clarkson, Helen. *The Last Day.* New York: Torquil, 1959.

Clum, John M. "'The Time before the War': AIDS, Memory, and Desire." *American Literature* 62.4 (1990): 648–67.

Cohn, Carol. "Sex and Death in the Rational World of Defense Intellectuals." *Signs: Journal of Women in Culture and Society* 12.4 (1987): 687–718.

Colter, Ephen Glenn, Wayne Hoffman, Eva Pendleton, Alison Redick, and David Serlin (a.k.a. Dangerous Bedfellows), eds. *Policing Public Sex.* Boston: South End Press, 1996.

Copjec, Joan. "*India Song/Son nom de Venise dans Calcutta désert:* The Compulsion to Repeat." In *Feminism and Film Theory.* Ed. Constance Penley. New York: Routledge, 1988. 229–93.

Corliss, Richard. "Chain Reactions." Review of *The China Syndrome,* dir. James Bridges. *Film Comment,* May 1979, 27.

———. Review of *The Incredible Shrinking Woman,* dir. Joel Schumacher. *Time,* 23 February 1981, 110.

Crain, Caleb. "Pleasure Principles." *Lingua Franca* 7.8 (1997): 26–37.

Creedon, Jeremiah. "Second Opinions on AIDS." *Utne Reader,* September/October 1992, 17–18.

Crimp, Douglas. "Introduction." In *AIDS: Cultural Analysis/Cultural Activism.* Ed. Douglas Crimp. Cambridge, Mass.: MIT Press, 1988. 3–16.

Cruising. Dir. William Friedkin. Lorimar, 1980.

Dawn of the Dead. Dir. George A. Romero. United Film, 1978.

Day of the Dead. Dir. George A. Romero. UFDC, 1985.

DeCurtis, Anthony. "'An Outsider in This Society': An Interview with Don DeLillo. In *Introducing Don DeLillo.* Ed. Frank Lentricchia. Durham, N.C.: Duke University Press, 1991. 43–66.

De Kerckhove, Derrick. "On Nuclear Communication." *Diacritics* 14.2 (1984): 72–81.

Delaney, Samuel. "Street Talk/Straight Talk." *differences: A Journal of Feminist Cultural Studies* 3.2 (1991): 21–38.

DeLillo, Don. *End Zone.* Boston: Houghton Mifflin, 1972.

———. *Libra.* New York: Viking Penguin, 1988.

———. *Mao II.* New York: Viking Penguin, 1991.

———. *White Noise.* New York: Viking Penguin, 1986.

Dellamora, Richard: *Apocalyptic Overtures: Sexual Politics and the Sense of Ending.* New Brunswick, N.J.: Rutgers University Press, 1994.

D'Emilio, John. *Sexual Politics, Sexual Communities: The Making of a Homosexual Minority in the United States, 1940–1970.* Chicago: University of Chicago Press, 1983.

Denby, David. Review of *The Incredible Shrinking Woman,* dir. Joel Schumacher. *New York,* 23 February 1981, 42.

Derrida, Jacques. *Of Grammatology.* Trans. Gayatri Chakravorty Spivak. Baltimore, Md.: Johns Hopkins University Press, 1976.

———. "No Apocalypse, Not Now (Full Speed Ahead, Seven Missiles, Seven Missives)." *Diacritics* 14.2 (1984): 20–32.

———. *The Post Card: From Socrates to Freud and Beyond.* Trans. Alan Bass. Chicago: University of Chicago Press, 1987.

———. "The Rhetoric of Drugs. An Interview." Trans. Michael Israel. *differences: A Journal of Feminist Cultural Studies* 5.1 (1993): 1–25.

Deutscher, Isaac. "The Mysticism of Cruelty." In *Nineteen Eighty-four: Text, Sources, Criticism.* 2d ed. Ed. Irving Howe. New York: Harcourt Brace Jovanovich, 1982. 332–43.

Dewey, Joseph. "Music for a Closing: Responses to AIDS in Three American Novels." In *AIDS: The Literary Response.* Ed. Emmanuel S. Nelson. New York: Twayne Publishers, 1992. 23–38.

Dickinson, Peter. "'Go-go Dancing on the Brink of the Apocalypse': Representing AIDS." In *Postmodern Apocalypse: Theory and Cultural Practice at the End.* Ed. Richard Dellamora. Philadelphia: University of Pennsylvania Press, 1995. 219–40.

Doane, Mary Ann. "Remembering Women: Psychical and Historical Constructions in Film Theory." In *Psychoanalysis and Cinema.* Ed. E. Ann Kaplan. New York: Routledge, 1990. 46–63.

———. "Woman's Stake: Filming the Female Body." In *Feminism and Film Theory.* Ed. Constance Penley. New York: Routledge, 1988. 216–68.

Dr. Strangelove; or, How I Learned to Stop Worrying and Love the Bomb. Dir. Stanley Kubrick. Columbia/Stanley Kubrick, 1963.

Dolan, Jill. "Introduction to Paula Vogel's *Desdemona.*" In *Amazon All Stars: Thirteen Lesbian Plays.* Ed. Rosemary Keefe Curb. New York: Applause Books, 1996. 437–40.

Dorris, Michael, and Louise Erdrich. "The Days after Tomorrow: Novelists at Armageddon." In *The Nightmare Considered: Critical Essays on Nuclear War Literature.* Ed. Nancy Anisfield. Bowling Green, Ohio: Bowling Green State University Popular Press, 1991. 52–57.

Dowling, David. *Fictions of Nuclear Disaster.* Iowa City: University of Iowa Press, 1987.

Duus, Peter. "Introduction." In *Japan Inc.: An Introduction to Japanese Economics: The*

Comic Book, by Ishinomori Shotaro. Trans. Betsey Scheiner. Berkeley: University of California Press, 1988.

Dworkin, Andrea. *Pornography: Men Possessing Women.* New York: Putnam, 1981.

Dyson, Freeman. *Weapons and Hope.* New York: Harper and Row, 1984.

Edelman, Lee. *Homographesis: Essays in Gay Literary and Cultural Theory.* New York: Routledge, 1994.

———. "The Plague of Discourse: Politics, Literary Theory, and AIDS." *South Atlantic Quarterly* 88.1 (Winter 1989): 301–17.

———. "Seeing Things: Representation, the Scene of Surveillance, and the Spectacle of Gay Male Sex." In *Inside/Out: Lesbian Theories, Gay Theories.* Ed. Diana Fuss. New York: Routledge, 1991. 93–116.

———. "Tea Rooms and Sympathy; or, The Epistemology of the Water Closet." In *The Lesbian and Gay Studies Reader.* Ed. Henry Abelove, Michèle Aina Barale, and David M. Halperin. New York: Routledge, 1993. 553–74.

Ellmann, Mary. *Thinking about Women.* New York: Harcourt Brace Jovanovich, 1968.

The Fantastic Voyage. Dir. Richard Fleischer. Twentieth-Century Fox, 1966.

Farber, Manny. Review of *Panic in the Streets,* dir. Elia Kazan. *Nation,* 9 September 1950, 213–14.

Ferguson, Frances. "The Nuclear Sublime." *Diacritics* 14.2 (1984): 4–10.

Ferro, Robert. *Second Son.* New York: Crown, 1988.

Fitzpatrick, Laurie. "Lesbians and AIDS." *Art and Understanding* 30 (March/April 1997): 22–25.

The Fly. Dir. Kurt Neumann. Twentieth-Century Fox, 1958.

The Fly. Dir. David Cronenberg, Twentieth-Century Fox/Brooksfilm, 1986.

Forte, Jeanie Kay. "Focus on the Body: Pain, Praxis, and Pleasure in Feminist Performance." In *Critical Theory and Performance.* Ed. Janelle Reinelt and Joseph Roach. Ann Arbor: University of Michigan Press, 1992. 248–62.

Foucault, Michel. *The Archeology of Knowledge.* Trans. A. M. Sheridan Smith. New York: Harper Colophon Books, 1972.

———. *The History of Sexuality.* Vol. 1. Trans. Robert Hurley. New York: Vintage/Random, 1990.

Fowler, Douglas. *A Reader's Guide to "Gravity's Rainbow."* Ann Arbor, Mich.: Ardis, 1980.

Frank, Pat. *Alas, Babylon.* 1959. Rpt., New York: Harper and Row, 1983.

Freibert, Lucy M. "Control and Creativity: The Politics of Risk in Margaret Atwood's *The Handmaid's Tale.*" In *Critical Essays on Margaret Atwood.* Ed. Judith McCombs. New York: G. K. Hall, 1988. 280–91.

Freud, Sigmund. "Female Sexuality." In *The Standard Edition of the Complete Works of Sigmund Freud.* 24 vols. Trans. James Strachey. London: Hogarth Press, 1953–66. 21:223–43.

Friedberg, Anne. "A Denial of Difference: Theories of Cinematic Identification." In *Psychoanalysis and Cinema.* Ed. E. Ann Kaplan. New York: Routledge, 1990. 36–45.

Friedman, Alan J., and Manfred Puetz. "Thomas Pynchon and *Gravity's Rainbow.*" *Contemporary Literature* 15.3 (1974): 345–59.

Fromm, Erich. *The Revolution of Hope: Towards a Humanized Technology.* New York: Harper and Row, 1968.

Fung, Richard. "Looking for My Penis: The Eroticized Asian in Gay Video Porn." In *How Do I Look? Queer Film and Video.* Ed. Bad Object Choices. Seattle: Bay Press, 1991. 145–68.

Garrett, Laurie. *The Coming Plague: Newly Emerging Diseases in a World Out of Balance.* New York: Penguin Books, 1994.

Gee, Maggie. *The Burning Book.* London: Faber and Faber, 1983.

George, Peter. *Dr. Strangelove; or, How I Learned to Stop Worrying and Love the Bomb.* 1963. Rpt., Oxford: Oxford University Press, 1988.

Giddins, Gary. "Vaporizing Midland City." Review of *Deadeye Dick.* In *The Critical Response to Kurt Vonnegut.* Ed. Leonard Mustazza. Westport, Conn: Greenwood Press, 1994. 251–53.

Gilbert, Sandra M., and Susan Gubar. *The Madwoman in the Attic: The Woman Writer and the Nineteenth-Century Literary Imagination.* New Haven, Conn.: Yale University Press, 1979.

Gilman, Sander L. *Disease and Representation: Images of Illness from Madness to AIDS.* Ithaca, N.Y.: Cornell University Press, 1988.

Glaser, Chris. "AIDS and A-Bomb Disease: Facing a Special Death." In *The AIDS Epidemic: Private Rights and Public Interest.* Ed. Padraig O'Malley. Boston: Beacon Press, 1989. 251–56.

Glenday, Michael K. *Norman Mailer.* New York: St. Martin's Press, 1995.

Golden, Robert E. "Mass Man and Modernism: Violence in Pynchon's *V.*" *Critique* 14.2 (1972): 5–17.

Goldman, Emma. *The Traffic in Women and Other Essays on Feminism.* New York: Times Change Press, 1970.

Goodheart, Eugene. "Some Speculations on Don DeLillo and the Cinematic Real." In *Introducing Don DeLillo.* Ed. Frank Lentricchia. Durham, N.C.: Duke University Press, 1991. 117–30.

Gordon, Andrew. *An American Dreamer: A Psychoanalytic Study of the Fiction of Norman Mailer.* London: Associated University Press, 1980.

Gray, W. Russel. "'That Frightful Torrent of Trash': Crime/Detective Fiction and *Nineteen Eighty-four.*" In *The Revised Orwell.* Ed. Jonathan Rose. East Lansing: Michigan State University Press, 1982. 117–30.

Halperin, David. *One Hundred Years of Homosexuality and Other Essays on Greek Love.* New York: Routledge, 1990.

Hardwick, Elizabeth. "Bad Boy." Review of *An American Dream. Partisan Review* 32 (1965): 291–94.

Harpham, Geoffrey Galt. *On the Grotesque: Strategies of Contradiction in Art and Literature.* Princeton, N.J.: Princeton University Press, 1982.

Henkle, Roger B. "Pynchon's Tapestries on the Western Wall." *Modern Fiction Studies* 17.2 (1971): 207–20.

Henriksen, Margot A. *Dr. Strangelove's America: Society and Culture in the Atomic Age.* Berkeley: University of California Press, 1997.

Hilgartner, Stephen, Richard C. Bell, and Rory O'Connor. *Nukespeak: Nuclear Language, Visions, and Mindset.* San Francisco: Sierra Club Books, 1982.

Hinds, Lynn Boyd, and Theodore Otto Windt Jr. *The Cold War as Rhetoric: The Beginnings, 1945–1950.* New York: Praeger, 1991.

Hite, Molly. "Feminist Theory and the Politics of *Vineland.*" In *The Vineland Papers: Critical Takes on Pynchon's Novel.* Ed. Geoffrey Green, Donald J. Greiner, and Larry McCaffery. Normal, Ill.: Dalkey Archive Press, 1994. 135–53.

Hoban, Russell. *Riddley Walker.* 1980. Rpt., New York: Touchstone/Simon and Schuster, 1992.

Hoffman, Wayne. "Skipping the Life Fantastic: Coming of Age in the Sexual Devolution." In *Policing Public Sex.* Ed. Ephen Glenn Colter, Wayne Hoffman, Eva Pendleton, Alison Redick, and David Serlin (a.k.a. Dangerous Bedfellows). Boston: South End Press, 1996. 337–54.

Hoffman, William. *As Is.* New York: Random House, 1985.

Holleran, Andrew. *Ground Zero.* New York: Plume/New American Library, 1988.

Hollinghurst, Alan. *The Swimming-Pool Library.* New York: Vintage International/Random House, 1989.

Holt, Terrence. "The Bomb and the Baby Boom." *TriQuarterly* 80 (1990–91): 206–20.

Houston, Bo. *The Dream Life.* New York: St. Martin's Press, 1992.

Howard, Gerald. "Publishing Paul Auster." *Review of Contemporary Fiction* 14.1 (1994): 92–95.

Howe, Irving. "*1984:* History as Nightmare." In *Nineteen Eighty-four: Text, Sources, Criticism.* 2d ed. Ed. Irving Howe. New York, Harcourt Brace Jovanovich, 1982. 320–32.

Hunt, John W. "Comic Escape and Anti-Vision: *V.* and *The Crying of Lot 49.*" *Critical Essays on Thomas Pynchon.* Ed. Richard Pearce. Boston: G.K. Hall & Co., 1981. 32–41.

Huxley, Aldous. *Brave New World.* 1932. Rpt., New York: Perennial Library, 1969.

The Incredible Shrinking Man. Dir. Jack Arnold. Universal, 1957.

The Incredible Shrinking Woman. Dir. Joel Schumacher. Universal/Lija, 1981.

Innerspace. Dir. Joe Dante. Warner/Amblin/Steven Spielberg/Guber-Peters, 1987.

Invasion of the Body Snatchers. Dir. Philip Kaufman. United Artists/Robert H. Solo, 1978.

It. Dir. Clarence Badger. Famous Players-Lasky/Paramount, 1927.

Jameson, Fredric. "Of Islands and Trenches: Naturalization and the Production of Utopian Discourse." *Diacritics* 7.2 (June 1977): 2–21.

———. *The Political Unconscious: Narrative as a Socially Symbolic Act.* Ithaca, N.Y.: Cornell University Press, 1981.

———. *Postmodernism; or, The Cultural Logic of Late Capitalism.* Durham, N.C.: Duke University Press, 1992.

———. "Progress versus Utopia; or, Can We Imagine the Future?" *Science Fiction Studies* 9.2 (1982): 147–58.

Johnson, Denis. *Fiskadoro.* New York: Vintage, 1986.

Johnson, Wayne L. *Ray Bradbury.* New York: Frederick Ungar, 1980.

Jones, James W. "The Plague and Its Texts: AIDS and Recent American Fiction." *Journal of American Culture* 16.1 (1993): 73–80.

———. "Refusing the Name: The Absence of AIDS in Recent American Gay Male Fiction." In *Writing AIDS: Gay Language, Literature, and Analysis.* Ed. Timothy F. Murphy and Suzanne Poirier. New York: Columbia University Press, 1993. 225–43.

Kael, Pauline. Review of *The Fantastic Voyage,* dir. Saul David. *New Republic,* 8 October 1966, 34–35.
———. Review of *The Incredible Shrinking Woman,* dir. Joel Schumacher. *New Yorker,* 9 March 1981, 110.
Klawitter, George. "Verse Letters to T. W. from John Donne: 'By you my love is sent.'" In *Homosexuality in Renaissance and Enlightenment England: Literary Representations in Historical Context.* Ed. Claude J. Summers. New York: Haworth Press, 1992. 85–102.
Knee, Adam. "The Metamorphosis of *The Fly.*" *Wide Angle* 14.1 (1992): 20–34.
Koestler, Arthur. *Darkness at Noon.* New York: Macmillan, 1941.
Kopit, Arthur. *The End of the World.* New York: Hill and Wang, 1984.
Kramer, Larry. *The Normal Heart.* New York: Plume/New American Library, 1985.
Kroker, Arthur, and Marilouise Kroker, eds. *Body Invaders: Panic Sex in America.* New York: St. Martin's Press, 1987.
Kruger, Steven F. *AIDS Narratives: Gender and Sexuality, Fiction and Science.* New York: Garland Publishing, 1996.
Kushner, Tony: *Angels in America: A Gay Fantasia on National Themes.* Part 1: *Millennium Approaches.* New York: Theatre Communications Group, 1993.
———. *Angels in America: A Gay Fantasia on National Themes.* Part 2: *Perestroika.* New York: Theatre Communications Group, 1996.
———. "On Art, *Angels,* and 'Postmodern Fascism.'" Interview by Michael Lowenthal. *Harvard Gay and Lesbian Review* 2.2 (1995): 10–12.
Leap, William L. "Language and AIDS." In *Culture and AIDS.* Ed. Douglas A. Feldman. New York: Praeger, 1990. 137–58.
LeClair, Tom. *The Art of Excess: Mastery in Contemporary Fiction.* Urbana: University of Illinois Press, 1989.
Leitch, Thomas M. "Twice-Told Tales: The Rhetoric of the Remake." *Literature/Film Quarterly* 14.3 (1990): 138–49.
Lemp, George F., et al. "HIV Seroprevalence and Risk Behaviors among Lesbians and Bisexual Women in San Francisco and Berkeley, California." *American Journal of Public Health* 85 (1995): 1549–52.
Lenzen, Dieter. "Disappearing Adulthood: Childhood as Redemption." In *Looking Back on the End of the World.* Ed. Dietmar Kampter and Christoph Wulf. Trans. Philip N. Hewitt. New York: Semiotext(e), 1989. 64–78.
Levine, George, and David Leverenz. "Mindful Pleasures." *Twentieth Century Literature* 21.2 (1975): iii–v.
Lifton, Robert Jay, and Richard Falk. *Indefensible Weapons: The Political and Psychological Case against Nuclearism.* New York: Basic Books, 1982.
Little Shop of Horrors. Dir. Frank Oz. Warner Bros., 1986.
The Living End. Dir. Gregg Araki. Mainline/Strand Releasing/Desperate Pictures, 1992.
Lonoff, Sue. "Composing *Nineteen Eighty-four:* The Art of Nightmare." In *The Revised Orwell.* Ed. Jonathan Rose. East Lansing: Michigan State University Press, 1992. 25–46.
Looking for Mr. Goodbar. Dir. Richard Brooks. Paramount, 1977.
Lyons, Donald. "The Trouble with 'Angels.'" *New Criterion* 11 (1993): 57–59.
MacCannell, Dean. "Baltimore in the Morning . . . After: On the Forms of Post-Nuclear Leadership." *Diacritics* 14.2 (1984): 33–46.

MacKinnon, Catharine A. *Feminism Unmodified: Discourses on Life and Law.* Cambridge, Mass.: Harvard University Press, 1987.

Macklin, Ruth. "Modifying Behavior, Thought, and Feeling: Can Big Brother Control from Within?" In *Reflections on America, 1984: An Orwell Symposium.* Ed. Robert Mulvihill. Athens: University of Georgia Press, 1986. 159–78.

Mad Max beyond Thunderdome. Dir. George Miller and George Ogilvie. Warner/Kennedy/Miller, 1985.

Magid, Ron. "*The Blob*—a Gelatinous Villain Comes Back." *American Cinematographer,* December 1988, 82–89.

Mailer, Norman. *Advertisements for Myself.* 1959. Rpt., New York: Putnam's/Berkeley Medallion, 1969.

———. *Barbary Shore.* New York: Rinehart, 1951.

———. *Cannibals and Christians.* New York: Dial Press, 1966.

———. *The Deer Park.* New York: Putnam's, 1955.

———. "The Homosexual Villain." In *Advertisements for Myself.* New York: G. P. Putnam's Sons, 1959. 222–27.

———. *The Naked and the Dead.* New York: Rinehart, 1948.

———. *The Presidential Papers.* New York: G. P. Putnam's Sons, 1963.

———. "The White Negro." In *Advertisements for Myself.* New York: G. P. Putnam's Sons, 1959. 337–58.

———. *Why Are We in Vietnam?* 1967. Rpt., New York: Holt, Rinehart, and Winston, 1977.

Maltby, Richard. *Harmless Entertainment: Hollywood and the Ideology of Consensus.* Methuen, N.J.: Scarecrow Press, 1983.

Mars-Jones, Adam. *Monopolies of Loss.* New York: Vintage International/Random House, 1994.

———. *Venus Envy: On the WOMB and the BOMB.* London: Chatto and Windus, 1990.

Martin, Emily. *Flexible Bodies: Tracking Immunity in American Culture—From the Days of Polio to the Age of AIDS.* Boston: Beacon Press, 1994.

Maslin, Janet. Review of *The Blob,* dir. Chuck Russell. *New York Times,* 5 August 1988, sec. 3, 6.

Mason, Marshall W. "Production Note." In *As Is,* by William M. Hoffman. New York: Random House, 1985. xx.

Maupin, Armistead. *Tales of the City.* Vol. 1. New York: Harper and Row, 1978.

———. *Tales of the City.* Vol. 2: *More Tales of the City.* New York: Harper and Row, 1980.

———. *Tales of the City.* Vol. 3: *Further Tales of the City.* New York: Harper and Row, 1982.

———. *Tales of the City.* Vol. 4: *Babycakes.* New York: Harper and Row, 1984.

———. *Tales of the City.* Vol. 5: *Significant Others.* New York: Harper and Row, 1987.

———. *Tales of the City.* Vol. 6: *Sure of You.* New York: Harper and Row, 1989.

May, Elaine Tyler. *Homeward Bound: American Families in the Cold War Era.* New York: Basic Books, 1988.

Maynor, Natalie, and Richard F. Patteson. "Language as Protagonist in Russell Hoban's *Riddley Walker.*" *Critique* 36.1 (1994): 18–25.

McCombie, S. C. "AIDS in Cultural, Historic, and Epidemiologic Context." In *Culture and AIDS.* Ed. Douglas A. Feldman. New York, Praeger, 1990. 9–27.

McGehee, Peter. *Boys Like Us.* New York: St. Martin's Press, 1991.

———. *Sweetheart.* New York: St. Martin's Press, 1992.
McHoul, Alec, and David Wills. *Writing Pynchon: Strategies in Fictional Analysis.* Urbana: University of Illinois Press, 1990.
McKay, Alwyn. *The Making of the Atomic Age.* New York: Oxford University Press, 1984.
Merril, Judith. *Shadow on the Hearth.* Garden City, N.Y.: Doubleday, 1950.
Messmer, Michael W. "Nuclear Culture, Nuclear War." *Minnesota Review* 30.1 (1988): 161–80.
———. "'Thinking It Through Completely': The Interpretation of Nuclear Culture." *Centennial Review* 32.4 (1988): 408–12.
Metz, Christian. "The Imaginary Signifier." *Screen* 16.2 (1975): 14–76.
Michael, Magali Cornier. *Feminism and the Postmodern Impulse: Post–World War II Fiction.* New York: State University Press of New York, 1996.
Midnight Cowboy. Dir. John Schlesinger. United Artists/Jerome Hellman, 1969.
Miller, D. A. "Sontag's Urbanity." *October* 49 (1989): 91–101.
Millett, Kate. *Sexual Politics.* 1970. Rpt., Urbana: University of Illinois Press, 2000.
Monette, Paul. *Afterlife.* New York: Avon Books, 1991.
———. *Becoming a Man.* New York: Harcourt Brace Jovanovich, 1992.
———. *Borrowed Time.* San Diego, Calif.: Harcourt Brace Jovanovich, 1988.
———. *Love Alone: 18 Elegies for Rog.* New York: St. Martin's Press, 1988.
Morgan, Speer. "*Gravity's Rainbow:* What's the Big Idea?" In *Critical Essays on Thomas Pynchon.* Ed. Richard Pearce. Boston: G. K. Hall, 1981. 82–98.
Mueller, Janet. "Lesbian Erotics: The Utopian Trope of Donne's 'Sappho to Philaenis.'" In *Homosexuality in Renaissance and Enlightenment England: Literary Representations in Historical Context.* Ed. Claude J. Summers. New York: Haworth Press, 1992. 103–34.
Muñoz, José Esteban. "Ghosts of Public Sex: Utopian Longings, Queer Memories." In *Policing Public Sex.* Ed. Ephen Glenn Colter, Wayne Hoffman, Eva Pendleton, Alison Redick, and David Serlin (a.k.a. Dangerous Bedfellows). Boston: South End Press, 1996. 355–72.
Murphy, Patrick D. "Reducing the Dystopian Distance: Pseudo-Documentary Framing in Near-Future Fiction." *Science Fiction Studies* 17.1 (1990): 25–40.
Nelson, Emmanuel S. "AIDS and the American Novel." *Journal of American Culture* 13.1 (1990): 47–53.
Night of the Living Dead. Dir. George A. Romero. Continental, 1968.
O'Brien, Tim. *The Nuclear Age.* New York: Knopf, 1985.
O'Connell, Shaun. "The Big One: Literature Discovers AIDS." In *The AIDS Epidemic: Private Rights and Public Interest.* Ed. Padraig O'Malley. Boston: Beacon Press, 1989. 485–506.
Offit, Avodah. *Virtual Love.* New York: Simon and Schuster, 1994.
Orwell, George. *1984.* 1949. Rpt., New York: Signet/New American Library, 1981.
O'Toole, Lawrence. Review of *The Incredible Shrinking Woman,* dir. Joel Schumacher. *Maclean's,* 9 February 1981, 58.
Ozier, Lance W. "The Calculus of Transformation: More Mathematical Imagery in *Gravity's Rainbow.*" *Twentieth Century Literature* 21.2 (1975): 193–210.
Panic in the Streets. Dir. Elia Kazan. Twentieth-Century Fox, 1950.

Patteson, Richard. "What Stencil Knew: Structure and Certitude in Pynchon's *V.*" In *Critical Essays on Thomas Pynchon.* Ed. Richard Pearce. Boston: G. K. Hall, 1981. 20–31.
Patton, Brian. "Cell Wars: Military Metaphors and the Crisis of Authority in the AIDS Epidemic." In *Fluid Exchanges: Artists and Critics in the AIDS Crisis.* Ed. James Miller. Toronto: University of Toronto Press, 1992. 272–86.
Patton, Cindy. *Inventing AIDS.* New York: Routledge, 1990.
———. *Sex and Germs: The Politics of AIDS.* Boston: South End Press, 1985.
Pearce, Richard. "Introduction." In *Critical Essays on Thomas Pynchon.* Ed. Richard Pearce. Boston: G. K. Hall, 1981. 1–12.
———. "Where They're At, Where They Going?: Thomas Pynchon and the American Novel in Motion." In *Critical Essays on Thomas Pynchon.* Ed Richard Pearce. Boston: G. K. Hall, 1981. 213–29.
Piercy, Marge. *He, She, and It.* New York: Knopf, 1991.
Poirier, Richard. "The Importance of Thomas Pynchon." *Twentieth Century Literature* 21.2 (1975): 151–62.
———. *Norman Mailer.* New York: Viking Press, 1972.
Porter, Jeffrey. "'Three Quarks for Muster Mark': Quantum Wordplay and Nuclear Discourse in Russell Hoban's *Riddley Walker.*" *Contemporary Literature* 31.4 (1990): 448–69.
Porter, Laurence M. "Psychomachia versus Socialism in *Nineteen Eighty-four.*" In *The Revised Orwell.* Ed. Jonathan Rose. East Lansing: Michigan State University Press, 1982. 61–74.
Preston, Richard. "Crisis in the Hot Zone." *New Yorker,* 26 October 1992, 58–81.
Prose, Francine. "Scent of a Woman's Ink: Are Women Writers Really Inferior?" *Harper's,* June 1998, 61–70.
Pynchon, Thomas. *The Crying of Lot 49.* 1966. Rpt., New York: Perennial Library, 1986.
———. *Gravity's Rainbow.* 1973. Rpt., New York: Penguin Books, 1987.
———. *V.* Philadelphia: J. B. Lippincott, 1963.
———. *Vineland.* New York: Penguin Books, 1991.
Quam, Michael D. "The Sick Role, Stigma, and Pollution: The Case of AIDS." In *Culture and AIDS.* Ed. Douglas A. Feldman. New York, Praeger, 1990. 29–44.
Radetsky, Peter. *The Invisible Invaders: The Story of the Emerging Age of Viruses.* Boston: Little, Brown, 1991.
Radford, Jean. *Norman Mailer: A Critical Study.* New York: Harper and Row/Barnes and Noble, 1975.
Rahv, Philip. "The Unfuture of Utopia." In *Nineteen Eighty-four: Text, Sources, Criticism.* 2d ed. Ed. Irving Howe. New York: Harcourt Brace Jovanovich, 1982. 310–16.
Rambuss, Richard. "Pleasure and Devotion: The Body of Jesus and Seventeenth-Century Devotion." In *Queering the Renaissance.* Ed. Jonathan Goldberg. Durham, N.C.: Duke University Press, 1994. 253–79.
Robinson, Kim Stanley. *The Wild Shore.* New York: Berkley Publishing Group, 1984.
Román, David: "'It's My Party and I'll Die If I Want To!': Gay Men, AIDS, and the Circulation of Camp in U.S. Theater." *Theatre Journal* 44 (1992): 305–27.
Rose, Jonathan. "Eric Blair's School Days." In *The Revised Orwell.* Ed. Jonathan Rose. East Lansing: Michigan State University Press, 1982. 75–96.

———. "The Invisible Sources of *Nineteen Eighty-four.*" In *The Revised Orwell.* Ed. Jonathan Rose. East Lansing: Michigan State University Press, 1982. 131–48.
Ross, Judith Wilson. "The Militarization of Disease Rhetoric: Do We Really Want a War against Aids?" *Soundings* 72.1 (1989): 39–58.
Rothbard, Murray N. "George Orwell and the Cold War: A Reconsideration." In *Reflections on America, 1984: An Orwell Symposium.* Ed. Robert Mulvihill. Athens: University of Georgia Press, 1986. 5–14.
Rowland, Craig. "The Examination Table." In *Personal Dispatches: Writers Confront AIDS.* Ed. John Preston. New York: St. Martin's Press, 1989. 104–13.
Rubin, Gayle. "The Traffic in Women: Notes on the 'Political Economy' of Sex." In *Toward an Anthropology of Women.* Ed. Rayna R. Reiter. New York: Monthly Review Press, 1975. 157–210.
Ruppert, Peter. *Reader in a Strange Land: The Activity of Reading Literary Utopias.* Athens: University of Georgia Press, 1986.
Safer, Elaine B. "The Allusive Mode and Black Humor in Pynchon's *Gravity's Rainbow.*" In *Critical Essays on Thomas Pynchon.* Ed. Richard Pearce. Boston: G. K. Hall, 1981. 157–69.
Sanders, Scott. "Pynchon's Paranoid History." *Twentieth Century Literature* 21.2 (1975): 177–92.
Sanderson, Richard K. "The Two Narrators and Happy Ending of *Nineteen Eighty-four.*" *Modern Fiction Studies* 34.4 (1988): 587–95.
Savoy, Eric. "Reading at Risk: The Mortification of AIDS." *Minnesota Review* 40 (1993): 65–83.
Savran, David. "Ambivalence, Utopia, and a Queer Sort of Materialism: How *Angels in America* Reconstructs the Nation." *Theatre Journal* 47 (1995): 207–27.
———. "Introduction." In *"The Baltimore Waltz" and Other Plays,* by Paula Vogel. New York: Theatre Communications Group, 1996. ix–xv.
Scarry, Elaine. *The Body in Pain: The Making and Unmaking of the World.* New York: Oxford University Press, 1985.
Schell, Heather. "Outburst! A Chilling True Story about Emerging-Virus Narratives and Pandemic Social Change." *Configurations* 5.1 (1997): 93–133.
Schell, Jonathan. *The Abolition.* New York: Knopf, 1984.
———. *The Fate of the Earth.* New York: Knopf, 1982.
Schley, Jim, ed. *Writings in a Nuclear Age.* Hanover, N.H.: University Press of New England, 1972.
Schulman, Sarah. *People in Trouble.* New York: Plume, 1991.
Schwenger, Peter. *Letter Bomb: Nuclear Holocaust and the Exploding Word.* Baltimore, Md.: Johns Hopkins University Press, 1992.
———. *Phallic Critiques: Masculinity and Twentieth-Century Literature.* London: Routledge and Kegan Paul, 1984.
Schweninger, Lee. "Ecofeminism, Nuclearism, and O'Brien's *The Nuclear Age.*" In *The Nightmare Considered: Critical Essays on Nuclear War Literature.* Ed. Nancy Anisfield. Bowling Green, Ohio: Bowling Green State University Popular Press, 1991. 177–85.
Sedgwick, Eve Kosofsky. *Between Men: English Literature and Male Homosocial Desire.* 1985. Rpt., New York: Columbia University Press, 1992.
———. *Epistemology of the Closet.* Berkeley: University of California Press, 1990.

———. "Paranoid Reading and Reparative Reading; or, You're So Paranoid, You Probably Think This Introduction Is about You." In *Novel Gazing: Queer Readings in Fiction.* Ed. Eve Kosofsky Sedgwick. Durham, N.C.: Duke University Press, 1997. 1–37.

Seed, David. "The Flight from the Good Life: *Fahrenheit 451* in the Context of Postwar American Dystopias." *Journal of American Studies* 28.2 (1994): 225–40.

———. "Further Notes and Sources for *Gravity's Rainbow.*" *Pynchon Notes* 16 (1985): 25–36.

Sharnik, John. *Inside the Cold War: An Oral History.* New York: Arbor House, 1987.

Showalter, Elaine. *Hystories: Hysterical Epidemics and Modern Culture.* New York: Columbia University Press, 1997.

Shute, Neville. *On the Beach.* New York: William Morrow, 1957.

Silkwood. Dir. Mike Nichols. ABC, 1983.

Silverman, Kaja. "Historical Trauma and Male Subjectivity." In *Psychoanalysis and Cinema.* Ed. E. Ann Kaplan. New York: Routledge, 1990. 110–27.

Simmon, Scott. "*Gravity's Rainbow* Described." *Critique* 16.2 (1974): 54–67.

Simmons, Todd. "The Glamorization of AIDS." *The Advocate,* 28 Nov. 1995, 29–35.

Singer, Linda. *Erotic Welfare: Sexual Theory and Politics in the Age of Epidemic.* New York: Routledge, 1993.

Slade, Joseph. "Communication, Group Theory, and Perception in *Vineland.*" In *The Vineland Papers: Critical Takes on Pynchon's Novel.* Ed. Geoffrey Green, Donald J. Greiner, and Larry McCaffery. Normal, Ill.: Dalkey Archive Press, 1994. 68–88.

Sontag, Susan. *"Illness as Metaphor" and "AIDS and Its Metaphors."* 1978. Rpt., New York: Anchor/Doubleday, 1989.

Stacy, Ryder. *Doomsday Warrior.* New York: Kensington Publishing, 1984.

———. *Doomsday Warrior No. 2: Red America.* New York: Kensington Publishing, 1984.

Stockinger, Jacob. "Homotextuality: A Proposal." In *The Gay Academic.* Ed. Louie Crew. Palm Springs, Calif.: ETC Publications, 1978. 143–51.

Stone, Albert E. *Literary Aftershocks: American Writers, Readers, and the Bomb.* New York: Twayne Publishers, 1994.

Strehle, Susan. "Pynchon's 'Elaborate Game of Doubles.'" In *The Vineland Papers: Critical Takes on Pynchon's Novel.* Ed. Geoffrey Green, Donald J. Greiner, and Larry McCaffery. Normal, Ill.: Dalkey Archive Press, 1994. 101–18.

Strieber, Whitley, and James Kunetka. *Warday: And the Journey Onward.* New York: Holt, Rinehart and Winston, 1984.

Tanner, Tony. *City of Words: American Fiction, 1950–1970.* London: Jonathan Cape, 1971.

———. "The Uncertain Messenger: A Reading of *Slaughterhouse-Five.*" In *Critical Essays on Kurt Vonnegut.* Ed. Robert Merrill. Boston: G. K. Hall, 1990. 125–30.

Taxi Driver. Dir. Martin Scorsese. Columbia/Italo-Judeo, 1976.

Teeuwen, Ruud. "Dystopia's Point of No Return: A Team-Taught Utopia Class." In *Teaching Atwood's "The Handmaid's Tale" and Other Works.* Ed. Sharon R. Wilson, Thomas B. Friedman, and Hannon Hengen. New York: Modern Language Association of America, 1996. 114–21.

Testament. Dir. Lynne Littman. Paramount, 1983.

Thompson, Howard. Review of *The Blob,* dir. Irving S. Yeaworth Jr. *New York Times,* 7 November 1958, 23.

Touponce, William F. *Ray Bradbury and the Poetics of Reverie: Fantasy, Science Fiction, and the Reader.* Ann Arbor, Mich.: UMI Research Press, 1984.

Treichler, Paula. "AIDS, Gender, and Biomedical Discourse: Current Contests for Meaning." In *AIDS: The Burdens of History.* Ed. Elizabeth Fee and Daniel M. Fox. Berkeley: University of California Press, 1988. 190–267.

———. "AIDS, Homophobia, and Biomedical Discourse: An Epidemic of Signification." In *AIDS: Cultural Analysis/Cultural Activism.* Ed. Douglas Crimp. Cambridge, Mass.: MIT Press, 1988. 31–70.

United States. Centers for Disease Control. *Women with AIDS—L264 Slide Series (through 1995).* 9 October 1996. Online. Technical Information Activity. Internet. 26 March 1997.

Vogel, Paula. *The Baltimore Waltz.* In *"The Baltimore Waltz" and Other Plays.* New York: Theatre Communications Group, 1996. 1–57.

Vonnegut, Kurt. *Cat's Cradle.* 1963. Rpt., New York: Delacorte Press, 1973.

———. *Deadeye Dick.* New York: Delacorte Press/Seymore Lawrence, 1982.

———. *Player Piano.* 1952. Rpt., New York: Avon Books, 1967.

———. *Slapstick; or, Lonesome No More!* New York: Delacorte Press/Seymore Lawrence, 1976.

———. *Slaughterhouse-Five.* New York: Delacorte Press, 1969.

Washburn, Katharine. "A Book at the End of the World: Paul Auster's *In the Country of Last Things.*" *Review of Contemporary Fiction* 14.1 (1994): 62–65.

Watney, Simon. *Policing Desire: Pornography, AIDS, and the Media.* 2d ed. Minneapolis: University of Minnesota Press, 1989.

Watt, Donald. "Burning Bright: *Fahrenheit 451* as Symbolic Dystopia." In *Ray Bradbury.* Ed. Martin Harry Greenberg and Joseph D. Olander. New York: Taplinger Publishing, 1980. 195–213.

Weart, Spencer. *Nuclear Fear: A History of Images.* Cambridge, Mass.: Harvard University Press, 1988.

Weber, Myles. "When a Risk Group Is Not a Risk Group: The Absence of AIDS Panic in Peter Cameron's Fiction." In *AIDS: The Literary Response.* Ed. Emmanuel S. Nelson. New York: Twayne Publishers, 1992. 69–75.

Weir, John. *The Irreversible Decline of Eddie Socket.* New York: HarperCollins, 1991.

Weisenburger, Steven. "The End of History? Thomas Pynchon and the Uses of the Past." In *Critical Essays on Thomas Pynchon.* Ed. Richard Pearce. Boston: G. K. Hall, 1981. 140–56.

———. "Pynchon's Hereros: A Textual and Bibliographic Note." *Pynchon Notes* 16 (1985): 37–45.

Weston, Susan B. *Children of the Light.* New York: St. Martin's Press, 1985.

White, Edmund. *The Beautiful Room Is Empty.* 1988. Rpt., New York: Ballantine-Random, 1992.

White, Edmund, and Adam Mars-Jones. *The Darker Proof: Stories from a Crisis.* New York: Plume/New American Library, 1988.

Whitfield, Stephen J. *The Culture of the Cold War.* Baltimore, Md.: Johns Hopkins University Press, 1991.

Whitmore, George. *Nebraska.* New York: Grove Press, 1987.

———. *Someone Was Here: Profiles in the AIDS Epidemic.* New York: New American Library, 1988.

Winterson, Jeanette. *Written on the Body.* New York: Knopf, 1993.

Wolfley, Lawrence. "Repression's Rainbow: The Presence of Norman O. Brown in Pynchon's Big Novel." In *Critical Essays on Thomas Pynchon.* Ed. Richard Pearce. Boston: G. K. Hall, 1981. 99–123.

Woods, Tim. "'Looking for Signs in the Air': Urban Space and the Postmodern in *In the Country of Last Things.*" In *Beyond the Red Notebook: Essays on Paul Auster.* Ed. Dennis Barone. Philadelphia: University of Pennsylvania Press, 1995. 107–28.

Wylie, Philip. *The Disappearance.* New York: Pocket Books, 1952.

———. *Tomorrow!* New York: Rinehart, 1954.

Zamyatin, Yevgeny. *We* (1972). Trans. Mirra Ginsburg. New York: Avon Books, 1987.

Index

Aaron, Daniel, 24
alterapocalyptic literature, 38, 52–68, 73; and *A Clockwork Orange,* 86
anal fixation, 180
Andriano, Joseph, 200n.17
Ansen, David: review of *Innerspace,* 215n.6; review of *The China Syndrome,* 215n.10
anxiety, 163
Araki, Gregg: *The Living End,* 157
Ashe, Frederick, 204n.36
Atwood, Margaret: *The Handmaid's Tale* as alterapocalyptic literature, 38, 58–61, 62, 63, 64; *The Handmaid's Tale,* gendered reading of, 112, 114
Auster, Paul, 38; *The Country of Last Things,* 54–56, 58, 60, 61, 63, 64
AZT (azidothymidine), 3

backward glance, 39–42, 187
Baker, Martin, 206n.53
Baker, Nicholson: *Vox,* 75–76
Barone, Dennis, 202n.25
Barthe, Roland: *Mythologies,* 182
Bartlett, Neil: *Who Was That Man?,* 49–52, 121
Bartter, Martha A., 152
Baudrillard, Jean, 203n.26; *Fatal Strategies,* 52–53
behindsight. *See* backward glance
Bendau, Clifford P., 208n.10
Berlin Wall, 1, 2
Bérubé, Alan, 23, 145, 213n.40
Best Years of Our Lives (Wyler), 164–65
Birkets, Sven, 203n.25
Biskind, Peter, 177
Blob, The (Russell), 162, 181–86
Blob, The (Yeaworth), 162, 181–86
Booker, M. Keith, 204n.33
Bradbury, Ray: *Fahrenheit 451* as alterapocalyptic literature, 38, 56–58, 61, 62, 64; *Fahrenheit 451,* gendered reading of, 132–36; *Fahrenheit 451* as preapocalyptic literature, 68–69, 72
Bray, Rosemary, 75
Brians, Paul: "Nuclear Family/Nuclear War," 152
Briggs, Raymond: *The Tin-Pot Foreign General and the Old Iron Woman,* 89; *When the Wind Blows,* 37, 81, 88–91
Bristow, Joseph, 200n.11, 210n.19
Brown, Gillian, 208n.11
Brown, Rita Mae: *Venus Envy,* 123–24
Brownworth, Victoria A., 209n.15
Buchanan Patrick, 16
Buckley, William F., 16
Bufithis, Philip H., 137, 212n.34
Bulletin of the Atomic Scientists, 1, 2
Burdick, Eugene: *Failsafe,* 88
Burgess, Anthony: *A Clockwork Orange,* 81, 86–87
Bush, George, Sr., 1, 9

Caldwell, Larry W., 294n.32
Cameron, Peter: *Leap Year,* 36, 70, 72; *One Way or Another,* 36, 70, 72; *The Weekend,* 78, 154–56
Carmichael, Virginia, 207n.7
Carpenter, Mary Wilson, 200n.17
castration anxiety, 164–65, 167, 170; and fetishism, 169, 181
Caws, Mary Ann, 27, 31–32, 34
Celmer, Paul W., Jr., 204n.36
Chaloupka, William, 20
Chambers, Ross, 200n.12, 210n.19
Chelsey, Robert: *Jerker; or, The Helping Hand,* 76–77
China Syndrome, The (Bridges), 175, 177–79
Clarkson, Helen: *The Last Day,* 152

Clum, John M., 41, 199n.9
cognitive mapping, 186–87
Cohn, Carol, 208n.11
Colter, Ephen Glenn, 189
Conant, James Bryant, 26
Corliss, Richard, 215n.10
Creedon, Jeremiah, 22
Crimp, Douglas, 194n.4
Cuban missile crisis, 195n.14

De Kerckhove, Derrick, 23, 32, 81
Delaney, Samuel, 29
DeLillo, Don, 23–25; *End Zone,* 24; *Libra,* 12, 16, 18; *Mao II,* 24; *White Noise,* 24
Dellamora, Richard, 200n.11
Derrida, Jacques, 201n.17; "No Apocalypse . . . ," 20, 33–34, 39, 52, 81, 190, 198n.24, 200n.16; *Of Grammatology,* 29, 30, 33 51, 197n.22; *The Post Card,* 39–41; "The Rhetoric of Drugs," 199n.5
desire: and identification, 180
Dewey, Joseph, 46, 200n.13
Dickinson, Peter, 196n.18
Dolan, Jill, 122
doomsday clock, 1–4
Dorris, Michael, 205n.45
Douglas, Mary, 196n.15
Dowling, David, 82
Dr. Strangelove (Kubrick), 146
Duke, David, 6
Duplechain, Larry: *Tangled Up in Blue,* 156–57
Duus, Peter, 91
Dworkin, Andrea, 193n.2
dystopian literature, 28; authors of, 53

Edelman, Lee: *Homographesis,* 48; "Plague of Discourse," 13, 96, 196n.18, 197n.21; "Seeing Things," 17, 40–42, 199n.7; "Tearooms and Sympathy," 194n.9
emerging viruses, 10
Enders, John, 22
environment, nuclear damage to the, 25–26, 112–14, 158–60, 208n.11
Erdrich, Louise, 205n.45
escapism, 73, 206n.47
espionage, 144; in films, 170
extraepidemic literature, 70–73

Fantastic Voyage (Fleischer), 146, 170–75
Farber, Mannie, 215n.9
Ferguson, Frances, 34, 198n.25
Ferro, Robert: *Second Son,* 79, 158–60
Fly, The (Cronenberg), 165
Fly, The (Neuman), 165
Forché, Carolyn, 26–27
Forte, Jeanie Kay, 27
Foucault, Michel: *The Archaeology of Knowledge,* 11, 12; *The History of Sexuality,* 18, 194n.10
Fowler, Douglas, 66
Frank, Pat: *Alas, Babylon,* 145–46
Franklin, H. Bruce, 193n.1
Freibert, Lucy M., 203n.29
Freud, Sigmund, 39–40, 181, 215n.4
Friedländer, Saul, 24
Friedman, Alan J., 99, 205n.38
Fromm, Erich, 69
Fung, Richard, 210n.20

Gee, Maggie: *The Burning Book,* 147, 149–54
George, Peter: *Dr. Strangelove,* 88
Giddins, Gary, 85–86
Gilbert, Sandra M., 140
Gilman, Sander, 216n.14
Glaser, Chris, 16
Glenday, Michael K., 212n.34
Goodheart, Eugene, 24
Gordon, Andrew, 137, 212n.33
Gray, W. Russel, 211nn.27–28
Grmek, Mirko D., 22
Gubar, Susan, 140

Halperin, David, 18
Harpham, Geoffrey Galt, 28–29, 31
Henriksen, Margot A., 1, 193n.1, 213n.39
hibakusha, 16, 149–50
Hinds, Lynn Boyd, 14, 19, 194n.7
Hite, Molly, 101–2, 140
Hoban, Russell, 88; *Riddley Walker* as post-apocalyptic literature, 37, 81, 87–88; *Riddley Walker,* gendered reading of, 103–7
Hoffman, Wayne, 189
Hoffman, William: *As Is,* 77; and Mason's production note to *As Is,* 80
Holleran, Andrew: *Ground Zero,* 157
Hollinghurst, Alan: *The Swimming-Pool Library* as pre-epidemic literature, 36, 42–44, 50, 51; *The Swimming-Pool Library,* gendered reading of, 116
Holt, Terrence, 205n.42, 206n.52

House Un-American Activities Committee (HUAC), 14, 19
Houston, Bo: *The Dream Life,* 47–48
HUAC. *See* House Un-American Activities Committee
Hunt, John W., 207n.4

identification: and desire, 180
Incredible Shrinking Man, The (Arnold), 164–69, 170, 174
Incredible Shrinking Woman, The (Schumacher), 164–69, 171, 174
information, circulation/value of, 175–79
Innerspace (Dante), 172–75
intraepidemic literature, 37, 38, 73–80
iron curtain, 194; in Churchill's speech, 14
islands. *See* metonymy

Jameson, Fredric: *Postmodernism,* 19, 186–87, 190, 199n.6; and the utopic, 189, 216nn.1–3
Japanese comics, 91–92
Jenkins, Walter, 194n.9
Johnson, Dennis: *Fiskadoro,* 81–83
Johnson, Wayne L., 203n.31
Jones, James W.: *The Gay Academic,* 206n.49; "Refusing the Name," 79

Kael, Pauline, 215
Kazan, Elia, 175
Knee, Adam, 165, 169
Kramer, Larry, 37, 48; *The Normal Heart,* 77, 80
Kroker, Arthur, 194n.8
Kroker, Marilouise, 194n.8
Kruger, Stephen F., 22, 97, 200n.14, 206n.50, 209n.18
Kunetka, James: *Warday,* 152
Kushner, Tony, 122; *Angels in America* as fantasy literature, 124; *Angels in America* as intraepidemic literature, 77–78, 80; *Angels in America,* gendered reading of, 119–22, 130–31, 154, 156

Leap, William L., 194n.3, 195n.12
LeClair, Tom, 37, 141
Leitch, Thomas M., 179–80
Leverenz, David, 99, 140
Levine, George, 99, 140
Lifton, Robert Jay, 16
Lonoff, Sue, 211nn.27–28
love triangles. *See under* triangularity
Lowenthal, Michael, 122

MacCannell, Dean, 26
MacKinnon, Catharine A., 193n.2
Macklin, Ruth, 201n.17
Mailer, Norman, 136; *Advertisements for Myself,* 138; *The Barbary Shore,* 138; *Cannibals and Christians,* 136–37, 138; *The Deer Park,* 138; "The Homosexual Villian," 138; *The Naked and the Dead,* 138; *The Presidential Papers,* 138; "The White Negro," 137; *Why Are We in Vietnam?,* 138–39
Mars-Jones, Adam: *The Darker Proof,* 37; *Monopolies of Loss,* 37, 78, 199n.2; "Remission," 79; "Slim," 79
Maslin, Janet, 215n.13
Mason, Marshall W., 80
Maupin, Armistead: *Tales of the City* as extraepidemic literature, 70–73; *Tales of the City,* gendered reading of, 116–18
May, Elaine Tyler, 142–43, 145, 196n.17, 213n.41
McCarthy, Sen. Joseph, 16, 213n.41
McCarthyism, 145, 194n.8, 215n.8
McCombie, S.C., 13
McGehee, Peter: *Boys Like Us,* 116, 156; *Sweetheart,* 116, 156, 214n.43
McHoul, Alec, 204n.36
McNally, Terrence, 122
Merril, Judith: *Shadow on the Hearth,* 152
Messmer, Michael W., 194n.10, 207n.9
metaphor, 5, 27–35, 85–86, 151; and the bomb, 32–33, 156–58, 161, 177–79; and "cordon sanitaire," 28; and the grotesque, 28; and illness, 27–31, 154–56, 175–77; and interpersonal connection, 76, 78, 80; and "metaphorization," 81, 85, 91; military forms of, 28, 30; and the nuclear sublime, 34, 198n.25; in supplemental relationship with metonymy/the literal, 29, 32, 34, 39, 49, 70–71, 95, 199n.7; and the surreal, 31; and "textuality," 33
metonymy, 5, 34–35, 95; and irrelevance to/removal from AIDS crisis, 154, 156; and "island," 28, 77, 82, 159–60, 190; and "the metonymic," 29, 55, 70–71, 73; and technologically constructed social barriers, 74–78, 81, 208n.12; and utopianism, 70–71, 72–73, 82, 88, 189–91

Metz, Christian, 215n.11
Michael, Magali Cornier, 201n.17
Miller, D. A., 197n.21
momism, 110, 146
Monette, Paul, 48; *Afterlife,* 37, 115, 118–19, 156; *Becoming a Man,* 49, 51; *Borrowed Time,* 115; "Current Status 1/22/87," 77; "Manifesto," 214n.44
More, Sir Thomas: *Utopia,* 5, 28
Morris, David B., 1, 6
Muñoz, José Esteban, 189
Murphy, Patrick D., 53, 201n.17, 203n.28

Nelson, Emmanuel S., 198n.1

O'Brien, Tim: *The Nuclear Age,* gendered reading of, 107–10, 130–31; *The Nuclear Age,* illness imagery in, 147–49, 150, 152–54
O'Connell, Shaun, 80
Oedipal relationships, 179–82
Offit, Avodah: *Virtual Love,* 74–75
oral fixation, 180
Orwell, George, 38; *1984* as alterapocalyptic literature, 61–64; *1984,* gendered reading of, 132–36

Panic in the Streets (Kazan), 175–77, 179, 215n.8
para-AIDS literature, 36, 70
Pattison, Richard, 65
Patton, Brian, 197n.21
Patton, Cindy: *Inventing AIDS,* 15, 22, 197n.19; *Sex and Germs,* 16, 23
Pearce, Richard, 141, 204n.36, 205n.38
phallic symbolism, 146, 165, 168, 173, 183; and fetish, 169; and woman, 140, 213n.38
Piercy, Marge: *He, She, and It,* 112–14, 208nn.12–13
plagues, 4–5, 9, 15
Poirier, Richard: "The Importance of Thomas Pynchon," 99, 140–41; *Norman Mailer,* 137–38, 212n.31
polio vaccine, 13; Salk's discovery of, 22, 195n.14
Porter, Jeffrey, 206n.51
Porter, Laurence M., 203n.31, 211n.28
postapocalyptic literature, 37–38, 73, 81–93
postepidemic literature, 5
postmodernism, 4, 5, 11–16
pre-AIDS novels. *See* pre-epidemic literature
preapocalyptic literature, 5, 68–70
pre-epidemic literature, 36, 37–38, 42–52, 53, 73; autobiography as, 49–52
Preston, Richard, 25
Prose, Francine, 212n.36
protease inhibitors, 2
Puetz, Manfred, 99, 205n.38
Pynchon, Thomas: *The Crying of Lot 49,* 65; *Gravity's Rainbow* as alterapocalyptic literature, 64–68; *Gravity's Rainbow,* gendered reading of, 99–100, 102–3, 104; *V.* as alterapocalyptic literature, 65; *V.,* gendered reading of, 100–102; *Vineland* as alterapocalyptic literature, 64, 65; *Vineland,* gendered reading of, 100–101, 140

Radetsky, Peter, 22, 29
Radford, Jean, 212n.32
Reagan, Ronald, 1, 2, 9
Reed, Paul: *Facing It,* 156–57
Reich, Wilhelm, 137, 212n.33
repetition and return, 39–40, 199n.7
Román, David, 199n.4
Rose, Jonathan, 211n.28
Rothbard, Murray N., 202n.20
Rowland, Craig, 78
Ruppert, Peter, 193n.3
Ryan White Act, 2

Sabin, Albert, 195n.14
Salk, Jonas, 22, 195n.14
SALT (Strategic Arms Limitation Talks), 1
Sanderson, Richard K., 204n.32
Savran, David: "Ambivalence, Utopia . . . ," 210nn.21–22; "Introduction" to *The Baltimore Waltz,* 123
Scarry, Elaine, 27
Schell, Heather, 197n.19
Schell, Jonathan, 10, 23, 25, 53, 193n.2
Schulman, Sarah: *People in Trouble,* 125–26, 130–31
Schwenger, Peter: *Letter Bomb,* 20, 52, 95–96, 213n.38; *Phallic Critiques,* 199n.8; reading *Riddley Walker,* 87, 104–7; reading *The Burning Book,* 213n.42; reading *The Nuclear Age,* 107, 207n.5; reading *The Post Card,* 39, 41, 199n.8; reading *When the Wind Blows,* 89
Schweninger, Lee, 149
Sedgwick, Eve Kosofsky: erotic triangles in *Between Men,* 97, 132, 140, 172–73,

211n.26; homosexual panic in *Epistemology of the Closet,* 16; open secret in *Epistemology of the Closet,* 215n.7; and paranoia in literature, 193n.1
Seed, David, 201n.18
Sharnik, John, 11–12, 14
shrinkage, 165, 170
Shute, Neville: *On the Beach,* 81–82, 152
Silko, Leslie Marmon: *Almanac of the Dead,* 212n.36
Silkwood (Nichols), 178
Silverman, Kaja, 164–65, 166, 168–69
Simmon, Scott, 141
Simmons, Todd, 205n.44
Singer, Linda, 199n.6
Slade, Joseph, 204n.35
Sontag, Susan: discussion based on *"Illness as Metaphor" and "AIDS and Its Metaphors,"* 5, 19, 20, 21, 26, 27, 28–29; antimilitary arguments of, 23, 158; criticism of, 196n.18, 197n.21
spatiotemporality, 5, 38–39, 92–93, 186–87, 189–91, 199n.6
Spillane, Mickey, 145, 213n.41
Sputnik, 193n.1, 195n.14
START (Strategic Arms Reduction Talks) treaty, 2
Stone, Albert E., 27, 201n.17
Strategic Arms Limitation Talks (SALT), 1
Strategic Arms Reduction Talks (START), 2
Strehle, Susan, 65
Strieber, Whitley: *Warday,* 152
Symbolic, the, 167, 181, 187

Tanner, Tony: *City of Words,* 197n.20, 207n.3; "The Uncertain Messenger," 84
Teeuwen, Ruud, 202n.22
Testament (Littman), 152
Thompson, Howard, 215n.9
Treichler, Paula, 21
triangularity, 6, 94–96; romantic, 96–98, 130–42
Truman, Harry S., 14, 19; and the Loyalty Program, 19

urinal politics, 194n.8
utopian literature, 5–6, 193n.3, 201n.17, 208n.12
utopianism. *See under* metonymy

violence: and illness, 30, 145, 152–54, 197n.22, 207n.9
Vogel, Paula, 122; *The Baltimore Waltz,* 123–25, 130
Vonnegut, Kurt: *Cat's Cradle,* 83–84; *Deadeye Dick,* 84–85; *Player Piano* as preapocalyptic literature, 69–70, 72; *Player Piano,* gendered reading of, 132–36; *Slapstick,* 84; *Slaughterhouse-Five,* 84

Washburn, Katharine, 202n.25
Watney, Simon, 14–15
Watt, Donald, 203n.27, 212n.29
Weber, Myles, 70–71, 205n.43
Weir, John: *The Irreversible Decline of Eddie Socket,* 80, 209n.18
Weisenburger, Steven, 64
Wheeler, Harvey: *Failsafe,* 88
White, Edmund: *The Beautiful Room Is Empty,* 49; *The Darker Proof,* 37; "An Oracle," 79; "Palace Days," 79; "Running on Empty," 214n.43
Whitfield, Stephen J., 145, 213n.41
Whitmore, George: *Nebraska,* 36, 44–47; *Someone Was Here,* 78, 206n.48
Wills, David, 204n.36
Windt, Theodore Otto, Jr., 14, 19, 194n.7
Winterson, Jeanette: *Written on the Body,* 126–31
Wolfley, Lawrence, 141, 205n.41
Woods, Tim, 202n.24
Wylie, Philip: *The Disappearance,* 110–12, 116; *Tomorrow!,* 143–44, 146–47, 196n.17

JACQUELINE FOERTSCH teaches English at Auburn University and is the editor of *Outlook,* the quarterly newsletter of East Alabama AIDS Outreach. She has published articles in *Genre* and *South Central Review* and contributed a chapter to *Straight with a Twist: Queer Theory and the Subject of Heterosexuality* (University of Illinois Press, 2000). She is working on a study of the relationship among gay, lesbian, and feminist schools of thought.

Composed in 10.5/13 Minion
with Minion and Helvetica Neue Extended display
by Celia Shapland
for the University of Illinois Press
Designed by Paula Newcomb
Manufactured by Thomson-Shore, Inc.

University of Illinois Press
1325 South Oak Street
Champaign, IL 61820-6903
www.press.uillinois.edu